**Dian Shepperson Mills**, CertEd (Nutrition), BA (Education and Psychology), DipION, MA (Health Education – Nutrition), was the Information Manager for Lamberts Library Trust, the largest medical/nutrition library in Europe. She is a tutor, governor and lecturer at the Institute for Optimum Nutrition (ION), London, and Morley College, London.

Her research interests included women's health issues, endometriosis, male and female infertility, premenstrual syndrome, endocrine disorders in males and females, and the menopause. She has published several papers, abstracts and book chapters, and has given lectures to scientific societies in Europe, the USA, Asia and South America.

A past trustee of the National Endometriosis Society of Great Britain, Dian has researched the relationship between endometriosis and diet, and works closely with several doctors in England, Denmark and America. She also has links with the American, Australian, New Zealand, Irish, Danish, Japanese and Brazilian endometriosis groups. She is an active member of the European Society of Human Reproduction and Embryology (ESHRE), the Association of Reproductive Medicine (ASRH) and the SHE Trust (Simply Holistic Endometriosis) and is an advisor to the International Endometriosis Association (EA) whose headquarters are in the USA. Dian runs nutrition clinics for one-to-one consultations at ▮▮▮▮▮▮▮▮▮▮▮▮▮▮▮▮▮▮▮▮▮▮, London, and in Sussex, England, and over her web page endometriosis.co.uk and makingbabies.com.

In addition to Dian's professional understanding of endometriosis, she has personal experience of the condition. For spells between 1981 to 1982 and 1987 to 1989, endometriosis caused her to suspend her career and she was bedridden, suffering from extreme, debilitating pain. She tried one drug treatment, which made her ill, and had laser surgery, but did not wish to have major surgery. She looked into complementary treatments, as the motto 'Let's try the least harsh method first and work up' was her main philosophy. The Optimum Nutrition route was a major part of her healing process. She consulted a Doctor in nutritional medicine in 1988 and, following the advice she had been given, regained her health and her energy. Since 1989 she has remained symptom-free. Dian has since retrained and has worked with hundreds of other women suffering from endometriosis and fertility problems. While following a healthy eating plan, these women have seen a regression of their symptoms. Dian now also works with Foresight – the Charity for Preconceptual Care – helping couples who have suffered from miscarriage and infertility to conceive – at ████████████████

Medicine and the California Center for Pelvic Pain and Fertility.

The Endometriosis & Fertility Clinic,
The Hale Clinic, London W1N
02076 373377

The Endometriosis & Fertility Clinic,
ION London SW15
02088779993

**Michael W Vernon,** PhD, HCLD is a reproductive physiologist and scientific director at the Woman's Hospital of Baton Rouge, Louisiana, USA. He previously held the post of Associate Professor at the University of Kentucky where he lectured on medical endocrinology. His research areas are uterine physiology, endometriosis and ART (assisted reproductive technology). He has published over 100 peer-reviewed papers, abstracts and book chapters, and has given plenary lectures to scientific societies in the USA, Europe, Asia and South America. Dr Vernon is an ad hoc member and past chair of the National Institute of Health (NIH), Washington DC, study sections in reproductive biology.

He is an active member of several societies, including the American Society for Reproductive Medicine (ASRM), the Society for Gynecological Investigation (SGI), the Society for the Study of Reproduction (SSR) and the Endometriosis Association of the USA.

Dr Vernon has an extensive background in in vitro fertilization treatment (IVF). He was part of the first research team at the Wisconsin Primate Center that successfully performed IVF in the rhesus monkey. He was the embryologist for the first babies born in Kentucky through IVF, GIFT, ZIFT, micromanipulation and cryopreservation.

Praise for

*Endometriosis:*
*A Key to Healing Through Nutrition*

'Many women with endometriosis have found that nutrition can play a major role in overcoming some of the most debilitating effects of the disease. Dian Mills has studied the role of nutrition in treating endometriosis and, together with Michael Vernon, has made this information available in an understandable and compassionate way in this very helpful book.'

Mary Lou Ballweg, President

INTERNATIONAL ENDOMETRIOSIS
ASSOCIATION

'This book fills the void left by the traditional treatment of endometriosis, and provides physicians and patients with additional options.'

Deborah A Metzger, PhD, MD

DEPARTMENT OF OBS AND GYNE
SCHOOL OF MEDICINE
YALE UNIVERSITY

'The book is simple, easy to comprehend and will be embraced by a large majority, particularly those afflicted with endometriosis. It will be essential reading for scientists and the general public interested directly or indirectly in endometriosis.'

Dr O A Odukoya

DEPARTMENT OF OBSTETRICS AND
GYNAECOLOGY
JESSOP HOSPITAL FOR WOMEN
SHEFFIELD

'Endometriosis has an effect on all aspects of the life of a woman who suffers from this debilitating and perplexing condition. Modern medicine has made great strides in bringing help and relief to many women. Unfortunately, to date, there is still no known cure.

'During my years as Chair to the NES it became obvious that women are more than willing to help themselves. Regrettably, the tools to do this have been few and far between. With the publication of this book women will now have the opportunity to try to help themselves without resorting to powerful drugs and/or surgery, or to use the information as complementary alongside orthodox medicine. I welcome a book that will give women a choice.'

Diane Carlton, SRN, D/N Cert
SENIOR PRACTICE NURSE
CHAIR TO THE NATIONAL
ENDOMETRIOSIS SOCIETY 1983–97,
FOUNDER AND CHAIR OF
THE SHE TRUST

# ENDOMETRIOSIS
## A Key to Healing Through Nutrition

Dian Shepperson Mills MA and
Michael Vernon PhD, HCLD

*May good health be yours,*

*Dian*

ELEMENT

Shaftesbury, Dorset • Boston, Massachusetts • Melbourne, Victoria

© Element Books Limited 1999

Text © Dian Shepperson Mills and Michael Vernon 1999

First published in the USA in 1999 by
Element Books, Inc.
160 North Washington Street
Boston, MA 02114

Published in the UK in 1999 by
Element Books Limited
Shaftesbury, Dorset SP7 8BP

Published in Australia in 1999 by
Element Books and distributed
by Penguin Australia Limited
487 Maroondah Highway, Ringwood,
Victoria 3134

Reprinted 2000

Cover design and imaging: Slatter - Anderson
Photography: R.S.A. photography Ltd
Text illustrations by Janice Sharp
Designed and typeset by Penny Mills
Printed and bound in the USA by Courier Westford

British Library Cataloguing in Publication
data available

Library of Congress Cataloging in Publication
data available

ISBN 1 86204 300 0

*Note*: The information contained in this book is true and complete to the best of the authors' knowledge and is given for the purpose of helping people who suspect or know that they suffer from endometriosis. This book is not to be used as a substitute for professional medical treatment. The ultimate decision concerning care should be between you and your doctor. The information in this book is general and is offered with no guarantees on the part of the authors or Element Books. The authors and Publisher disclaim all liability in connection with the use of this book.

# Contents

# Acknowledgements

Thanks must go to those who have been supportive through the research and writing of this book:

To Mike Vernon for suggesting that we write this book together, for all his encouragement and guidance throughout its inception. From our chance conversation in Houston in 1989 a book has grown and its production has been tremendous fun. We should thank all the people who created cyberspace and e-mail which has made communication so easy.

To G J Mills, Bev Martin and Matthew Vernon and other family members and friends who gave us the support to lock ourselves away. To Dian's father and grandfather who gave her an enquiring mind through all her childhood games with physics and chemistry experiments.

Guidance and encouragement came from friends and staff at the University of Brighton and from the Institute for Optimum Nutrition. Dian's ION students were always supportive and gave great encouragement.

Inspiration was received from Mary Lou Ballweg of the International Endometriosis Association of America, and from Mrs Peter Barnes of Foresight – their dedication to endometriosis and infertility research made this book possible. Admiration for the ongoing work of Margaret and Arthur Wynn in pulling together so much research on preconceptual care from around the world should be an inspiration to us all.

To Karen Robinson for her editing, support and friendship and to Margaret Washington for reading through the book as we were writing it and for all their suggestions. To Janet Thomson, a fellow author, for her encouragement to write the book. And especially to Janice Sharp who, with her understanding of the subject, created such beautiful drawings to adorn this book.

To the gynaecologists who have aided our quest – Stephen Kennedy of Oxford University for all his time in reading the book in draft form and for his support and belief in us; to Deborah

Metzger of Yale University and Mr Odukoya of Sheffield University for their encouragement along the nutrition highway.

To all the women who have had faith to try the nutrition path and especially to those who have persevered and have taken the time to write their story for this book in the hope that they may inspire others to follow their lead. To all those women with endometriosis around the world who are suffering – we hope to give them a path back to good health.

The authors and publisher wish to thank the ASRM for permission to reproduce the ASRM Revised Classification of Endometriosis form in Appendix A (reprinted with permission from the American Society for Reproductive Medicine, Fertility and Sterility, 1997, 67 (5): 817–21), Arnold Kresch MD for permission to reproduce the Kresch Pain History Forms and Pain Mapping Forms in figures 3.1 and 3.2 and P Holford of ION for permission to reproduce the Food Pyramid in figure 9.1 and the supplement charts in Table 9.1.

# Foreword

Women with endometriosis commonly complain that doctors do not take their symptoms seriously. There is a feeling that if doctors did listen and if only doctors knew more about endometriosis, women would not have to suffer years of pain without a definitive diagnosis. The frustration is justified as recent research has shown that it usually takes about ten years from the onset of symptoms for the diagnosis to be made.

I think that this apparent indifference to symptoms, such as painful periods and painful sex, merely reflects the lack of interest shown by society in general to health problems that are specific to women. I also think that sufferers themselves should be trying to raise awareness about endometriosis among both the medical profession and the general public. Endometriosis should be as well known as asthma or diabetes given how many women it affects and how much misery it creates.

The principal problem, however, is that not enough is known about the condition. Despite over 20 years of intensive research, we still do not understand what causes endometriosis; why there is such discrepancy between the intensity of symptoms and the severity of disease, or how best to treat patients. When doctors struggle in the dark because they do not comprehend a condition, it is inevitable that patients will receive care that they perceive to be unsatisfactory.

The other common complaint I hear is that sufferers feel restricted by the inability of many doctors to explain, using language that can be understood, the nature of the disease and the treatment options available. It is clear from recent research in Oxford that the failure to meet the information needs of sufferers leads to disillusion and a sense of disempowerment.

I believe that it is vital to provide women with high quality information, especially about treatment, to enable them to make the kind of important decisions that may potentially have a profound effect upon their lives. The reality, however, is that the treatment options are limited and the medications currently available rarely provide a cure. Therefore it is understandable that sufferers should seek complementary therapies that allow them to take control over their own bodies.

This book is unique because, for the first time, a highly respected scientist has teamed up with a nutritionist who uses complementary medicine, to give women a better understanding of the scientific basis for the use of nutritional therapies that many women around the world have found helpful. It should give encouragement to those in despair because conventional treatments have failed or produced unacceptable side effects. Eating healthily produces only good side effects.

The authors provide considerable evidence illustrating the role of basic nutrients in metabolic pathways involved in the normal menstrual cycle and pain-associated inflammation. Generally speaking, the medical profession has been slow to appreciate the importance of nutrients in the prevention and treatment of disease. For example, it has only recently been accepted that folic acid should be given to all women planning to conceive, so as to prevent neural tube defects. Much of what is said in this book, however, is common sense: eat well and your body will benefit. What is new is that Dian Mills and Michael Vernon provide the rationale for doing so in a condition that traditionally has been treated only with hormonal drugs and surgery. A holistic approach to endometriosis is vitally important because of the limitations of conventional medicine, and the authors are to be congratulated for providing the reader with a number of novel strategies for coping with this debilitating condition.

Stephen Kennedy

SENIOR FELLOW IN REPRODUCTIVE MEDICINE

UNIVERSITY OF OXFORD

*'I would like to emphasize maternity as the frontier of human welfare and that the defence of mothers is the defence of nations. There is no place in the public health field that offers greater opportunity for service to mankind and the welfare of the human race than the application of newer and ever increasing knowledge of nutrition at the human frontier.'*

Ina May Hobbler, 1952

*'This human body, at peace with itself, is more precious than the rarest gem. Cherish your body, it is yours for this one time only. The human form is won with difficulty; it is easy to lose. All worldly things are brief, like lightning in the sky. This life you must know was the tiny splash of a raindrop. A thing of beauty that passes away even as it comes into being. Therefore set your goal, and make every day and night a time to obtain it.'*

Lama Tsong Khapa
14th-Century Tibetan Scholar and Yogi

# 1 What's happening to me?

The body has a miraculous capacity
to heal itself
*Live and Learn and Pass it On,*
*quote from the Central Baptist Hospital*
*1997 calendar*

You have a key to good health. Your body wants to be well, that is its natural state.

Endometriosis is a jigsaw puzzle of symptoms. You need to fit all the pieces together to provide clues as to what is happening within your body. This book will try to give you some of the pieces of the jigsaw, but you have to put them together yourself. This book will guide you to a truth. As you will read in the following chapters, some pioneering women have taken this path before and they share their success with you. Let them lead the way. They have found that, by giving the body the building blocks it needs, health can be regained.

That is the key, which you must always remember. Your body wants to be well. If you cut or burn your hand, you heal. If endometrial cells are growing in the wrong place, rest assured the body is trying to heal that area by whatever means it has available. Many women try drug and surgical treatments, and for some women they suppress some symptoms, but do not heal. Some people do get well, but many need other remedies or treatments.

Endometriosis is the second most common gynaecological complaint recognized by reproductive endocrinologists, affecting one out of every ten women. Endometriosis is everywhere and does not discriminate between women, race, colour, social status, body size, or colour of hair (although some women with red hair may have a greater incidence of endometriosis as they are more inclined to have allergies). It is possible that many women may have symptoms of endometriosis at some point in their lives, as every woman has the potential to develop endometriosis, but they do not always get a correct diagnosis. You are never alone with this disease – it is shared by many other women.

The term 'endometriosis' means that some of our body cells are growing in the wrong place, like weeds in a garden. Instead of staying inside the womb where they belong, to form the womb lining, these cells have spread outside the womb to infiltrate the ovaries and other areas of the body. If we knew exactly why these cells move around, it would be easier to find a cure. The endometrium normally grows only inside the womb. It is a nutrient-rich tissue designed to act as a food source and 'nest' for a fertilized egg. It also sets the stage for building the placenta which protects the baby as it develops in the womb.

For some unknown reason these endometrial cells migrate in endometriosis and seek other areas to grow. These areas are known as 'endometriotic implants' in medical terms, as they appear to seed themselves onto other organs in the peritoneal cavity (the abdominal area). Only cells from the spleen and endometrium in the human body are known to behave like this and migrate to other areas, and we need to understand why this happens in order to find a cure.

Women with endometriosis often ask 'Why me?' when they look around at their seemingly healthy friends. Endometriosis can be very distressing, and self-confidence may evaporate, but good health is not an impossible dream.

If you understand what is happening to you, it is easier to fight endometriosis and win. This book will look at how endometriosis manifests itself, how the body behaves, and how to approach drug and surgical treatments. It is important to look at how women as individuals can work with their bodies to help themselves heal, and to strengthen the immune and reproductive systems naturally using the nutrients which we ingest daily. The aim is to get the feel better factor!

We are all unique. No other person in the known universe is like you. People are meant to be different. Just look around in the street or your place of work at all the variables of face, hair colour, eyes, noses, height and weight. These differences are what make the strong gene pool of humankind. Orthodox medical and infertility treatments treat women as though they are all exactly the same. They take no account of your uniqueness. A 7-stone woman will be given the same dose tablet as a 14-stone woman. Treatments which work perfectly for you may not work as well for someone else because his/her body is slightly different. Moreover, many illnesses keep evolving, like the symptoms of ovarian/vaginal endometriosis, increasing levels of anxiety in those who suffer from them.

The purpose of this book is to outline the steps you can take to maximize your body's ability to fend off endometriosis. Although there is no known proven medical cure for endometriosis, nutrition may suppress the symptoms which are perceived as being due to endometriosis, and thus help to prevent them from interfering in your daily life. The book will review some of these options, especially the benefit of proper nutrition in the battle against endometriosis. Women who have tried these options and succeeded in combating endometriosis share their experiences.

Nutrition is not an alternative approach like herbal medicine or homeopathy. It is essential to life. *Eating is something we do every day. It sustains us and keeps us healthy, or it can make us unhealthy.* Unfortunately nutrition is no longer taught in schools. It is now assumed that we have a good choice of foods in the shops. But it is the quality of the foods you choose to eat which can make all the difference to your body's ability to heal itself. Nutrition is certainly very low on the list of doctors' priorities, many of whom may have had only a few hours of lessons in nutrition, and do not understand how nutrients relate to body biochemistry. It is a rare doctor who shows any interest in your food intake.

The 52 known nutrients in our foods are vital to all of us; they make our bodies work as nature intended. Vitamins, minerals and essential fatty acids and the actions of phytochemicals in plants are the body's building blocks to produce healthy new cells and to renew damaged tissue. For example, the mucous membrane which lines the digestive tract is renewed rapidly every 72 hours. New tissue can be formed very quickly on damaged organs, given the right building blocks of life. So the food you eat each day can help heal endometriosis.

Good quality, nutrient-rich food can improve the functioning of the body cells. This book will guide you through the selection of foods which will increase your intake of much-needed nutrients, especially those required by the reproductive and immune systems. It will give advice on which nutritional supplements may be helpful in the short term to boost body cells and correct hormone production, while you assess and improve your dietary intake.

The digestive system is the key to your healthy intake of nutrients, and improvement in this area can be a major factor in recovery from endometriosis. The gut flora and membranes must be healthy in order for all the nutrients from foods to be absorbed, so that they can reach the cells via the bloodstream. If your digestion is poor, it must be corrected before you can begin to get well. This is another key to your healing process. Once your digestion works efficiently, then the body can begin to heal itself.

Endometriosis can cause terrible pain, and adhesions which can stick organs together, possibly causing infertility in some women. The authors will inform you how the phytochemicals and nutrients in foods and herbs may work to reduce inflammation and pain. The known reasons for pain and infertility will be discussed, to help demystify endometriosis.

By understanding and improving the workings of your immune system, you can help to heal the reproductive system and improve fertility naturally, and the book looks at how assisted fertility works when endometriosis is present.

---

### Gwenneth B of Sussex

*The nutrition path was absolutely brilliant. I was so well while continuing it. Unfortunately I stopped. I have to go camping and go away with other groups from time to time. It then becomes impossible to follow the diet. I wish I had more self-control so that I could do it all over again. Any chance of a new start with some supplements again? Thank you for all your help in the past.*

• C A S E  S T U D Y •

---

The incidence of endometriosis is high and many women may never even have heard of the condition, let alone be aware that their abdominal pain is due to it. Much of our society remains blissfully ignorant of endometriosis and of all its ramifications. All those with endometriosis need to teach everyone around them to understand this disease. The word endometriosis itself is disconcerting and cumbersome: 'endo-me-tree-osis'. This book will attempt to explain exactly what endometriosis is, and how you can try to reduce its symptoms by using the body's natural healing ability.

Furthering research is a main aim of the endometriosis groups all over the world, in America, Britain, Australia, New Zealand, Japan, India, Poland, Germany, Hong Kong, Singapore and Brazil. Women in the international endometriosis associations are pulling together around the globe to encourage governments to provide more funding for studying this disease, while also trying to raise money for research from their supporters. Research into endometriosis should continue apace to help improve diagnosis and treatment. Future research into how cells behave and how their basic physiology relies upon nutrients should lead to new ideas about endometriosis treatments. All women suffering from endometriosis should encourage new research to find a cure, and to prevent the next generation having to endure this disease and its traumatic treatments. We can all see hope for a future cure. Drugs and surgery are not the only answer, as we shall see. Healing from within is an important concept.

If you use this book wisely, it may help you to find the real you again – minus the symptoms of endometriosis. Feeling like a shadow of your former self is not a pleasant experience. Endometriosis leaves you with no energy to do anything. You feel so very tired from fighting the pain. You hope that the pain will just go away, but it doesn't. The body needs help in order to attempt to rid itself of the 'rogue' tissue of endometriosis. Seeking such help requires information and understanding, and in this book the authors hope that everyone will find the support they need to help them begin their healing process. Understanding is the key. Once you properly understand what you are fighting, it becomes easier. It helps to have all the information at your fingertips. If information is withheld from you, always be suspicious. Where your own body is involved you have a right to know what is being done and why. Always ask questions and only act when you feel satisfied with the answers. Truth is important to developing trust between practitioner and patient, so if information is withheld it prevents healing.

Everyone wants to be happy and healthy and to enjoy life. Endometriosis hurts our lives. It stops us in our tracks. It prevents us living the life we want to lead. The pain associated with endometriosis can at times be so intense that women grow desperate to find a cure. When the body suddenly lets us down, the shock of feeling disabled is stunning and frightening. One feels out of control. Suggestions for treatments are made and you try them all. You just want to be well again; but fighting illness day in, day out causes despondency and great sadness for the lost time.

The medical profession has no absolute cure for endometriosis. It can support the patient and suppress the disease symptoms, but often the drug and surgical treatments do not get to the root of the problem and promote healing. Research shows that symptoms usually return within 18 months, after drug treatments are stopped. It is not uncommon for women to have taken five or six different drugs, one after another, and to have had several operations and still be in pain. Once all the reproductive organs have been removed, some members of the medical profession assume that endometriotic implants can no longer grow and women's symptoms can be dismissed and even ridiculed. Your local endometriosis group can advise you who is the right practitioner for you, and who is the most caring and compassionate.

So what is this book going to do for you, the reader? Hopefully it will inspire you to know how magical your body can be. Both authors want to help you to find ways to let your body begin to heal itself. If you can give it the tools and the fuel it needs to fight the disease, that is a good start. Chapters 8, 9, 10 and 12 are a basic guide to the practical steps you can take as you attempt to heal yourself.

## Barbara B of Kent

*The first benefit was the mental boost from feeling that I was actually taking control, doing something about my endometriosis. Within a very short time I had more energy and people stopped telling me how dreadful I looked! I also lost weight which was great. I took the vitamin supplements and generally worked hard to improve my diet. My endometriosis was extremely severe and yet even now, four years after a laparoscopy to remove cysts and reposition my womb, I remain totally free from endometriosis. My surgeon finds it unbelievable and constantly tells me how lucky I am. Thank you for all the support at the worst time in my life.*

• C A S E S T U D Y •

The keys to well-being are all around us. It is like a treasure hunt, but the treasure is not precious gems or gold; it is even more precious – health. For without that we can do nothing. Health is something which money cannot buy, but effort and willpower can take us a long way towards our goal. Strive to make it happen.

Feeling healthy and well is a right. Life without health can be intensely distressing. But it is important to fight to stay well, and one of the ways to help yourself heal is simply through eating good quality food. It is hoped that this book will inspire all women with endometriosis, and give you an insight into an area of self-help that is not difficult to follow. It will act to guide you, to choose food wisely, to enable you to absorb all the nutrients from your daily food intake, without making a meal of it.

Take your health into your own hands and work with your body. Look after it. After all, it is designed to last almost a century, according to the latest research on ageing. At least a lifetime, and we all want that lifetime to be full to the brim.

Good luck on the road to recovery. There is light at the end of the tunnel. As Mary Lou Ballweg of the International Endometriosis Association, headquartered in the USA says 'Better to light one candle than to curse the darkness'.

It is up to you. There are many paths back to health – nutrition, gentle exercise and relaxation all have their part to play. Bring them together in your own life. Be gentle with yourself and learn to pace yourself. When the body has been ill for some time, it takes a while to get it back on track. There is a need to nurture yourself back to health. Take your life in both hands and let's go!

> Too much of a good thing can be wonderful.
> *Mae West, Actress*

## SUMMARY

1  This book gives you the information about how endometriosis behaves and how nutrition may help you to combat the disease. Each chapter has a summary of all the key factors for you to follow, should you so wish.

2  Your body wants to be well. You are giving it a fighting chance to good health through choosing good quality food, fresh air, natural daylight and gentle exercise.

3  You are unique. Your body biochemistry is individual to you and needs treating as such. What works for one person may not work in the same way for you. Find out what suits you. Use your intuition. What feels right? Use this book wisely as a guide.

4  Your body cells use nutrients as building blocks to renew damaged tissues. These nutrients come from the freshest foods.

5  You can use your food choice to reduce inflammation and pain.

6  Arm yourself with a wide range of information which will enable you to choose wisely which treatments you feel are right for you. Never allow anyone to coerce you into having a treatment which feels wrong to you.

7  You can take control over what is happening to you by trying some self-help techniques, and working with your body, which is giving you signals that it needs help. Be gentle with yourself.

8  The medical profession has no cure for endometriosis and drugs and surgery can only suppress symptoms. Nutrition can help to speed up healing after surgery and, in some cases, can reduce the side effects of drug treatments.

9  Orthodox and complementary medicines can work alongside one another and enhance healing.

# 2 How endometriosis affects your body

All is flux, nothing stays still
*Heraclitus, 540–480BC*

## OH NO! MY PERIOD HAS STARTED AGAIN – SO SOON?

How many times have these words been uttered by women? The menstrual period has a way of appearing at the most awkward time and interfering with daily life. In women with endometriosis menstruation can be worsened, and may lead to severe, sometimes excruciating, pain and possible infertility. It can interfere with normal daily activity, and we can shy away from learning about the biology of endometriosis when the cycle provokes such distress. When the monthly cycle includes pain or lack of a hoped-for pregnancy time after time, it becomes physically and emotionally draining. Other women seem to have no period pain and to fall pregnant so easily – it all seems so unfair. We stand aghast and become angry with our own body and its failings.

The reproductive system is the core of our feminine identity and its many subtleties and biological intricacies could be better understood. It should be celebrated as the focus of the origin of new life and menstruation should *never* be painful. By understanding the reproductive system you will be better able to understand endometriosis and how proper nutrition can help you in your fight against this disease.

Our bodies are wondrous things, and understanding the amazing ways in which they work will help us to see more clearly what should be happening and just how endometriosis affects our whole body. Understanding can place us more in touch with the miracles going on within our cells each day. Endometriosis has the ability to mess up what should be a perfectly normal reproductive system, causing the wrong hormonal messages to be sent. The body always tries to get things right, so we have to enhance what it is attempting to do by natural means wherever possible.

# THE REPRODUCTIVE SYSTEM

The menstrual or reproductive cycle of women is a complex process that involves many different endocrine glands and the hormones they secrete. These hormones all work together in a 28-day menstrual cycle that prepares the uterus for a possible pregnancy.

The major organs of the reproductive system are the hypothalamus, pituitary gland, thyroid, ovary, uterus (womb), endometrium and Fallopian tubes. To understand how the menstrual cycle works, we need to look at where the various endocrine glands are located (figure 2.1). The glands control the whole reproductive cycle. People often assume that only the uterus and ovaries are involved. However, several endocrine glands control the system and they trigger the menstrual cycle. After we have familiarized ourselves with the reproductive system, this chapter will discuss how the glands and the hormones they produce interact during the reproductive cycle, and how endometriosis interferes with this cycle.

## THE HYPOTHALAMUS AND PITUITARY GLAND

The control centre for the reproductive cycle is the hypothalamus and the pituitary gland in the brain. The hypothalamus secretes hormones (chemical messengers) which control the timing and the amount of hormone produced by the pituitary (figure 2.1). The pituitary gland can be viewed as the 'master gland' of the endocrine system, since its hormones orchestrate the activity of most of the other endocrine glands of the body, including the ovaries and testes in men. Think of the pituitary gland as the conductor of the orchestra, wielding the baton, telling the other glands what to do and when.

The pituitary gland nestles in a bony cavity at the base of the skull; it is the size of a pea (figure 2.2). It has a rich blood supply that allows it to distribute its hormones rapidly throughout the body. The pituitary gland is divided into two parts: the anterior and posterior pituitary.

1  The anterior pituitary secretes several protein hormones which affect a variety of glands and tissues of the body. However, the two major hormones of the anterior pituitary that affect the reproductive system are follicle-stimulating hormone (FSH) and luteinizing hormone (LH). These two hormones control the activity of the ovaries, and are very important controls for fertility.

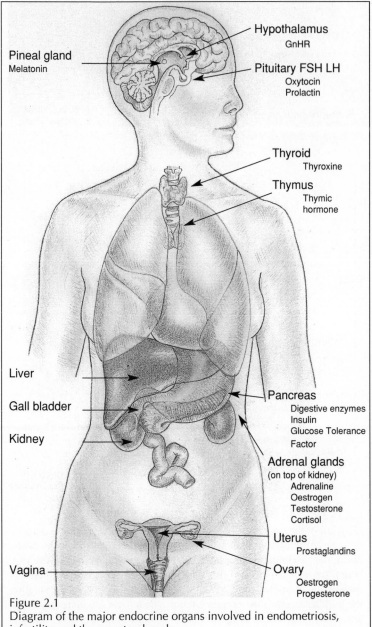

Figure 2.1
Diagram of the major endocrine organs involved in endometriosis, infertility and the menstrual cycle.

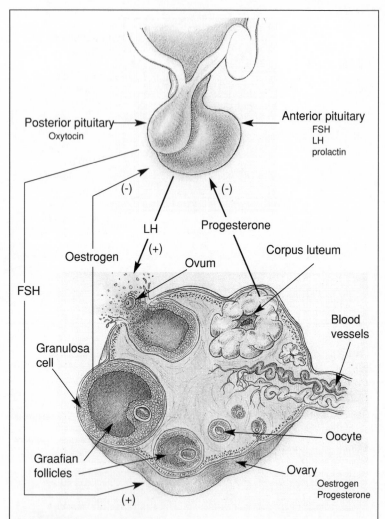

Figure 2.2
Diagram of the endocrine (hormone) relationships between the anterior pituitary and ovary. The pituitary secretes FSH (follicle-stimulating hormone) to stimulate the growth of the follicle which contains the egg. When the egg is ripe and the follicle large, the pituitary secretes LH (luteinizing hormone) and the egg is expelled (ovulated). After ovulation the follicle becomes the corpus luteum. The follicle produces oestrogen and the corpus luteum progesterone. (+) means stimulates and (-) means inhibits.

2  The posterior pituitary also secretes several protein hormones. Oxytocin is the hormone that most directly affects the reproductive system. Oxytocin causes the smooth muscle of the uterus to contract during the birthing process. Oxytocin production is dependent on sufficient levels of the mineral manganese. It is thought to be important for bonding at birth and oxytocin levels are known to be increased in the brain when we fall in love.

## THE THYROID

The thyroid is dealt with in detail in chapter 8. This gland can have an effect upon fertility; and lower than normal thyroid hormone levels (hypothyroid) cause infertility in both men and women.

## THE OVARIES

The ovaries contain the female sex cells, also known as oocytes or eggs (*see* figures 2.2 and 2.3). All of the eggs that a woman has in her ovaries were produced while she was developing as a fetus in her mother's womb. The health of each egg inside a baby girl is therefore dependent upon the health of the mother. When a female fetus develops in her mother's uterus, her eggs increase in numbers until the seventh month of pregnancy, and then their numbers decline throughout the remainder of the pregnancy and throughout her life. As many as seven million eggs are present in a female fetus by the seventh month of pregnancy, but there are fewer than one million eggs at birth.[1]

From birth to puberty, the number of eggs declines further, from one million to about 400,000, which is the total number of eggs available to a woman during her reproductive years. During the reproductive years one egg is selected every month to develop to a stage that allows for ovulation, fertilization *and* conception. When a woman reaches 50 to 55 years of age, the supply of eggs is exhausted and the reproductive cycle stops. This is, of course, the time of natural menopause.

At any given time, two major structures can be seen within the ovary – the follicle and the corpus luteum (figures 2.2 and 2.3). Each follicle contains an egg surrounded by granulosa cells or 'nurse cells'. During the menstrual cycle the follicle becomes filled with follicular fluid and looks like a small cyst, about one centimetre in diameter. The granulosa cells of the follicle secrete the steroid hormone oestrogen; the corpus luteum produces the hormone progesterone. Oestrogen has several roles:

1  It stimulates the endometrium to grow and replace the endometrial cells that were shed during menstruation.

2  It enhances the contractions of the uterus and is required during the birthing process.

3  Too much oestrogen acts as an abortant. Too much produced very early in the pregnancy and not balanced by sufficient progesterone from the corpus luteum could trigger the loss of the pregnancy.

Progesterone, on the other hand, has different roles from oestrogen. Progesterone will:

1  Stimulate the endometrium to become nutrient-rich, in preparation for a pregnancy.

2  Enhance relaxation of the uterus and prevent contractions of the uterus.

3  Inhibit oestrogen from stimulating contractions of the uterus and is required for the maintenance of a pregnancy.

The follicle produces oestrogen from day 1 to day 14 of the cycle; then the corpus luteum produces progesterone from day 15 to day 28 of the cycle. These steroid hormones are both oil-based, therefore the health of these hormones depends upon the quality of the oils you eat.


THE UTERUS

The uterus or womb is a little smaller than a woman's clenched fist, but during pregnancy it can expand to over 45cm (18in) in length (*see* figures 2.1 and 2.3). It consists of a well-developed muscular wall (the myometrium) and an inner mucus-like membrane (the endometrium). The smooth muscles of the myometrium are required to expel the baby during the birthing process, and it is the contractions of these muscles that also cause menstrual cramps. These muscles require a balance of calcium and magnesium to help

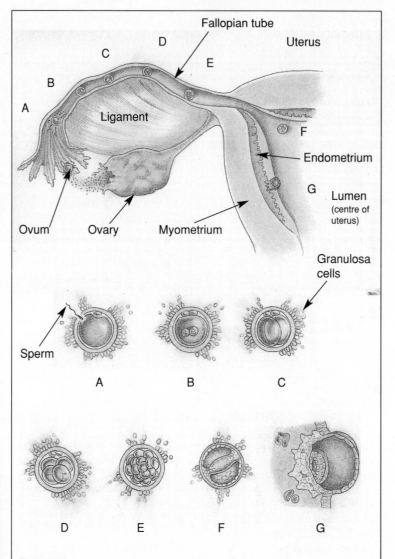

Figure 2.3
Cross-section of the uterus and Fallopian tube and diagrams of the development of the egg to embryo. (A) Fertilization of ovum. (B) Fertilized egg with pronuclei. (C) Two-cell embryo. (D) Four-cell embryo. (E) Multicellular embryo (100 cells) – a morula. (F) Early blastocyst embryo. (G) Blastocyst invading the endometrium.

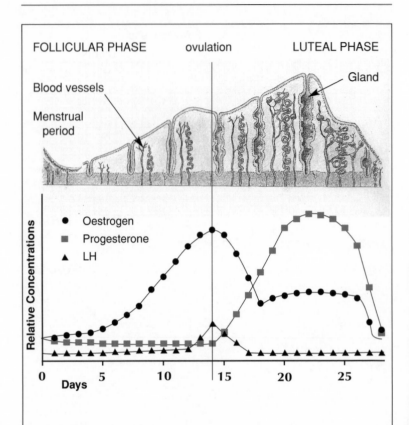

Figure 2.4
Graph of the day-to-day changes in the reproductive hormones during the menstrual cycle and the appearance of the endometrium during these changes. Note the endometrium gets thick and develops numerous blood vessels and glands because of the increase in oestrogen. The progesterone continues this build-up and makes the glands secretory, and prepares the endometrium for pregnancy. When the steroids decline at the end of the cycle, the endometrium sloughs off (menstrual period) and the cycle starts over again at day 1.

them function correctly. Calcium tenses muscles and magnesium allows them to relax. Magnesium-rich foods should be eaten when muscular cramps are a problem.

## THE ENDOMETRIUM

The endometrium (tissue lining the womb) plays a vital role in the reproductive process (*see* figures 2.3 and 2.4). The endometrium is brownish-red in colour with a fluffy appearance and slimy texture. The brownish-red colour is due to its nutrient-rich blood supply, and the slimy texture is due to the large amount of protein contained in its secretions. In order for a woman to conceive, the embryo must physically implant into this 'lush' endometrium. The endometrium is the sole source of nutrients and oxygen for the newly formed embryo. If nutrients are in poor supply, the womb lining will be unable to support the embryo's development. The growth of the embryo places a heavy nutrient demand on the endometrium, and this tissue needs to develop a rich blood supply. As we will see later, the quality of food eaten greatly influences the nutrients that are available to the endometrium.

The endometrium is also an important endocrine gland and secretes a family of hormones called prostaglandins (PG). Prostaglandin F (PGF) can stimulate strong uterine contractions (cramps) and prostaglandin E (PGE) can cause pain. These prostaglandins are the hormones directly responsible for most of the cramps and pain associated with endometriosis and menstruation. PGF also inhibits the development of the corpus luteum in the ovary and therefore reduces progesterone production. Therefore PGF has been used clinically to initiate abortions. If higher levels than normal of PGF are produced, miscarriages may occur.

As an endocrine gland, the endometrium is very responsive to the levels of hormones circulating in the blood. The balance of oestrogen and progesterone greatly affects the growth and activity of the endometrium. In chapter 9, the effects on the balance of what you eat will be clearly explained.

## FALLOPIAN TUBES

The womb has two tube-like extensions called the oviducts or Fallopian tubes, which are the transport system (rather like a highway) for the sperm to reach the egg and for the embryo to reach the uterus (*see* figure 2.3). The process of fertilization takes place in the upper third of the Fallopian tubes, so the sperm have to be robust enough to be propelled from the uterus up two-thirds of the Fallopian tube in order to fertilize the egg. Contractions in the uterine muscle during orgasm are believed to assist this process.

## ENDOCRINE COMMUNICATION

How does the body know when the embryo will be entering the womb? The womb must have a precise line of communication to the ovary, where the eggs are manufactured and released. This is accomplished through endocrine communication. The pituitary and ovaries communicate with each other by sending 'chemical messengers' (hormones) through the blood system to tell each other what to do and when. The major hormones involved in the reproductive system are listed in table 2.1.

### Table 2.1
### The major reproductive hormones of the menstrual cycle

| ORGAN | HORMONE | ACTION |
|---|---|---|
| Hypothalamus | Gonadotrophin-releasing hormone GnRH | Stimulates the pituitary gland to produce FSH and LH |
| Anterior pituitary | Follicle-stimulating hormone (FSH) | Stimulates ovarian follicles |
| | Luteinizing hormone (LH) | Initiates ovulation |
| | Prolactin | Stimulates lactation |
| Posterior pituitary | Oxytocin | Stimulates uterine contraction |
| Ovary | Oestrogen | Stimulates endometrial growth and uterine contractions |
| | Progesterone | Maintains pregnancy |
| Uterus | Prostaglandins (PGE/PGF) | Stimulates uterine contractions, menstrual pain and birth |

Establishing the correct levels of these hormones is the key to getting the right message to the right place at the right time. When we say that the hormones are 'out of balance', the wrong messages are being sent and received, and things can begin to go awry.

# THE REPRODUCTIVE CYCLE

The bottom line of the reproductive system is to make a healthy bouncing baby through the processes of sexual intercourse, conception and pregnancy. One of the more formidable tasks of the female reproductive system is to prepare the lining of the womb (the endometrium) to feed and nurture the embryo. However, it is not possible for the body to maintain the endometrium in a continuous, heightened 'ready state' for pregnancy. Thus the body follows a monthly cycle of slowly building up the endometrium so that it will be in a nutrient-rich state only when a fertilized embryo may be around. Think of the endometrium as fresh food for the embryo; if it gets old (past its sell-by date) it is less nutritious and is less likely to sustain the pregnancy. This 'food for the fetus' is renewed each month, so the quality of food you eat is crucial to the health of this tissue. If a fertilized egg fails to appear, then the body flushes away the existing endometrium, and starts all over again. This flushing away of the endometrium is, of course, the menstrual period.

## THE MENSTRUAL CYCLE

The menstrual cycle in most women lasts approximately 28 days, with the first day of blood flow (the menstrual period) usually designated as day 1 of the cycle (*see* figures 2.2 and 2.4). Around day 1 the hypothalamus secretes gonadotrophin-releasing hormone (GnRH) and, in response to this hormone, the pituitary gland secretes increasing amounts of FSH (follicle-stimulating hormone). FSH stimulates the granulosa cells of the follicle of the ovary to grow and produce oestrogen and stimulates the egg to ripen. Oestrogen also sends a message to the womb to tell it to produce more endometrial cells, so that a healthy thickened endometrium will be present to accept the egg should it be fertilized by a sperm in the Fallopian tubes. Unfortunately, oestrogen also has some bad effects. It is responsible for the water retention between cells, which is why some women can feel bloated before a period, and for stimulating uterine contractions (menstrual cramps).

When the follicle reaches 15mm to 17mm in diameter (around day 14–15 of the cycle), the pituitary produces a surge of luteinizing hormone (LH). This surge stimulates the egg to mature and also signals the ovary to expel the mature egg (ovulate) out towards the Fallopian tubes. The mature egg is then sucked up by the Fallopian tube so that the sperm can fertilize it. Ovulation usually occurs on the 15th day of the cycle. If the body does not ovulate, then the LH surge may not be happening as it should, implying that the hypothalamus is not functioning efficiently. The hypothalamus requires vitamin B6 and zinc to produce GnRH. If it is not working efficiently, the right message is not passed to the pituitary gland for the LH release. All these hormones and the health of the egg are nutrient-dependent.

After ovulation, the empty follicle undergoes a dramatic physical change. It turns a yellow colour (because of its oil-rich tissue) and is called the 'corpus luteum' (which means yellow body). The corpus luteum is very important as it secretes the hormone progesterone which sends the message to the endometrium of the uterus to become receptive for a possible pregnancy (*see* figure 2.4). As its names implies, progesterone (which means for gestation) is required for the pregnancy to be maintained. In response to the progesterone, the endometrium starts to produce the nutrients the embryo will need for its development, and the myometrium (muscle) layer of the uterus relaxes. Without sufficient levels of progesterone and magnesium, the uterus would start to contract and expel the developing embryo. Therefore, if the corpus luteum is poorly developed, a pregnancy may fail. Again, oils are implicated here. Studies show that 'Vitamin B6 (pyridoxine 5 phosphate) is necessary for the formation of the hormone progesterone' and the same source indicates that 'vitamin B6 is also required after ovulation when the body has a high level of oestrogen. B6 acts as a natural diuretic and helps alleviate some of the bloating associated with PMS. It is a precursor to progesterone'.[2] Moreover, 'the action of steroid hormones is balanced by B6 – it has an effect on endocrine diseases'.[3]

The fate of the egg is dependent upon whether or not it will meet up with a sperm in the Fallopian tube (figure 2.3). If no sperm are present, both the unfertilized egg and the corpus luteum will degenerate (die). The slow destruction of the corpus luteum leads to a decrease in progesterone and oestrogen secretion (*see* figure 2.4). Without these steroids, blood flow to the endometrium decreases and the lush endometrium cannot be maintained. The endometrium starts to degenerate from a lack of oxygen and nutrients, and it begins to separate physically from the uterus and is shed. This withdrawal of oestrogen and progesterone is the cause of the menstrual period (blood flow). With the onset of the menstrual period, a new menstrual cycle starts all over again and a new lining of endometrium is made for another attempt at pregnancy.

Women often accept a very heavy menstrual flow as the norm because that is what they have come to expect. Dr Casmir Funk, the man who isolated vitamin B1 in 1912, described the effect of vitamin B complex in reducing a woman's menstrual flow from five or six days to three or four days. He reported that menstruation came on 'completely without warning' (i.e. with no symptoms of premenstrual syndrome, or PMS) while these women were on B complex vitamin therapy. He treated PMS successfully through nutrition, rather than drugs.[4] Large blood clots can be prevented when vitamins C and E are used together with evening primrose and fish oils as 'these all have oestrogenic properties, and certain oestrogens produce changes in blood clotting'.[5] The amount of blood lost is usually about 60ml (2 fl oz).[6] At the beginning of the menstrual cycle rich red blood should be the norm, whereas brown granular blood with chopped-liver-like clots implies poor nutrient uptake. The nutrients used to improve periods include iron EAP2, vitamin B6, B complex vitamins, magnesium, chromium, vitamins C and E, and evening primrose and fish oils.

## FERTILIZATION

If sperm are present in the Fallopian tube, then the egg may be fertilized (*see* figure 2.3). A fertilized egg, called a zygote, sends a hormonal message to the reproductive system that conception has occurred and the corpus luteum is prevented from degenerating. The corpus luteum of pregnancy continues to produce progesterone and the endometrium gets even more lush. As the zygote passes down the Fallopian tube its cells begin to divide to form the embryo. It keeps dividing, first into a two-cell embryo, then a four-cell embryo and then an eight-cell embryo, up to about 100 cells, at which point it is called a 'morula' (*see* figure 2.3).

At this stage of development, the cells of the embryo begin to develop into specific different types of body cells, and a fluid-filled area forms in the middle of the embryo. The embryo is now called a blastocyst and it implants into the endometrium, a process dependent on vitamin E and zinc. It takes about seven days for a fertilized egg to develop into a blastocyst and to implant in the endometrium. A woman is totally unaware of these important events. She will not know that she is pregnant for another week when she misses her period.

Once the sperm has entered the egg, how does the body recognize that a conception has occurred? A message comes from the embryo that prevents the shedding of the endometrium. Within two weeks of conception the level of progesterone produced by the corpus luteum is maintained, and this protects the pregnancy. This progesterone enhances the ability of the endometrium to produce nutritious fluids that the embryo will need during its very early development.

Just imagine, from the tiny egg in the ovary and the minute sperm from the testes a whole new person can grow. The beauty of it is that each egg and sperm contain totally unique blueprints so that the baby developed from them will be a totally unique individual. We all began from this miracle of nature, we are the stuff that stars are made of.

As complicated as the reproductive process is, it is easy to see that human procreation is a miracle. In fact, the incidence of infertility in human beings is high, and as many as 15 to 20 per cent of all couples may be infertile. Some of this infertility may be the result of 'hiccups' in the reproductive process or a result of anatomical deformities in the reproductive system. As you will see in chapter 4, endometriosis may adversely affect many parts of the reproductive processes. What we have to do is make the body less tolerant of endometriosis and get the right messages to the right place at the right time, to enhance the reproductive and immune systems. The correct choice of food will help our bodies to work efficiently as the nutrients help to trigger the correct hormonal messages.

## CERVICAL MUCUS

The uterus is connected to the vagina through a small opening called the cervix, which acts as a physical barrier to protect the female reproductive organs from germs in the external environment. The state of the cervical mucus within the vagina is very important in achieving fertilization, and it is also dependent on the correct hormonal messages. Oestrogen makes the mucus runny and slippery, rather like egg white, making it easy for the sperm to swim through in order for conception to take place. Progesterone, on the other hand, thickens the mucus to stop sperm or bacteria from entering the womb during the second half of the cycle when the uterus could contain a pregnancy, which needs protection from the external environment. By watching for a clear mucus, like egg white, from the vagina, you will have a good indication as to when ovulation takes place.

# ENDOMETRIOSIS

## ENDOMETRIUM VERSUS ENDOMETRIOTIC IMPLANTS

The endometrium of the womb plays a vital role in the reproductive process. It is a dynamic tissue that undergoes continuous changes in the preparation for and maintenance of pregnancy. But although the endometrium is required for normal reproduction, it is also the major culprit in endometriosis. In this disease, pieces of endometrium grow and develop in areas outside the uterus. These rogue pieces of the normal endometrium are called 'endometriotic implants' by gynaecologists and scientists, and they can be found throughout the body. In general, however, endometriotic implants are usually found in the lower abdomen with the greatest number occurring in the base of the pelvis or the cul-de-sac/Pouch of Douglas and on the outer surface of the womb, ovary and the bowel, bladder and intestines (figure 2.5).

To a lesser extent endometriotic implants are found in the upper parts of the abdomen, including the small intestine, stomach, liver, gall bladder, kidney, pancreas and diaphragm, and also in the vagina and on the external genitalia. Implants have also been noted in lungs, skin spots, joints, the brain, gums and in the lining of the nose, but these locations are, thank goodness, fairly rare. They have even been observed in the scar tissue in women who have had hysterectomies or Caesarean sections. A bizarre location for endometriotic implants is in the joints of elderly men.[7] Three men in Australia were found to have endometriotic implants on their bladder as a result of taking oestrogenic drugs for cancer of the prostate.[8, 9] As men do not have a uterus, this is a true medical

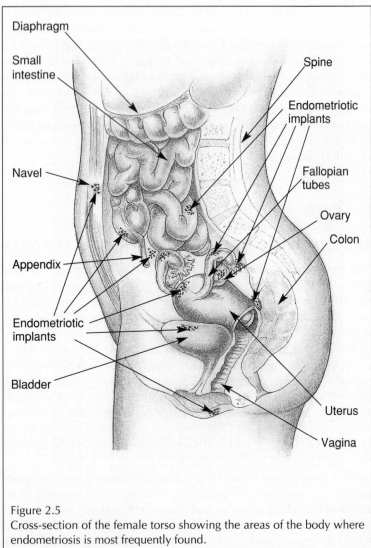

Figure 2.5
Cross-section of the female torso showing the areas of the body where endometriosis is most frequently found.

curiosity. Some scientists believe that as a fetus develops, some of the cells migrate to the wrong place and are triggered by a hormonal message at some later date. Endometriosis is so curious and very difficult to live with, but fascinating in its bizarre behaviour.

## WHAT CAUSES ENDOMETRIOSIS?

Although we do not have definitive proof of the true origin of this disease, several theories have been proposed as to what causes endometriosis. Dr Sampson in the early 1920s developed the theory of 'retrograde menstruation'.[10] He reported that endometrial tissues, in addition to flowing out of the vagina at the time of menstruation, also move up into the Fallopian tubes, from where they pour into the peritoneal cavity (abdomen). These backward-flowing fragments of endometrium then attach to the cells lining the abdomen and grow in a similar fashion to the uterine endometrium.

Sampson's theory has received the most support from the scientific community, since it agrees with the observation that the numbers of endometriotic implants increase with proximity to the opening of the Fallopian tube. As the endometriotic tissue flows out of the tubes, it would bathe the outer surface of the ovary and uterus, and large amounts would settle at the base of the pelvis in the cul-de-sac/Pouch of Douglas area. As mentioned above, these are the areas of highest occurrence of the disease. Recent research by Dr Jouko Halme of North Carolina University, USA, also supports Sampson's theory. Dr Halme examined the abdomen of his patients at the time of their menstrual flow. He observed the presence of endometrial fragments in the peritoneal (abdominal) fluid of 90 per cent of those who had normal, open tubes, compared with no endometrial fragments in the peritoneal cavity of the patients who had their tubes tied.[11]

These studies confirm that endometrial tissue can make its way through the tubes into the abdomen. Research performed by Dr Michael Vernon on monkeys has also shown that endometrial tissue placed on the surface of the cells lining the abdomen readily supports the growth and development of endometriotic implants.[12]

Thus it seems that Sampson's theory of retrograde menstruation provides a workable explanation of how endometriosis starts. However, it does not explain how endometriosis can develop in the bladder of men, so some additional theories have been suggested over the past 60 years. A second theory proposes that endometrial fragments work their way into the blood circulation or lymphatic system at the time of the menstrual period. The uterus has a rich supply of blood and lymphatic vessels (*see* figure 7.1 p. 136). As the endometrium is sloughed off, some pieces may enter open blood vessels or the lymphatic system and travel around the body. The lymphatic system is a part of the immune system and is explained in detail in chapter 7. It is similar to the blood circulation system, except that there is no heart to act as a pump. The body's movements aid the flow of the lymph, which is an oil-like fluid through which the white blood cells can flow. This theory offers an explanation for endometriosis in lungs, since endometrial fragments entering the circulatory system at the uterus would flow freely until they reach the small blood vessels in the lungs. It also may explain the presence of endometriosis in joints.

Another theory, noted by Meyer in 1927, proposed that epithelial tissue (the cells on the surface of most tissues) has the ability to transform into different types of epithelial tissue. Meyer proposed that some epithelial tissue (for example, joint epithelial cells) is converted into endometrial cells, thus explaining how men may develop endometriosis.[13] Quite perplexing, isn't it? The important question is 'Why does this happen in some women, but not in others?' Once we can find the answer to this we will be nearer the cure.

As the endometriotic implants are composed of a tissue very like that of the endometrium, the implants behave like the endometrium, and they respond to the same endocrine hormone messages. In fact, when Sampson first described the disease in the 1920s, endometriotic implants were sometimes referred to as 'mini-uteri'. Using microscopic observations, Dr Deborah Metzger of Yale University has closely examined the response of the endometriotic implant to ovarian hormones. She noted 'a correlation between morphological features (physical appearance) and the ability of endometriotic implants to respond to endogenous gonadal hormones (oestrogen and progesterone) in a manner similar to intrauterine endometrium'.[14] So the two tissues behave in an almost identical manner; one having a life-giving function and the other causing misery and pain.

Women with endometriosis in their noses actually have nose-bleeds at the same time as their menstrual period. When the oestrogen of the ovary stimulates the cells of the uterine endometrium to proliferate, the cells of the endometriotic implant also increase. Therefore, endometriosis may 'spread' in response to the oestrogen produced during the menstrual cycle.

It has also been suggested that endometriotic implants may be fuelling their own growth by producing their own supply of oestrogen.[15] Such an 'intracellular' source of oestrogen could help to explain why some women's endometriosis does not respond to the standard drugs which reduce oestrogen production from the ovaries. It could be said that endometriotic tissue is very devious. It could be perpetuating its own growth by making its own home-grown supply of oestrogen.[16]

When the progesterone produced by the corpus luteum in the ovary stimulates the cells of the womb endometrium to become more secretory, the endometriotic implants also start to secrete large amounts of proteins, carbohydrates, fats and oils (lipids) and hormones. However, the big difference with endometriotic implants is that its secretions are not contained safely within the womb, but are dumped into the abdomen or other areas of the body. The delicate organs and tissue inside the abdomen would not normally come in contact with these secretions.

Some of these chemical secretions can be quite harmful to abdominal function and possibly to the ova and sperm. For instance, large amounts of prostaglandin E (PGE) and prostaglandin F (PGF) are produced by the endometrium and the endometriotic implant. PGE stimulates excruciating pain. Laboratory technicians who accidentally expose a cut or the mucous membrane of their nose to prostaglandin E feel severe pain for hours, and sometimes days, after the contact. Prostaglandin F can cause increased gut motility (causing irritable bowel syndrome) and stimulates diarrhoea. Prostaglandin F can also shut down the function of the corpus luteum and interfere with the reproductive cycle by reducing progesterone output. Balancing the anti-inflammatory and pro-inflammatory prostaglandins seems to be another of the keys on the road to reducing inflammation and pain. This balance is dependent on the quality of fats and oils which we take into our body, and on our absorption of zinc, magnesium, vitamin B6 and biotin, as these four nutrients are all involved in the metabolism of oils.

There is no medical cure for endometriosis. The primary reason for this is owing to the fact that the cells of the endometriotic implant respond to the same cues and chemical messengers as the uterine endometrium. If researchers developed a chemical or physical agent that destroyed the cells of the endometriotic implant, it would also destroy the endometrium lining the womb which would have very serious consequences for fertility. What we need to do is find the differences between womb endometrium and endometriotic implants so that we can destroy the endometriotic implants without harming the endometrium.

## APPEARANCE OF ENDOMETRIOSIS

Not only does endometriosis appear in multiple sites within the body, it can also have a different physical appearance depending on its biochemical status. Several researchers have attempted to classify endometriosis by the appearance of the implant and some classification systems list over 30 types of endometriosis! Dr M W Vernon of the Woman's Hospital of Baton Rouge, Louisiana, USA, has developed a simplified classification system of endometriosis to explain the different physical appearance and biochemical status of the endometriotic implants.[17] In this system the implants are divided into three types:

1  *Red or petechial implants.* The first type owe their bright red appearance to a rich blood supply and look rather like a blood blister. These implants are the most biochemically active implants and may be the major culprit in the symptoms of endometriosis (i.e., pain and infertility), as they appear to secrete prostaglandins and oestrogens.

2  *Brown or intermediate implants.* These endometriotic implants look exactly like the fluffy, reddish-brown endometrium of the womb. They are less biochemically active than the red implants and are therefore called intermediate implants.

3  *Black or powder-burn implants.* These implants are virtually biochemically inactive. They have a poor capacity to secrete hormones, and they are associated with the formation of connective tissue that causes adjacent organs to become attached to each other (i.e., adhesion formation).

Adhesions can literally tie up organs, like the intestine, and cause serious gastrointestinal problems. Stretching these adhesions may also stimulate pain receptors on nerve endings. The triggering of pain impulses and the production of the PGE proinflammatory prostaglandins directly by the implants may be the major cause of the pain associated with endometriosis, especially where the bowel may be attached to the ovary or uterus. Many women reading this book will understand exactly how excruciating that pain can be.

When a woman has endometriosis, the endometriotic implants are usually found in multiple locations in the body and all three types of endometriotic implants can be present at the same time. To help physicians determine the relative severity of the disease, the American Society for Reproductive Medicine (ASRM) has developed a classification system for endometriosis that has been used worldwide. This classification is based upon a scoring system that reflects the size, number and location of the endometriotic implants. Dependent upon the final score, the severity of a patient's disease is classified into one of four stages (*see* Appendix A):

- Stage I or minimal disease
- Stage II or mild disease
- Stage III or moderate disease
- Stage IV or severe disease

The ASRM classification system has recently been revised by a group of international scientists, and the new revised system also incorporates the three types of endometriotic implants into disease assessment (*see* Appendix A). It also records the percentage of the three types of implants, as well as the size, number and location of the implants.

In the future, most physicians who directly examine endometriosis through surgery will be able to classify the severity of the disease by ascertaining the stage of disease and the percentage of the incidence of the various types. Your gynaecologist should be able to tell you exactly what your implants look like. Ask about this! It is important that this information is in your notes if you change consultants.

The question arises as to how can such an important tissue as the endometrium turn into such a villain when it grows outside the womb and what can we do about it. The best way to elicit change is by helping the endocrine glands to send the right message.

## DIAGNOSING ENDOMETRIOSIS

The two major symptoms of endometriosis are pain and infertility. Unfortunately, to many doctors these symptoms sound vague and in themselves do not present definitive evidence of the presence of endometriosis. The pain that most women with endometriosis feel may be similar to the pain from a long list of medical problems, including extreme uterine cramps, gastrointestinal bloating (causing painful distension), childbirth contractions, stomach ulcers, pelvic inflammatory disease, kidney dysfunction, irritable bowel disease, diverticulitis, cystitis and bladder infections and many others. Similarly, it is difficult to determine from a physical examination whether a patient is infertile due to endometriosis or some other reproductive problem (unless large lumps of endometriosis are palpable, but these could also be mistaken for fibroids or ovarian cysts). The only definitive proof of the presence of endometriosis is through direct observation, which means surgery.

To diagnose endometriosis, a doctor can look surgically for the disease via laparoscopy or laparotomy (*see also* chapter 5 for information on these procedures). Laparotomy is a surgical procedure involving a 10–12cm (4–5in) abdominal incision and exposure of the peritoneal cavity. This is a very invasive procedure and is often unnecessary. The second and preferred surgery is laparoscopy or 'belly-button surgery' (*see* figure 5.1, p. 104). In this procedure a fibre-optic device, called a laparoscope, is inserted through a small incision in the navel and the abdomen is examined and photographed or videoed. This procedure requires anaesthesia but can be done in one day as an out-patient service. Some general practitioners can perform a mini-laparoscopy in their surgeries. As we will see in chapter 5, laparascopy has the added advantage of allowing the doctor not only to diagnose the disease, but also to perform a simultaneous laser treatment, to 'burn' away visible endometriotic implants. If a woman consents to having a laparoscopic examination, she should confirm with the physician that in addition to diagnosing her disease, the endometriosis will be classified and photographed, and removed (by ablation, cauterization or laser). This saves a second operation and the information will be very helpful in determining subsequent treatments. It would also prevent repeating the procedure if the patient changes doctors. Chapter 5 will discuss consent issues.

During laparoscopy gases are pumped into the peritoneal cavity to increase the viewing area and to enable the consultant to move organs around in order to locate the endometriotic implants. Usually this form of surgery is successful in locating and ablating troublesome implants. The gases may dissipate to the four corners of the body, causing aching shoulders. Very occasionally the spine may need correcting by a chiropractitioner or osteopath as when the body is tilted for several hours the lumbar and cervical vertebrae may become misaligned. In order to speed up the healing of wounds after operations it has been shown that vitamin C and zinc supplements help as they are essential to the formation of collagen.

(Both Guy's and St Thomas's Hospitals in London, England use this treatment for their patients after operations.)

## CELLULAR BIOLOGY AND ENDOMETRIOSIS

Endometriosis happens at a cellular level; the implant attaches to the cell wall and hangs on for dear life. The important questions to ask are: Is something in the body weakening the cell membrane so that the endometriotic implants can take hold? How can we maintain the integrity of our cell membrane? If the cell membrane can remain strong, will it prevent the endometriotic implants from taking hold? Is a 'balanced' diet sufficient when we are so ill, or do we need nutritional supplements to help our bodies 'kick start' the healing process?

Knowing how our cells work helps us understand why this may be essential in the short term.

### CELL STRUCTURE AND FUNCTION

There are many different types of cell in the human body – sperm cells in semen, bone-forming cells, red and white blood cells, cells forming connective tissue to hold us together, cells secreting acid in the stomach to help us digest food, cells storing fat in adipose tissue so that we are ready to survive a famine or drought, and the germ cells which form the ova. The list is endless. The basic structure is the same, but the function is very different for each cell. Together, cells make up the body in which we live. Each type of cell relies upon the nutrients in our diet to be fully functional. Low levels of essential nutrients cause cellular function to begin to fail.

Our bodies are about 70 per cent water. The cells also contain many minerals, trace elements and vitamins, often linked with sugars, fats or proteins. You are made up from what you eat.

The basic cell structure (figure 2.6) consists of the outer layer or cell membrane, and the inner area which contains a fluid called cytoplasm. Within the latter are mini-organs rather like factories where proteins, fats, enzymes and hormones can be built. The centre of the cell contains the nucleus. This is the brain of the cell which controls how the cells behaves and how it will pass on its code to a new cell. The nucleus contains deoxyribonucleic acid (DNA),

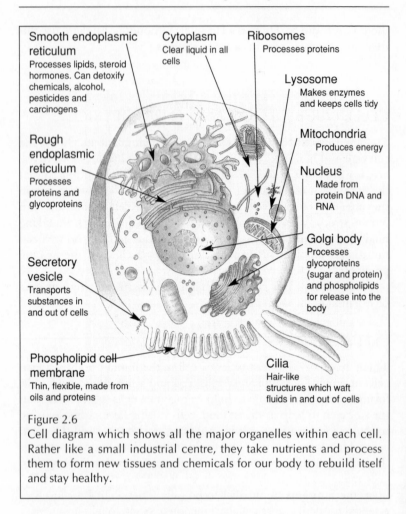

Smooth endoplasmic reticulum
Processes lipids, steroid hormones. Can detoxify chemicals, alcohol, pesticides and carcinogens

Rough endoplasmic reticulum
Processes proteins and glycoproteins

Secretory vesicle
Transports substances in and out of cells

Phospholipid cell membrane
Thin, flexible, made from oils and proteins

Cytoplasm
Clear liquid in all cells

Ribosomes
Processes proteins

Lysosome
Makes enzymes and keeps cells tidy

Mitochondria
Produces energy

Nucleus
Made from protein DNA and RNA

Golgi body
Processes glycoproteins (sugar and protein) and phospholipids for release into the body

Cilia
Hair-like structures which waft fluids in and out of cells

Figure 2.6
Cell diagram which shows all the major organelles within each cell. Rather like a small industrial centre, they take nutrients and process them to form new tissues and chemicals for our body to rebuild itself and stay healthy.

the genetically coded information that we have inherited from our parents.

The cell membrane consists of phospholipids (compounds made up of cis-oils and phosphorus). In chapter 3 we look at the role of prostaglandins (which are oil-based hormones), and how the quality of the oils we eat is very important for fertility and pain reduction. The cis-fats found in natural oils can keep the cell membrane strong, whereas the trans-fats from manufactured or processed oils cannot lock into the membrane very well and leave the cell wall more likely to be breached by harmful substances. (Trans-fats may be made within the body or they could be from the environment.) The cell membrane is permeable, to allow nutrients and substances used for rebuilding the body cells to pass in and out.

A cell is rather like a little powerhouse, or production line. There are factories making proteins from amino acids, phospholipids from fats and oils, and glycoproteins from sugars and proteins. The structures called mitochondria take from your diet iron, vitamins C, B1, B2, B3, and coenzyme-Q10, and with glucose, water and oxygen make all the energy the body needs. Magical stuff goes on in the twinkling of an eye.

We know that the amount of magnesium in the body is important for the integrity of the cell membrane. Research has shown that magnesium on the cell membrane can prevent the changes that cause cancer. Research shows that: 'Magnesium on the cell membrane helps cells stick together in a normal fashion. Magnesium is required in more than 30 enzyme systems that deal with cell growth and division, which are disordered in cancers.'[17] Endometriosis cells appear to mimic the way cancer cells grow and this may be important to understanding the disease. Endometriosis is thought to have nothing to do with cancer, but the way in which the endometrial cells can implant themselves in other tissues and travel all over the body has some resemblance to the attachment and movement of cancers. By understanding more about the mechanism of transport, it may help us understand better how we can prevent the disease from taking hold. As magnesium is required for DNA replication and is involved with the enzymes affecting cell growth and division, we know that this mineral could be vital for reproduction and possibly for prevention of endometriotic implants. More research is necessary to show how magnesium levels affect endometriosis.

Production of skin, mucous membranes, cell membranes and tissue renewal are dependent on vitamins A, C and E, zinc, manganese, choline and essential oils (fatty acids). The mitochondria are protected by manganese and choline. Deficiency of manganese leads to alterations in cell tissues. So our nutrient intake can make the skin, mucous membranes and cell membranes throughout our body much stronger. Our bodies can only use what we put into them. If we are stressed, take in too many anti-nutrients (such as coffee, chocolate, alcohol, refined sugars, fizzy pop and cigarettes), if we are surrounded by pollution (lead, cadmium, mercury, aluminium, food additives, pesticides and fungicides), or eat processed foods low in essential minerals (such as zinc, magnesium, manganese, chromium and selenium) and essential fatty acids it becomes more difficult for our poor bodies to cope.

## FREE OXIDIZING RADICALS

Alex Comfort, the gerontologist, says 'FoRs are highly reactive chemical agents that will combine with anything that is around – like conference delegates.' To add insult to injury, 'free radical damage' to the cell membrane could be another problem. Free oxidizing radicals (FoRs) occur naturally in the body and are formed when glucose is burned to produce energy. Free oxidizing radical means that the molecules are incomplete; they have an electron missing, giving them an uneven, negative electric charge. As a result, the FoRs will rush around the body like mad things trying to steal an electron from an already complete molecule in order to make themselves whole.

However, changes in our diets and the environment have also caused an increase in the number of free radicals produced. FoRs are present in burnt food, fried food, sunshine, smog, industrial factory fumes, pesticides, tobacco smoke, upholstery and carpet treatments, barbecued food, and chemicals used in the building and paint trade. The high levels of FoRs can cause the body to become overwhelmed so that it can no longer make them all safe.

FoRs can cause injury, inflammation and mayhem to cell membranes, collagen (the building block of all human tissue) and to the DNA in the nucleus. Wherever they have been, they leave behind a compound which has been denatured and can no longer function as it should. For example, proteins are rather like tight curly hair; once they have been denatured, the proteins uncurl and lose their power. Protein-based hormones, such as oxytoxin and prolactin, can be damaged in this way. The FoRs also damage the fats and oils in our bodies, including those oils making up the cell membrane, the steroid hormones, prostaglandins and the immune cells of the lymphatic system. All this thieving of electrons causes a domino effect, cascading through localized tissues and causing untold damage, as the cell loses control of its internal and external biochemistry.

FoRs cause damage in four main areas:

1 *Double bonds and DNA.* FoRs love the double bonds of DNA

molecules and are attracted to them because of the electrons they contain. If DNA function is impaired it can no longer reproduce itself faithfully. Cellular mutations may occur, and the production of new enzymes, hormones and proteins can become faulty.

2 *Immune cells.* Because immune cells are so complex, they are susceptible to FoR damage. If the immune cells are damaged by FoRs they can no longer identify and attack invading 'aliens' effectively, thus leaving our body tissues open to more damage than would normally have taken place. This damage may lead cells to attack 'self' tissue as in auto-immune diseases, which could be the case in endometriosis.

3 *Cell membranes.* The cell membrane is made up of lipids (oils) and the FoRs attack the lipids' double bonds allowing harmful chemicals into the cell that may damage its working. Arachodonic acid from animal fats may trigger the cell walls to secrete prostaglandins which cause a flammatory reaction in the surrounding area, as happens with endometriotic implants.

4 *Proteins.* These are most susceptible to free radical damage. Once the electrons have been stolen from proteins they lose all their normal activity. This is very serious as all protein-based hormones, such as oxytoxin and prolactin, and enzymes suffer irreparable damage. Collagen (the substance which holds cells together) is affected and wrinkles in skin can result. Skin and internal mucous membranes age more rapidly.

The question is, therefore, how to reduce the amount of damage caused by FoRs? There are several enzymes in the body which exist in order to 'mop up' FoRs.

1 Super oxide dismutase (SOD) releases an electron to neutralize the FoR. In order for SOD to work it needs regular supplies of copper, zinc and manganese from the diet. SOD forms part of a vital collection of genes which influence the repair of damaged DNA.

2 Glutathione peroxidase neutralizes FoRs by giving them an electron and stopping the damage before it begins. The amount of glutathione peroxidase present in the body is entirely dependent upon our absorption of selenium and vitamin B2 (riboflavin).

3 Catalase can only work when iron is present in sufficient quantity. It is an enzyme which plays an important role in the body's metabolism and it also neutralizes the effects of FoRs.

*Antioxidants*

Antioxidants are specific nutrients which can disarm the FoRs by adding an electron to the FoR and balancing the electric charge. The best-known antioxidants are vitamins A, C and E, and the mineral selenium. But coenzyme Q10, Quercetin (a flavinoid, *see* Glossary), and the amino acids taurine, glutathione and cysteine are also involved. Other substances which help support antioxidant activity are copper, manganese, iron, sodium and the vitamins B1, B2, B3, B5, B6, para-amino benzoic acid, choline and inositol. If our digestive systems are poor at absorbing these vital nutrients or our diets do not contain them in sufficient quantities, then we will sustain more FoR damage to our cells.

Does this mean that the damaged cell membranes may be prone to developing endometriosis? We don't know. More research is needed, but we can try to protect ourselves through our diet.

**SUMMARY**

1 The menstrual cycle is a complex mixture of interactions between the pituitary, the ovaries and the uterus.

2 The pituitary secretes the hormones FSH and LH which stimulate the ovary to produce mature eggs and steroid hormones (oestrogen and progesterone). The ovarian steroids, in turn, prepare the uterus for a possible pregnancy by stimulating the uterine endometrium to become a lush tissue that secretes the nutrients required by a developing embryo.

3 Endometriosis is a disease that is characterized by the presence of uterine endometrium in areas outside of the uterus, primarily within the abdomen. These rogue patches of endometrial tissue are known as endometriotic implants.

4 Endometriotic implants interfere with the menstrual cycle in a subtle fashion that is not fully understood. But they can lead to

pain and infertility in some women. The hormonal messages get mixed up in endometriosis.

5  Weakened cell membranes may make it easier for endometriotic implants to take hold.

6  Magnesium and natural cis-vegetable and fish oils are known to improve the integrity of cell membranes.

7  By reducing free radical damage the cell membrane may sustain less injury. Antioxidants such as selenium and vitamins A, C and E help to disarm free radicals. (A daily portion of fruit and vegetables will help to improve the dietary intake of these.)

8  Optimum nutrition and a healthy digestive system help to ensure that all cells work efficiently.

# 3 Coping with the pain of endometriosis

Nothing is too wonderful to be true, if it be consistent with the laws of nature.

*Michael Faraday, Physicist*

Pain is defined in the *Concise Oxford Dictionary* as 'suffering, distress, of body or mind'. The *Oxford American Dictionary* defines it as 'an unpleasant feeling caused by injury or disease of the body'. Endometriosis pain is dire, described by many as 'exquisite', because it takes over your life and colours your whole being, often leaving you stunned or unable to breathe. Pain is a signal that something is wrong within the body. Pain makes us adapt and do something to gain relief; it makes us react. Chronic intractable pain, such as that from endometriosis, is exhausting. It saps our vitality and robs us of our pleasure in life. Doctors often diagnose and attempt to treat the cause of the pain, but they often fail to discuss the meaning of this pain, so that we do not know what to expect in terms of our general well-being or our prospects for recovery. It is crucial that pain is taken seriously and not dismissed as being in the mind. Most women have great difficulty trying to explain to a sceptical doctor what is actually happening inside them. This adds to the anxiety, causing more tension and more pain.

Chronic pain is defined as pain which lasts for longer than one month and cannot be relieved by conventional treatment methods. With endometriosis the pain may be intermittent, but the pain is real and it causes much unhappiness and anxiety. Sometimes it becomes so overwhelming that death would actually seem a welcome relief. When ovarian cysts burst, the pain can be so unreal, so breathtaking, one almost wonders how the body can survive it. Being kept awake night after night by extreme pain wears out the nerves and leaves one feeling frail and battered. Struggling through day after day of pain wears down the soul.

## Jo R of London

*I can happily say that over the past few months since seeing the nutritionist many of my symptoms have subsided and I can now carry on a normal life. I was getting all the typical endometriosis symptoms, the bloating, abdominal pain, heavy periods and bad indigestion. After being careful with the foods I eat and cutting out wheat and reducing dairy foods, it has made an amazing difference. The fatigue has gone and period pains are a thing of the past. Really at first it sounded that cutting out some foods would be hard, but once you feel the effects, it is easy to keep to as you never want to feel so bad again. If to be well means I can't eat bread again, I can live without the bread. What I can't live with is the pain. I now take supplements on and off. Occasionally I lapse with the food if I'm eating out, but generally it is easy, and the way I feel now I do not want to give up and go back to those dark days.*

## WHAT CAUSES PAIN AND INFLAMMATION?

Pain is caused by inflammation. This is a protective mechanism in the body which is a local response around an area of damage to prevent or delay the spread of infection. It happens at a site of injury from stress, chemicals, heat, bacteria or trauma. The first reaction is for the blood vessels to dilate in order to increase the flow of blood to the site of injury. This gives the red appearance and feeling of warmth (with endometriosis this seems nearer to boiling point), which we feel after a cut to the skin. The mast cells (large cells in connective tissue) release histamines and prostaglandins which cause the inflammation. Histamine is a compound formed from an amino acid histidine and is found in all tissues of the body. It causes dilation of blood vessels and contraction (tightening) of muscles.

Small capillaries (blood vessels) in the area become permeable and fluids leak into the spaces between the cells, causing fluid retention (oedema) and localized swelling which puts pressure on the nerve endings, increasing the pain. At the site of the wound, zinc and vitamins C and A are always found as they are required for collagen production in order to build healthy new skin. The blood at the site of the inflammatory response clots (this uses vitamin K) in order to seal off the area and to prevent us from bleeding to death.

Clotting also stops the infection or damage from spreading into other areas of the body.

If bacteria are involved, chemotaxic chemicals (those which are on watch for danger) call for the 'immune army'. These include the blood cells called neutrophils, macrophages and lymphocytes which come to the injury site to fight the 'alien' danger. A pus-filled cavity may be formed, acting as a holding bay for dumping debris into, so that the white blood cells (macrophages) can come along and gobble it up.

With endometriosis much of the pain may be due to inflammation around the endometriotic implants. Once the immune army is called in and their chemical warfare begins, healthy tissue around the endometriosis may be bombarded with chemicals produced by immune cells – lymphokines, interleukins and interferons (*see* chapter 7 on the immune system). These white cells dump their chemical weapons onto the damaged tissues in an effort to remove the danger and to allow the body to heal the damage. The histamine release around the site also triggers more inflammation.

## COPING WITH PAIN

Chronic pain is often frightening, debilitating and excruciating. When it subsides there is always a terror that it may return. Prolonged mild pain is totally fatiguing; it stops you from enjoying the normal things in life and leaves you feeling in despair. What do you do with pain? Do you go with it, fight against it or just learn to live with it? Fighting pain can be counter-productive as it causes us to tense up, when the best form of action is to try to relax. When we are relaxed the brain is able to produce endorphins, which are natural painkilling hormones.

We all have different ways of trying to cope with pain. When it goes on unabated for months on end, we take a battering. It is almost as if the psyche goes into hibernation in order to protect us. Getting through each day becomes a major achievement. Trying to find the energy to take a shower or prepare a meal can be exhausting and you may have to rest afterwards. It can be terrifying to be so ill and to discover there is no known cure. You either have to learn to live with it, which is not an option, or you have to take the bull by the horns and try everything which instinct tells you is right for you, at your own pace. Let this time become useful by reading and learning new things, making something good come out of the bad. That way positive things can happen. Not giving in to the illness, but turning it to your own advantage, stops it from ruling and ruining your life. Build on other skills you have developed over the years from hobbies or interests. With careful management on your part, you can take positive steps to regain your health. Apply the principles of relaxation, exercise and healthy eating.

Pain management treatment can be useful, but what works for one person may not work for another, so you need to persevere to find a strategy which works for you. Perhaps some of the following strategies may help you, as they have helped other women:

1   Gentle exercise
2   Acupuncture
3   Manipulation by an osteopath or chiropractor
4   Weight loss or improved nutrition
5   Hypnotherapy
6   Relaxation techniques
7   Counselling
8   Distracting hobbies or activities
9   Self-help support groups
10  TENS (transcutaneous electrical stimulation) machines from your GP. (These work best to reduce pain of medium intensity, such as period pain. They work for 10 per cent of patients and can help to reduce the need for medication.)
11  Medication
12  Surgery

The British Endometriosis Society (founded by Ailsa Irving in 1982) asked its members how they coped with pain. Ninety per cent of the women who responded used a wide variety of over-the-counter or prescribed painkillers. Many women used them constantly, although the majority took them only when the pain began to increase. Painkillers work more effectively if they are taken when the pain begins. Once extreme pain has taken hold, it becomes too intractable to shift. A few women took more than the recommended dose of painkiller, which can be very damaging to the liver and stomach. The women's most common complaint was that no painkiller ever took the pain away completely; it was merely dulled. A few women had been taking anti-depressants, some for several years. Non-steroidal anti-inflammatory drugs (NSAIDs) which may cause bleeding of the stomach lining; anti-spasmodics

**What does your pain feel like?**

Some of the words below describe your *present* pain. Circle ONLY those words that best describe it. Leave out any category that is not suitable. Use only a single word in each appropriate category – the one that best applies.

| 1 | 2 | 3 | 4 | 5 |
|---|---|---|---|---|
| Flickering | Jumping | Pricking | Sharp | Pinching |
| Quivering | Flashing | Boring | Cutting | Pressing |
| Pulsing | Shooting | Drilling | Lacerating | Gnawing |
| Throbbing | | Stabbing | | Cramping |
| Beating | | Lancinating | | Crushing |
| Pounding | | | | |

| 6 | 7 | 8 | 9 | 10 |
|---|---|---|---|---|
| Tugging | Hot | Tingling | Dull | Tender |
| Pulling | Burning | Itchy | Sore | Taut |
| Wrenching | Scalding | Smarting | Hurting | Rasping |
| | Searing | Stinging | Aching | Splitting |
| | | | Heavy | |

| 11 | 12 | 13 | 14 | 15 |
|---|---|---|---|---|
| Tiring | Sickening | Fearful | Punishing | Wretched |
| Exhausting | Suffocating | Frightful | Grueling | Blinding |
| | | Terrifying | Cruel | |
| | | | Vicious | |
| | | | Killing | |

| 16 | 17 | 18 | 19 | 20 |
|---|---|---|---|---|
| Annoying | Spreading | Tight | Cool | Nagging |
| Troublesome | Radiating | Numb | Cold | Nauseating |
| Miserable | Penetrating | Drawing | Freezing | Agonizing |
| Intense | Piercing | Squeezing | | Dreadful |
| Unbearable | | Tearing | | Torturing |

Figure 3.1
Laparoscopic appearance of endometriosis, vol 1, 2nd ed, Resurge Press, Memphis,TN,1991, p. 33. Reproduced with kind permission from Arnold J. Kresch, D C Martin, D B Redwine and H Reich.

and analgesics were also mentioned. Some women drank alcohol with their painkillers, which is extremely dangerous.

## DESCRIBING AND MEASURING PAIN

It is very important to find a general practitioner who will listen to your description of your level of pain and who will work with you to find the right type of painkiller. The chart shown in figure 3.1, drawn up by the American gynaecologist Arnold Kresch, may be used to show your GP the type of pain you suffer. Circle the words which closely describe your pain, to explain the type of symptoms which are present, and photocopy them for your doctor.

The diagram of three women (figure 3.2) was also developed by Arnold Kresch, can be used to indicate where the pain is most severe. Write a 10 in the square where the pain is at its worst and

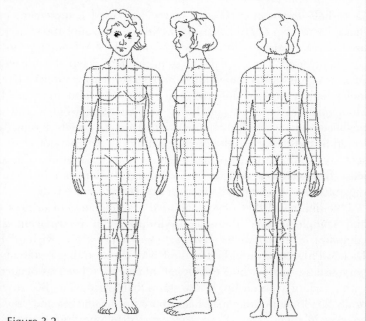

Figure 3.2
Laparoscopic appearance of endometriosis, vol 1, 2nd ed, Resurge Press, Memphis,TN,1991, p. 34. Reproduced with kind permission from Arnold J. Kresch, D C Martin, D B Redwine and H Reich.

radiate 9s around it. This way your GP can see exactly where the seat of the chronic pain lies, and this may help more effective pain-killing drugs to be prescribed.

Taking control into your own hands can help you cope. Endometriosis is so difficult to explain to sceptical individuals who have the philosophy 'Oh no, it's a woman's problem', and anxiety often can arise when you are unable to describe how the pain is creating problems for you. Certainly doctors need to be made aware of just how your pain affects your everyday life. When you are in the full throes of pain at 4 a.m. it is vital for the doctor to see you then. It is no good waiting until the next day when you are in recovery and crawling along to the surgery. The doctor needs to see the full effect of the pain in order to treat it correctly. If a doctor is unavailable, call an ambulance or get a taxi to the local casualty department.

## COMPLEMENTARY THERAPIES

Over half the women in the survey had used complementary therapies to help control their pain. Nutritional supplements were used by the majority, with DL phenylalanine (DLPA) being the most commonly used. These are discussed in chapter 9. Herbal medicines such as agnus castus, blue cohosh, raspberry leaves, slippery elm, violet leaves, peppermint and garlic oils were also mentioned. Homeopathic remedies had been used by some women and a qualified homeopathic practitioner can advise you on which remedy would be most appropriate for your symptoms. A variety of elixirs, such as camomile tea, raspberry leaf tea, arnica ointment, royal jelly, Bach Flower Rescue Remedy and Indian brandy, were suggested, and yet others used prayer and laying on of hands.

One-quarter of the women had used a combination of orthodox and complementary therapies. Winthrop, the pharmaceutical company, in their booklet *Managing Danazol Patients* by Richard P Dickey, PhD, MD (published in the USA), mention that irritability, nervousness, anxiety and emotional lability have been associated with a lack of vitamin B6. It also states that 'pyridoxine (B6) given orally 25–30mg per day may help to prevent headaches and visual changes in some cases'. So it is recognized by one drug company that a mixture of therapies may help. (Chapter 5 discusses the use of the drug Danazol as a treatment for endometriosis.)

A favourite way to treat pain was to curl up with a hot water bottle. Various techniques, like visualization, reading, having a warm

months to totally heal, although some people feel much improved after a couple of weeks. We are all different.

At 4 a.m. when things look bleak and you feel very alone, remember that there are many women all over the world feeling the same at that very moment, and that you are not alone. Think of each other (mind meld) and pull each other through.

The treatment strategies chosen depends upon each person's physical make-up, medical condition, their personality and other factors, such as where the pain is seated. We hope that some of our suggestions will be of help to you. Remember that anxiety, anger and guilt can make pain worse; they are negative emotions, so try to be positive. It has been known for over a century that our emotional state influences our physical health. There is a new field of study looking into the mind–brain–immune connections, psychoneuro-immunology. It is known that the activities of the white blood cells of the immune system are influenced by the brain and nervous system, as there are receptors on each which receive messages from the others. What we think and feel are likely to influence the way our immune cells respond. It is not understood how these areas influence each other and, as everyone is individual, it will differ from person to person. How we respond to the world and the pollution around us may affect our physical well-being. If we feel in control our bodies may cope better than if we feel out of control. Self-help is important because it makes us try to do something for ourselves and regain control over our health.

> The two foes of human happiness are
> pain and boredom
> *Arthur Schopenhauer, Philosopher*

## HOW TO COPE WITH CHRONIC PAIN

Some of the following ideas are suggested by the Chronic Pain Outreach Association in America:

1  Relax – listen to a relaxation tape or imagine a pleasant scene.
2  Do a distracting activity – reading, craftwork, etc.
3  Tell yourself that the pain is temporary and that it will pass.
4  Place a hot water bottle or bag of frozen peas on the pain site.

5   Make yourself laugh, watch a funny film.
6   Hold an involved conversation in your head.
7   Listen to your favourite music.
8   Try deep breathing or meditation.
9   Avoid stressful situations wherever possible.
10  Reduce tension by whatever means (even crying or shouting).
11  Notice the control that you do have (in whatever areas of your life).
12  Take a relaxing bath or shower.
13  Spend time in a very quiet room.
14  Use disassociation – become an 'observer' of your pain rather than feeling it as a 'participant'.
15  Use visual imagery to transform your pain into something different – a shape or colour, for example.
16  Focus your attention on a part of your body which has a different sensation.
17  Ask for the support of others.
18  Adjust your activity level gradually. Increase towards normal activity level over 3–4 days.

## NUTRITION TO REDUCE PAIN AND INFLAMMATION

### Linda C of Surrey

*After much trial and error I have changed my eating pattern to suit me, i.e. not combining foods and not eating foods that over a period of time have proved not to suit me (dairy, pastry, meats). I take vitamins and minerals every day and most of all I believe that a positive mental attitude to this condition has, along with the supplements, proved vital. I have had NO pain now for several years.*

CASE STUDY

### WHY CAN NUTRIENTS REDUCE PAIN?

Often diseases which are the result of vitamin deficiency are associated with unspecific pains. Changes in the central nervous system, and mucous membrane and skin inflammation are often

highlighted in these conditions. While researching into endometriosis and nutrition, several research papers surfaced which
showed that certain vitamins do possess analgesic (pain-relieving)
and anti-inflammatory properties which correspond to those of
orthodox medicines, but without the side effects. Pain is perceived as
the body's alarm signal, showing that all is not well. For instance,
severe vitamin C deficiency causes scurvy, manifested by bleeding
gums, and considerable pain in the joints. If the need for vitamin C
is corrected, then the symptoms diminish. Vitamin C combats
inflammation and pain by inhibiting the secretion of prostaglandins
which contribute to the symptoms.[2] Pain and inflammation which
has its origin in a vitamin deficiency is best treated with that
particular vitamin. Various other nutrients are known to play a role
in relieving pain; these are the essential fatty acids from fats and
natural cold-pressed oils, vitamins C, E and K and some of the B
complex vitamins, and DL phenylalanine (DLPA), zinc, selenium
and magnesium. If the body is subclinically deficient in certain
combinations of vitamins and minerals, our responses to 'normal'
pain could be heightened. By becoming optimally nourished we
may be able to protect ourselves from the intensity of pain.

## THE USE OF ANTI-INFLAMMATORY OILS

Use of good quality natural oils may be a vital key to our disease.
The choice of fats and oils used in cooking, for spreading and within
pre-prepared foods, may have the most profound impact on our
health and perception of pain. Most people know about saturated
and polyunsaturated fats, but the key is the form in which they are
found. Every cell membrane, all the steroid hormones and most
brain cells depend upon oils (lipids) which our bodies process from
the fatty foods we eat. In foods, oils can be found in two forms, cis
oils and trans oils.

### Cis fatty acids

In nature oil molecules are shaped rather like a horseshoe. This
shape of molecule fits tightly with other phospholipids to form a
strong cell membrane which protects the processes going on inside
each cell. The membrane maintains the integrity of each cell and
stops harmful chemicals from entering and damaging the
powerhouses inside, which are working to produce proteins,

prostaglandins, steroid hormones, enzymes and phospholipids. As these good quality cis oils make up almost one-third of brain tissue and every cell membrane, they are crucial to your state of health.

Your choice of these cis oils is therefore important. Look around your local health food shop for jars of extra virgin cold-pressed olive oils, organic butter and vegetable oils, such as sunflower, safflower and sesame, that are labelled 'unrefined', 'unhydrogenated' or 'cold-pressed'. Cold-pressed olive oil and butter are fine for light, shallow frying. For salad dressings use a mixture of extra virgin olive oil and some cold-pressed, unrefined sunflower or safflower oils. Keep the opened jar in the fridge. Oils in tins are best, as light causes oil to go rancid. Fresh nuts and seeds are also an excellent source of cis oils. A handful of nuts and seeds or a tablespoon of cis oils each day will help to balance your intake of good quality oils. They aid your metabolism and used in moderation do not make you fat. However, if you have poor digestion (heartburn, constipation or diarrhoea) (*see* chapter 8) or poor diet to start with so that you are unable to absorb enough of the nutrients needed to metabolize these essential fatty acids, then the digestion must be corrected and a digestive enzyme taken with each meal (*see* p 168).

### Trans fatty acids

Trans fatty acids are found when oils have been processed, hydrogenated or refined. They are often found in biscuits, cakes, pastries and margarines. Most vegetable oils on supermarket shelves have been processed, and so contain trans oils, which are implicated in breast cancer formation. Women with high levels of trans fatty acids in body cells have about a 40 per cent higher risk of getting breast cancer.[3, 4] When fats are processed, the molecule shape becomes more like a kink than a horseshoe. This fits loosely into the cell membrane, weakening it so that it is no longer effective at stopping harmful chemicals from entering the cell. This may damage the production of energy in the mitochondria and weaken defences against cancers. This may be why endometrial implants take hold.

Heat changes cis oils into trans oils, so deep frying is not advisable. You should avoid all oils which have been processed (hydrogenated), all oils which are rancid, and never use the same oil twice for frying. It is very important to read the label on oil jars and to buy only unhydrogenated, unrefined, cold-pressed oils. These are usually available only from your local health food store. It is in your best interest to avoid processed foods whenever possible, or to use convenience foods occasionally, but not every day. Being realistic, you will eat some trans fats, but you can try to keep them to a minimum.

*Using and choosing good quality oils*

There are three main fatty acids which the body uses:

1  Linoleic acid – series one prostaglandins.
2  Arachidonic acid – series two prostaglandins.
3  Alpha-linolenic acid – series three prostaglandins.

Series one and three fatty acids have anti-inflammatory properties, and series two can cause inflammation if not in balance with the other two. The body can make arachidonic acid from dairy products and the fat in meat, but it needs constant daily, fresh supplies of linoleic and alpha-linolenic acids from vegetable and fish oils as it cannot make series one and three vital fatty acids. If the daily diet is poor, the body supplies of these fatty acids will be extremely low.

### Jane WJ of Kent

*I remember that the nutritional programme did make me feel much better. I still rely on the evening primrose oil. I really feel the difference in pain and PMT if I run out or forget to take it before a period. I take 1,000mg a day, upping it to 2,000mg a day in the immediate days before the period.*

*I conceived straight away after the nutrition programme, and since then my endometriosis has been in remission.*

•
C
A
S
E

S
T
U
D
Y
•

*Essential oils – the precursors to prostaglandins*

Prostaglandins (PGs) are lipid (oil-based) hormones that have very important effects upon such body tissues as cell membranes in the reproductive system. The precursors to prostaglandins are the essential fatty acids (EFAs), arachidonic linoleic acid and alpha-linolenic acid. Cis fatty acids should be the preferred source of oils in our diet.

The conversion of prostaglandins from EFAs depends upon enzymes, which are in turn nutrient dependent. If an excess of the wrong types of prostaglandins are produced by our tissues, this may lead to internal inflammation. Often the actions of one group of the PG system are in direct opposition to those of another.

There are three types of prostaglandins (*see* figures 3.3 and 3.4):

1  Series 1 prostaglandins are derived from vegetable oils and they have anti-inflammatory properties. (Linoleic acid.)

2  Series 2 prostaglandins from dairy foods and fats within meat can cause inflammation to occur. (Arachidonic acid.)

3  Series 3 prostaglandins are metabolized from fish and linseed oils and have anti-inflammatory properties. (Alpha-linoleic acid.)

The three different types of PGs need to be kept in balance (*see* figure 3.3), because they have a role in maintaining body homeostasis. (Homeo means same; stasis means standing still; homeostasis is the harmony within the body). The body has an internal environment which has to be maintained within certain limits, for example, temperature control and the acid/alkaline balance, and it is constantly making adjustments to maintain this stable state. The body requires a rich mixture of gases, nutrients and water to control the temperature balance (here the thyroid gland in the neck is involved). It also needs fresh water to maintain health within cells. Health can deteriorate rapidly when this homeostatic balancing act is disturbed.

Thus PGs possess both pro-inflammatory and anti-inflammatory properties. It has been suggested that more evidence 'appears to indicate that PGs from series 1 conceivably dominantly have an anti-inflammatory property, whereas the series 2 PGs may have mainly pro-inflammatory qualities depending on their local concentrations'.[5] Series 3 PGs are also anti-inflammatory. If you absorb enough linoleic and alpha-linolenic series 1 and 3 groups from good quality cis oils, you should be able to produce sufficient prostaglandin PGE1 which reduces the production of series 2 arachidonic acid (arachidonic triggers inflammation and pain in the body). Thus you can help to control internal inflammation just by

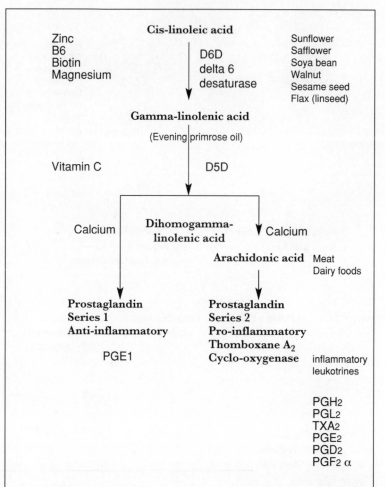

Figure 3.3 Metabolic pathway of the prostaglandin pathways for series 1 and series 2 prostaglandins

Linoleic acid, which the body cannot make, comes from safflower, sunflower, hemp, soya bean, walnut, pumpkin seed, sesame seed and flax (linseed) oils. You need a fresh daily supply of this cold-pressed oil. Linoleic acid is the precursor of series 1 and series 2 prostaglandins. In your body linoleic acid is changed using nutrients into gamma-linolenic acid (evening primrose oil). This is then changed again to dihomogamma-linolenic acid, which is the anti-inflammatory form, and also to arachidonic acid which is pro-inflammatory. The vitamins and minerals which are required for their formation are listed.

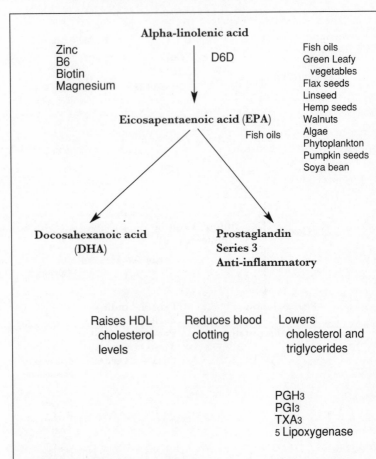

Figure 3.4 Metabolic pathway of the series 3 fatty acids down to prostaglandins

Alpha-linolenic acid is found in flax seeds, hemp seeds, pumpkin seeds, dark green leafy vegetables, soya bean, walnut and fish oils. The body cannot make this fatty acid so fresh supplies are required daily. Alpha-linolenic acid is the precursor of series 3 prostaglandins, which are anti-inflammatory. It is changed in the body to eicosapentaenoic acid. The enzymes require zinc, B6, magnesium and biotin to make series 3 prostaglandins. These are known to decrease blood pressure, reduce blood clotting, lower cholesterols and reduce internal inflammation. The vitamins and minerals involved in the process are listed.

eating the right sorts of oils. Evening primrose oil can be beneficial for some people; it tips the balance.

'Only the natural horseshoe shape cis form of linoleic and linolenic acids are able to contribute to the formation of PGs.'[6] Trans fatty acids which have been changed by chemical processing known as hydrogenation form a kink shape are not as effective in the formation of prostaglandins. Macrophages, often the predominant immune cells present during chronic inflammatory conditions, release PGs in response to inflammatory stimuli. In women with endometriosis the macrophage count is often higher than normal. If they release PGE2 more inflammation may occur (see chapter 7).

As an added bonus, PGE1 is able to stop blood cells becoming sticky; it can help to remove fluid from the body and can improve the functioning of nerves. It also has been shown to help immune cells in their work of clearing up cell debris in the abdominal cavity. These immune cells also need vitamin B6, iron and selenium.

Researchers think that an imbalance in the three different types of prostaglandins may be one of the causes of premenstrual syndrome and endometriosis pain. One piece of research shows that women with severe period pain, infertility and endometriosis had raised levels of prostaglandins series 2 (from arachidonic acid) in their peritoneal fluid, which could be the trigger for the inflammation. Therefore making the effort to ensure these oils are balanced in the diet is a good practical step to take.

*Daily oil intake*

How can you assess the daily intake of good quality oils in your diet and improve it where necessary? If your diet is very low in the oils from fresh nuts, seeds, good quality cold-pressed oils and oily fish, and very high in dairy foods and fatty meats, then the series 2 prostaglandins will outweigh those from series 1 and 3. The result may be internal inflammation and pain. A change in your eating pattern may be able to reduce this effect. Standard prostaglandin inhibitors (such as Ibroprufen) reduce all three types of prostaglandin, thus stopping the beneficial anti-inflammatory ones from working effectively.

Your body cannot take the steps to convert linoleic acid into gamma-linolenic acid (GLA) unless zinc, magnesium, vitamin B6 and biotin are absorbed from your diet. Vitamin C and calcium are then necessary for the final change into series 1 PGE1 and series 2 arachidonic acid. Evening primrose oil is very useful for some people as it bypasses the second stage of conversion, if the five nutrients (magnesium, B6, zinc, biotin, folic acid) are missing from the diet or being malabsorbed. Taken as a supplement, evening primrose oil can help to rebalance the three types of prostaglandins. The usual dose is four 500mg capsules per day. Too much stress, saturated animal fats, trans fatty acids and alcohol, can prevent the enzymes being able to change linoleic acid into a form the body can use to dampen down inflammation.

---

### Barbara G of Essex

*My endometriosis and period pains and periods in general are much better since being on a yeast-free diet and taking nutritional supplements, including GLA. I also eat oily fish (herring and mackerel), fresh 3–4 times each week. You can't beat fresh. Now I am recovered I will follow the same wholefood diet with a few extras such as a little bread. Efamol Marine has been extremely useful to me.*

CASE STUDY

---

Practical steps you can take include increasing your intake of fish and cold-pressed cis vegetable seed oils, while reducing the amount of dairy foods and meats. This helps to reduce the levels of arachidonic acid produced which causes inflammation. By eating oily fish twice a week and having one tablespoon of cis oils each day in salad dressing, soup or yogurt, the body may obtain sufficient oils to aid formation of the anti-inflammatory PGs. These good quality oils are essential in a well-balanced diet, and contrary to previous thought, they do not lead to an increase in weight. The fats which cause weight increase are the 'bad' saturated fats and trans fatty acids. The 'good' cis fatty acids aid body metabolism. Researchers have observed that 'the more linoleic acid in the fat tissue, the less obese the person'.[7]

### Fish oils

Fish oils are very important so long as they come from a reliable unpolluted source. Research on the effect of fish oils on endometrial implants in rabbits with surgically induced endometriosis showed the sites of endometrial tissue shrank when the rabbits were fed fish oils: 'Pro-inflammatory prostaglandins in the peritoneal fluid were significantly lower in the fish oil group versus the controls. Total endometriotic implant diameter eight weeks after induction was significantly smaller in the experimental group versus the controls.'[8] The researchers concluded 'that dietary supplementation with fish oils can decrease the peritoneal pro-inflammatory prostaglandin production and retard implant growth in animal models'. Studies on the use of fish oils in women with severe period pains showed that

## Best quality oils to choose (all fresh cold-pressed)

| | | |
|---|---|---|
| Flax (linseeds) | Pumpkin seeds | Soya beans |
| Fish | Walnuts | Seaweed |
| Sunflower seeds | Evening primrose oil | Sesame seeds |
| Almonds | Game birds | Hazelnuts |
| Cold-pressed oils in tins | | |

## Reasonable oils

| | | |
|---|---|---|
| Venison | Chicken | Mechanically cold-pressed oils in glass bottles |
| Eggs | Roasted fresh nuts and seeds | Organic butter in moderation |

## Oils to use in very small amounts

| | | |
|---|---|---|
| Bottled hydrogenated vegetable oils | Dairy products | Pork |
| Beef | Fried foods | Lamb |
| Butter | Hydrogenated margarine | |

Table 3.1 The quality of oils
Alcohol, sugars and refined starches all metabolize in the body to form fats which are stored in the body fat (adipose tissues). Fat cells produce oestrogen which helps endometriosis to grow. Therefore using only the good oils in moderation and cutting out saturated and trans oils will help to control and normalize oestrogen production.

the fish oils were effective at reducing pain. If you are vegetarian, you can use fresh edible food grade linseeds each day; grind and eat them with breakfast cereal.

The metabolism of essential fatty acids in the body to form anti-inflammatory prostaglandins is crucial. Essential cis fatty acids from both fish oils and unrefined, unhydrogenated cis vegetable oils are able to alleviate pain and inflammation in the peritoneal cavity and joints if taken for a sustained period at the right dose. People with arthritis or pelvic inflammatory disease can benefit from dietary supplementation with evening primrose oil, linseed oil (edible food grade), borage and starflower oil and fish oils. Always buy cold-pressed capsules from a reputable source. Some of the cheaper tablets can be ineffective and a waste of money.

## THE ROLE OF VITAMINS IN PAIN RELIEF

### Jo R of Slough

*Having suffered for years with extremely painful periods, mood swings, lethargy etc., I eventually sought complementary therapies. (After being diagnosed as having endo and being told that I needed a hysterectomy at 22 years of age.) Through cutting out all gluten foods, red meats and alcohol I found 110 per cent change for the better. Not only in my pain symptoms, but my monthly bleed would not be as heavy. My hair and nails became stronger and my overall health improved dramatically. Although I do feel the diet is difficult at times and slightly inconvenient, my whole attitude towards nutrition and health has changed. I think my mental health has improved too as I now feel stronger, more energetic and in control of my body. Thank you!*

•
C
A
S
E

S
T
U
D
Y

•

### Vitamin C

Vitamin C, when combined with bioflavinoids and digestive enzymes, has been shown in research to be more effective at reducing inflammation than non-steroidal anti-inflammatory drugs. An article about the research describes how 'Animal model trials looked at histamine-induced wheals in the peritoneal cavity. When given vitamin C, with bioflavinoids and digestive enzymes they reduced the effect of the histamine. It was felt that this was due to the nutrients strengthening cells against agents which were causing the inflammation'.[9] Bioflavinoids and vitamin C are known to have a beneficial effect upon immune cells. Vitamin C given to seriously ill cancer patients in a double blind controlled study showed that pain could be reduced significantly. Relief of pain using vitamin C has been shown in several other diseases. The way in which it works is not clear, but it may inhibit dopamine binding to membranes and inhibit prostaglandin levels. Low dietary levels of vitamin C in animal tests promoted the development of osteoarthritis. Relationships between vitamin E and vitamin C suggest that vitamin E may also be implicated in helping to reduce pain and inflammation. Together they thin blood, causing blood platelets to be less sticky. It has also been suggested that vitamin C 'has the property of a natural antihistamine and it reduces the severity of histamine attacks from internal inflammation, and may be able to detoxify excess histamine produced when the body is under stress'.[10]

*Vitamin E*

Vitamin E has an analgesic effect because it is able to inhibit pro-inflammatory prostaglandin production. In the 1970s research showed that '300 iu per day reduced muscle cramps and pains in the lower back'.[11] Studies also suggest that 'vitamin E has anti-inflammatory action as it protects lysosome membranes (internal cell particles which produce enzymes) from histamine and serotonin damage. It acts slowly to limit inflammation so needs to be taken regularly'.[12]

*B complex vitamins*

Some vitamins are used alone, but often their synergy means that when they are combined they are more powerful. B complex vitamins (B1, B6 and B12), when working together, have also been shown by research to exhibit an anti-inflammatory effect combined with an analgesic action: 'When vitamin B12 is taken with vitamin B1 and B6 they can together produce significant dose-dependent pain relief and inhibition of inflammation, comparable to the action of standard treatments in orthodox medicine, but without the side effects'.[13] Vitamin K seems to strengthen these effects; it has an anti-inflammatory and analgesic effect in animal models.

It is known from research that high doses of thiamin (vitamin B1) can suppress pain transmission, studies suggesting that there 'appears to be some relationship between thiamin and morphine'.[14] Vitamin B6 (pyridoxine) also has analgesic effects. If B6 is deficient, the amount of serotonin in the brain decreases and this can lead to depression. B6 helps to relieve the pain associated with premenstrual syndrome. It should always be taken with other B complex vitamins as they work synergistically. The best absorbed form of vitamin B6 is pyridoxal-5-phosphate, which acts as a coenzyme in transforming tryptophan into serotonin. (Serotonin is a neurotransmitter which exists is high concentrations in the hypothalamus, a major gland in the reproductive system – people with insufficient levels show signs of depression.)

'Vitamin B12 was shown in three independent trials to have an analgesic effect when injected intramuscularly'[15] and when combined with vitamins B1 and B6, they produce an even stronger therapeutic anti-inflammatory and analgesic effect.

---

## Tina R of Sussex

*Before starting the nutritional programme I suffered with excruciating painful periods, back pain, heavy bleeding, bloating, extreme fatigue and mood swings. The pain could be described as worse than being in labour. Conventional drugs were unsuccessful. I have now been on the diet for three months. Almost immediately I felt an improvement in my health. As well as following a healthy diet I try to avoid wheat and dairy foods which I have discovered result in bloating and cause more pain. My last period was lighter and almost pain-free. I no longer suffer with bloating caused by allergies and intolerances. I have an increased level of energy and a feeling of well-being, and I now have a 'zest' for life and it feels great. My health is of paramount importance and I know I shall always have to take care. Nutritional support and advice has been invaluable.*

• C A S E   S T U D Y •

---

MINERALS AGAINST PAIN

*Magnesium*

Magnesium is known to be necessary to the relaxation of muscles. It works to produce adenosine triphosphate (ATP), which produces energy in each cell. Without magnesium we would be plagued with cramps, spasms and convulsions. An adult needs 450–600mg of magnesium per day to maintain health. Magnesium plays a vital role in synthesizing myelin around the nerves, without which they become sensitive to pain. (Myelin is the protective fatty deposit which coats and protects nerves.) Magnesium also has an anaesthetizing effect on the central nervous system; therefore adequate magnesium 'is an important preventative against miscarriage and painful contractions of the uterus muscle'.[16] Magnesium malate is the best form to help with muscle relaxation and chronic fatigue; magnesium taurate is good for mental exhaustion and control of oestrodiol; and magnesium EAP2 is beneficial for the heart. All of these nutritional supplements are available in health food shops and by mail order.

## *Zinc*

Zinc sulphate was given to 24 patients with rheumatoid arthritis in one trial in Washington University, USA. It is known from research that zinc has anti-inflammatory effects in the knee joint. An article reports: 'In a 12-week double blind trial using a placebo, patients taking zinc sulphate showed significant improvement for joint swelling and morning stiffness, and their personal impressions of their overall condition was high. Zinc is known to inhibit the immunologically induced histamine and leukotrine release from mast cells. Thus it can dampen down inflammation'.[17] The good cis oils require zinc in order for the body to metabolize them to form anti-inflammatory prostaglandins.

## AMINO ACIDS

### *DL phenylalanine (DLPA)*

DL phenylalanine (DLPA) has been well researched and its potential to reduce chronic pain is well documented. Its effects can last for months, even after treatment ceases. Some people experience a marked relief from pain in the first few days of taking it, but others find that it can take up to three weeks before chronic pain dies down. Phenylalanine is a naturally occurring amino acid. In nature this amino acid is found as the 'L' form, and the mirror-image 'D' form is man-made, and when both the natural and man-made forms are combined they can relieve pain. DLPA also acts as an anti-depressant and an appetite suppressant. It should not be taken as a occasional painkiller; it must be taken consistently over a period of time. DLPA works in 60 per cent of people. If it has had no effect after taking it for three weeks, then it is probably not going to work for you. But when it does work, the results can be excellent.

How does DLPA work? When we are injured in some way our brain begins to produce endorphins, hormones whose properties mimic those of the most powerful analgesic drugs. They are the body's own pain control system. For example, in people injured in road accidents endorphins can prevent serious pain for several hours after the accident. DLPA works by reducing the levels of enzymes which normally break down endorphins, thus prolonging their effects in the body. The enzymes can also block the inflammatory effects of the pro-inflammatory prostaglandins.

Two DLPA tablets should be taken three times a day until the pain is reduced. The tablets can then gradually be reduced to a maintenance dose of one to two per day. The tablets should be taken 15 minutes before each meal if your blood pressure is normal (120 over 80 or below) or 15 minutes after each meal if your blood pressure is high (140 over 90 or above). Tablets are usually 375mg strength combined with vitamins C and B6 to act in synergy. They are available on prescription from the NHS. Contraindications would be pregnancy, breastfeeding, phenylketonuria, if you are taking monoamine oxidase (MAO drug) antidepressants or if you suffer extreme hypertension (high blood pressure).

Why do nutrients have this effect upon pain? It is probable that they activate certain enzymes and neurotransmitters involved with the perception of pain. Trying to achieve enzyme saturation point in all cells may be of benefit in promoting this anti-inflammatory and analgesic effect. (Saturation point occurs when the cells have the exact levels of vitamins, minerals and essential oils they need to work efficiently.) All enzymes use nutrients as co-factors in order to work effectively, so if the nutrient is in short supply, the pain control mechanism will not be able to work effectively.

Vitamins can be seen as keys to metabolic pathways. The gate to each pathway within the body is shut unless that specific vitamin comes along with its key. All the enzyme and hormone reactions on the other side of the gate cannot take place unless that vitamin is present. If you eat well and your digestive system is able to absorb properly, you remain healthy. But if you 'snatch and grab' meals of dubious quality foodstuffs or you have a poor digestive system, then you may require supplementary nutrients to help you in the short term while your diet, digestion and absorption are improved.

## USING NUTRIENTS TO CONTROL PAIN

### Helena G of London

*I would like to thank you for all your help. I have been keeping to my diet and taking the vitamins and minerals you prescribed for me. I must admit that I was sceptical at first about this kind of treatment, although I felt that it was worth a try since the treatment at hospital had not helped me at all. The diet did, however. It made me feel more positive as I felt that I had some kind of control over my health. Then, following the treatment for just over a month, I began to see a vast improvement. I felt more energetic and suffered less pain. Gradually over the second month I felt better than I had in years. Not only had the pain decreased greatly and the stomach upsets ceased, but I had greater concentration and did not feel as weak. My relationship with my family and friends, and especially my husband, has improved as I am no longer as quick-tempered, irritable and depressed as I had been. Also since following your treatment, I have not had to take any time off work, and have found it easier to deal with the stress of my job. I was sure that I would lose my job. Thank you.*

•

C
A
S
E

S
T
U
D
Y

•

Research into other conditions shows poor nutrition plays an important role in the development of other diseases and the sensible choice of good quality food could pay you dividends. We are all biochemically unique, therefore it is important for the individual to understand that what helps one person may not work in the same way for another. It has to be a trial and error approach. There are many treatments, orthodox and complementary, which others have found helpful. In chapter 9 we will look at which supplements can be taken safely and why they may be required. In chapters nine and ten we will discuss the type of healthy eating programme you could follow and which foodstuffs you should eat regularly.

## SUPPLEMENT PROGRAMME TO COMBAT PAIN

We have seen how important individual nutrients are in controlling degrees of pain within the body; how essential fatty acids can reduce inflammation and how vitamin C reduces histamine release. By maintaining a steady supply of good nutrients from food the body should be able to mute pain responses. Supplements may assist for a time to improve the body's fortitude. A selection of the following nutrients may help the body to cope with pain (*see* p 232):

- Multivitamin/mineral
- DL phenylalanine (DLPA)
- Essential fatty acids: omega 3 fish oils; omega 6 evening primrose oils (200mg per day)
- Magnesium malate
- Zinc citrate or amino acid chelate
- Selenium (non-yeast form)
- Vitamins A, C, E (antioxidants)
- Vitamins B1, B6, B12 (non-yeast form)
- Vitamin C with bioflavinoids and protein-digesting enzymes

### SUMMARY

1 Regardless of what anyone tells you, the pain from endometriosis is REAL. Get your pain taken seriously. Try to reduce the pain symptoms through nutrition and use any method which helps to distract you whenever possible.

2 Photocopy and fill in the pain charts from Arnold Kresch and use them to teach your GP the extent of this very real pain. You can also chart your pain and see how it changes over time.

3 Take painkillers early on to reduce pain. Once it takes hold it is much harder to control.

4 Exercising at a level with which you can cope helps to increase endorphin levels in the brain. These are the body's natural painkillers. Do exercise such as gentle walks or pleasurable swims when you feel able, to build up endorphin levels.

5 Use relaxation and visualization techniques to aid your control

of pain. Whatever works for you as an individual is the most important route to take. Feel comfortable about the techniques you try. If they feel wrong, stop using them.

6   Ask your GP or hospital for a TENS machine to try out.

7   Stay positive. You are going to beat this. At times when pain is overwhelming, this can feel nigh on impossible. Being positive helps to strengthen your immune cells to fight the endo-metriosis, which is essentially what is needed.

8   Let the time when you are incapacitated work for you. Use hobbies and skills you have acquired; you may be able to develop another career direction.

9   Vitamins and minerals possess some analgesic and anti-inflammatory properties which may help combat pain. If you are very ill the effort of preparing and cooking food is almost impossible, but try to eat fresh nutritious food. As you begin to absorb the vitamins and minerals, the body can work more effectively to combat pain.

10  Vitamins C, E, K, A, and B complex and the minerals selenium, zinc, magnesium, amino acids and DL phenylalanine and evening primrose and fish oils all aid in the suppression of pain. Ensure that you are eating and digesting these nutrients from foods in your diet. Remember that correcting the digestive tract is the first step. Consult a nutritionist for individualized advice.

# 4 Why is my fertility threatened?

All truth passes through three stages
First, it is ridiculed,
Second, it is opposed
Third, it is accepted as being self evident.
*Arthur Schopenhauer, Philosopher*

How many infertile couples do you know? One? Maybe two? The rate of infertility among couples of reproductive age in England and the USA is an amazing 15 to 20 per cent, about 1 in every 5 couples.[1] More than 2.4 million people in America alone have been robbed of the opportunity to conceive and have a family. It has been estimated that 30 per cent of infertile couples may be infertile as a result of endometriosis.[2] One in fifteen men and one in ten women are thought to be struggling with their fertility – you are not alone. Infertility is defined as lack of conception after at least 12 months of unprotected intercourse. Infertility is a major health issue, often due to an illness, yet it receives very little attention from our society or from Parliament and Congress. Fortunately, over 65 per cent of these infertile couples can be helped by drugs and surgery to achieve a pregnancy. And by following the correct nutritional advice that rate of success can be increased to 86 per cent if Foresight – the Association for Preconceptual Care's figures are taken into account. Thus help is available for the couple struggling with their fertility. By contrast, IVF only has a 10 per cent success rate in endometriosis patients.

Endometriosis is a complex disease that appears to have several different mechanisms through which it may trigger infertility. It is not clear if one or more of these mechanisms is the cause of the infertility associated with endometriosis, but endometriotic implants have several different effects on the reproductive system.

## ABDOMINAL ADHESIONS AND INFERTILITY

As the endometriotic implants grow and develop in the abdomen, where they do not belong, the body tries to surround them with fibrous connective tissue (scar tissue). The body does this in an attempt to isolate the implants and prevent them from doing harm. Adhesions can also be formed during surgery when abdominal tissue is traumatized. This fibrous tissue develops like moss growing on a stone and behaves like a Band-Aid on a wound.

These fibrous growths also have the effect of making the implants stick to adjacent tissues. Remember that blood is sticky and internal bleeding from the implant also forms adhesions, such that an implant may be stuck to several different tissues like a cat's cradle, as if we placed some very sticky glue-like gum in the abdomen and several organs became stuck to each other by the very sticky strands. For example, an endometriotic implant on the top of the uterus may cause the ovary and small intestine to become attached at the site of the implant. If the adhesions pinch off the Fallopian tube or if they cause a blockage of the opening of the Fallopian tube, they could obstruct the union of egg and sperm and prevent fertilization and conception, or cause an ectopic pregnancy, if the embryo can't travel to the womb. This type of obstruction can be easily diagnosed and surgically corrected.

However, this does not explain how patients with just a few implants and no adhesions can become infertile. Adhesions can also cause pain, as internal organs which normally slip and slide are firmly glued together. For example, if the bowel is stuck to a tender, painful ovary, flatulence could cause pain.

## SECRETIONS FROM ENDOMETRIOTIC IMPLANTS

As we have already seen, the endometrium within the womb is a dynamic tissue that secretes a wide variety of nutrients and hormones required for normal conception. The endometriotic implants also secrete these same substances, but instead of depositing them into the lumen (centre) of the womb as normal, the implants release their chemical secretions into the abdominal cavity. Some of these substances, which are in effect strong hormones, could interfere with fertility.

## PROSTAGLANDINS

One major group of hormones secreted by the normal endometrium is that of the prostaglandins. Prostaglandins are oil-based hormones found in nearly all the tissues of the body and are required for many bodily processes, including several stages of the menstrual cycle and pregnancy. Prostaglandins are required for ovulation, regression of the corpus luteum (i.e., ending the monthly menstrual cycle), sperm motility, immune interactions, contraction of the uterus at birth and menstrual cramps. Endometriotic implants and the endometrium of the uterus are the richest source of prostaglandin production in the body.

However, the problem with endometriotic implants is two-fold:

1   Prostaglandins are released into the abdomen instead of inside the womb.

2   Prostaglandin release by the implants seems to be out of phase with their release by the uterus. Prostaglandins are produced at the wrong time sending the wrong message.

For instance, there is a natural surge in prostaglandin F production at the end of the menstrual cycle, causing the effects of the corpus luteum of the ovary to die down and signalling the start of a new menstrual cycle. The endometriotic implants produce their prostaglandin surge several days after that of the womb lining. This may be one of the main causes of very early miscarriage. If a woman is a few days pregnant then the implant-produced prosta-glandin F would wrongly tell the ovary to start a new menstrual cycle, causing the womb lining with the implanted egg to be sloughed off – an early miscarriage. Prostaglandins are messengers and like all messengers they sometimes get it wrong.[4]

Prostaglandins also play an important role in the contractions of the womb and Fallopian tubes. During the normal menstrual cycle the gentle contractions of the womb and Fallopian tubes aid the movement of egg and sperm to the outer third of the Fallopian tube where fertilization occurs. High concentrations of endometriotic im-plant prostaglandins at the wrong time could interfere with this and may prevent fertilization. An excess of PGF2 and PGE2 could cause contractions that are too strong and expel the egg too quickly. Series 2 prostaglandins are produced from the fats in dairy and meat products, and it is recommended that intake of these foods be kept to a minimum.

Prostaglandins are also responsible for the contractions of the uterus at the end of pregnancy, stimulating the powerful uterine muscle contractions required for the birthing process. Inappropriate concentrations of implant-produced prostaglandins could stimulate forceful uterine contractions (cramps) at the time of embryo implantation and lead to early expulsion of the embryo. Indeed, in both humans and domestic animals, prostaglandin F is used clinically to induce abortion or to hasten the birthing process.

Series 1 and 3 prostaglandins, enhance the immune response and, as we will discuss in chapter 7, they may even modify normal immune interactions that could prevent conception. Prostaglandins also stimulate sperm motility, and high levels of pro-inflammatory series 2 prostaglandins could lead to early 'burn-out' of the sperm, preventing fertilization.

Although prostaglandin secretion into the peritoneal cavity is required for the reproductive process, it is clear that too much of the wrong type of prostaglandin in the wrong place, or prostaglandin production at the wrong time, could easily interfere with fertility. Exactly how or even whether prostaglandins play a role in the infertility associated with endometriosis is not known, but they do seem to be involved.

PROTEIN PRODUCTION

The endometrium of the uterus and endometriotic implants have 'a prolific ability to produce hundreds of different types of proteins'.[5] Although the roles of all these proteins are not known, some of them are used by the body as nutrition for the developing embryo, and some function as hormones or trigger hormone release. Various laboratory studies have shown that most of these proteins are produced by both the implants and womb endometrium. However, two proteins have been discovered that are produced only by the endometriotic implants.[6] They are called Endo I and Endo II. These two unique proteins may interfere with fertility. It is also possible that the proteins that are common to both the uterus and implant, like prostaglandins, may be inappropriately produced by the endometriotic implants, and are having a bad effect on the reproductive system.

## ABNORMAL OVULATION

The monthly maturation of eggs and the process of ovulation may be altered in the patient with endometriosis: 'Women with endometriosis have been shown to have smaller, but many more, follicles maturing at the time of ovulation than controls'.[7] This suggests that the chemical secretions from endometriotic implants hamper the ability of the ovary to respond correctly to the message from the pituitary hormones.

Under the influence of the pituitary luteinizing hormone, the follicular wall of the ovary close to the Fallopian tube thins and ruptures. Endometriosis may prevent the completion of this ovulatory process. This inability to ovulate is called 'luteinized unruptured follicle syndrome' (LUF). In LUF syndrome, women have the normal sequence of endocrine events and a normal menstrual period, but their ovaries do not release any eggs. This syndrome is difficult to diagnose since from all external measurements (hormone concentrations and menstrual flow), nothing appears to be wrong. As the egg is but a single cell and the ovary wall repairs itself almost immediately after ovulation, the absence of ovulation usually goes unnoticed. However, some researchers have tried meticulously to check for ovulation with laparoscopic examination of the ovary at the presumed time of ovulation.[8] They found the incidence of signs of ovulation was lower in endometriosis patients than in fertile control patients. The exact means by which endometriotic implants adversely affect the development of the egg within the ovary is not yet known, but it is suggested that implant secretions, such as prostaglandins and excess natural oestrogens or even oestrogens from outside the body (xeno-oestrogens), are damaging to conception.

## IMPAIRED FERTILIZATION

In addition to an alteration in follicular development and ovulation, the actual quality of the eggs in women with endometriosis may be different. Various *in vitro* fertilization (IVF) programmes have observed that the presence of endometriosis in the abdomen, and especially in the ovary, adversely affects the appearance of the egg and decreases its ability to fertilize. Normally the eggs have a yellowish appearance with a smooth oatmeal texture. The eggs of the endometriosis patient are sometimes dark brown in colour and have a granular texture. In 1985 Wardle noted that the fertilization rate of eggs from endometriosis patients was significantly lower than in patients who had unexplained infertility or blocked Fallopian tubes.[9] Again, this could be explained by the chemical secretions from the endometriotic implant which surrounds the ovary. Certainly it would seem that from observation, women who have ovarian cysts should have them removed before undergoing ART (assisted reproductive technology). The quality of the ova is poor if 'chocolate' cysts are present and improves after they have been removed. More research is needed to look at this phenomenon. But it implies that women with endometriosis stand a better chance with ART techniques when their health has been improved.

## EARLY MISCARRIAGE

The most common time for a miscarriage to occur is during the first three months (trimester) of pregnancy. At this time, the embryo is developing into a fetus and is undergoing truly amazing and dramatic changes, including the formation of most of its internal organs. This is a critical period of development that requires an appropriate nutrient-rich environment, a healthy placenta and a very delicate balance between the various hormones of pregnancy. It has been suggested that women with endometriosis have a greater chance of miscarriage than women with other types of reproductive dysfunction: 'Miscarriage rates as high as 46 per cent have been reported in the scientific literature'.[10] This area is currently being examined by other researchers who have not seen as dramatic an increase in the miscarriage rate of endometriosis patients.[11] A high miscarriage rate among women with endometriosis would offer another explanation for endometriosis-associated infertility.

However, the real enigma of a first trimester miscarriage is that if it occurs during the first six weeks of the pregnancy, there is a good chance that you may not even be aware that you are pregnant. You may think your period is late. It is very difficult to determine pregnancy rates in normal healthy women and in endometriosis patients. In fact, this lack of pregnancy information is one of the main reasons for the confusion in the scientific literature.

Regardless of whether or not there is a high miscarriage rate in endometriosis patients, it is imperative that you eat the right sort of nutrient-rich foods to try to ensure the maintenance of your pregnancy. Nutrition in both parents even before pregnancy has a profound effect on the state of the egg and sperm, as well as on the nature of the secretions within the peritoneal cavity. Your choice of foods, particularly fats and oils, may be a crucial factor as these affect the production of prostaglandins, cell membranes, steroid hormones, and neurotransmitters etc. (*see* chapter 3).

Thus, there are many reproductive problems associated with endometriosis, and scientific investigations have yet to determine exactly how endometriosis causes infertility. However, 40–60 per cent of women with endometriosis do appear to become pregnant. There are many positive ways that we can successfully attempt to correct the problem of infertility.

## FERTILITY AND THE ALERT IMMUNE SYSTEM

'The leading question we should be asking here is whether or not the presence of antibodies can cause infertility and early miscarriage, by interfering with implantation'.[12]

In order to achieve pregnancy, sperm has to enter the body. This sperm can be judged as 'alien' by a woman's immune cells, because it is 'non-self'. If pregnancy is achieved, the woman's immune system has to adapt to the presence of 'alien' tissues growing inside her for nine months. However, there must be some mechanism which tells the female immune system that this alien tissue is not a danger, in order to avoid damage to the embryo. Perhaps when the immune system is malfunctioning in endometriosis, this mechanism fails and causes an immune attack on the embryo and sperm, thus leading to infertility. Correcting or strengthening the immune system may help to achieve fertility.

Scientists at University College London have discovered a protein (iscollin) inside sperm which is released as egg and sperm fuse, and starts a chain reaction that causes the embryo to form. Chemical interactions trigger calcium deposits inside the egg to vibrate and begin the cell-splitting process that leads to formation of the embryo. Defective sperm or eggs could not begin this chain reaction. This exciting area may lead to more research into egg quality in women with endometriosis.[13]

## YOUR FERTILITY: NUTRITIONAL EFFECTS

Healthy parents usually have healthy babies. Once conception has happened, there is no changing what will be. We think of conception as the beginning of life, the time when sperm and egg collide and the magic of life begins. However, the egg and the sperm are not made in an instant; the parents' bodies have been working hard to prepare them for the previous three months. Women are born with all their eggs ready and waiting inside their ovaries (*see* p. 13). At birth female babies have around one million eggs, but by puberty only about 400,000 are still viable. Each month five to ten eggs begin to ripen, but only two or three fully mature. Over the normal 28-day menstrual cycle the mature eggs 'pop' out at ovulation to be sucked up by the Fallopian tubes, to begin their journey to reach a healthy sperm. The ripening of the egg is supported by the mother-to-be eating a diet rich in essential nutrients.

Many ethnic groups have a period of time when a new bride is well fed, before becoming pregnant; an early study on nutrition mentions how 'the Masai tribe had specific times for marriage to ensure that the bride had a few months on a nutritious diet'.[14] Even Queen Esther in the Bible had a special diet for a year before her wedding.[15] Leah became pregnant after eating mandrakes, which were believed to promote fertility.[16] In the book of Judges, an angel gave preconceptual advice to Samson's mother: 'Take care not to drink any wine or beer, or eat any forbidden food'.[17]

If the mother has a poor diet, consisting of highly refined foods, containing excessive sugar, fat and processed carbohydrates, the amount of nutrients available to the developing egg, or embryo, will be low. Poor nutrition at this time may lead to miscarriage.

Think of the womb lining as a nest. Birds build their nests to keep their young safe and warm; a place where they can be nurtured, fed and watered. A woman's womb plays a similar role. Each month the womb lining develops a lush, nutrient-rich, blood-engorged tissue; the womb is ready to receive the embryo and build a healthy placenta to supply all the nutrients the embryo needs to grow strong and healthy. If the mother's diet that month is poor, the womb lining will be poor, and a weak placenta is less likely to sustain an embryo. So the eggs and womb lining are both dependent upon a good diet.

*Wendy M of London*

*Years of undiagnosed endometriosis had led to the removal of a large ovarian cyst. Conventional treatments for the endometriosis and infertility had been to no avail. A visit to the nutritionist meant a substantial change to my diet and some vitamin supplements were taken. Within a few months period pains and bloating were less severe, PMS had virtually gone and I became pregnant. Yippee!*

C
A
S
E

S
T
U
D
Y

## WHY IT TAKES 12 MONTHS TO MAKE A BABY

We have touched upon the nutritional needs of the mother, but what of the man, the father? He is not going to nurture the baby inside his body, but the health of his sperm is also dependent upon his diet for the three months before conception. That is how long it takes the testes to make healthy sperm. Too much alcohol, cigarettes and drugs, working with certain harmful chemicals, eating too many processed foods and too few vegetables and fruits may lead to sad-looking and possibly defective sperm. A low sperm count may be due to environmental factors, such as oestrogenic pesticides, but a poor diet will also lead to weakened or deformed sperm.

Research has shown that some chemicals can cause mutations to the sperm. Instead of the head of the sperm being oval, it can be too large or too small, or become pear-shaped, and these changes also cause chromosomal abnormality. Moreover, 'it takes 120 days for sperm production to recover after exposure to chemicals'.[18]

*Putting a sorry-looking sperm into a starving egg and implanting the resulting embryo into a sick womb is a recipe for disaster.* In the UK about 750,000 babies are born each year, but more than 40,000 are born early and are too small. One in 150 babies is lost through stillbirth, and one in four pregnancies ends in miscarriage, up to 60 per cent of which are due to defective sperm.[19] Every miscarriage is a bereavement, the loss of a loved one. It is a very unhappy and traumatizing experience for everyone involved. Time can heal the grief, but there is always a part of the sad experience which lingers on.

For a healthy pregnancy, a healthy diet and digestive system are essential. Your diet counts. Let that be the message to remember.

Healthy babies are what everyone wants most of all. All children deserve the best start in life and by eating nutritious food for at least three months before you contemplate becoming pregnant, you are making a start.

---

*Mary F of Chicago*

*I cannot for the life of me remember exactly what nutritional measures I made and what supplements I took (outside of evening primrose oil) when I was trying to conceive; it was three years ago. I wish I could be of more help because you certainly helped me! All that I can tell you is that I believe that the nutritional measures you suggested played an integral role in my conceiving my second child.*

*I did have surgery for my endo, but very little was found. After being on your suggested regime for three months, I conceived naturally and eventually bore a beautiful daughter. I only wish I had known more about nutrition and the role it plays in endo when I was trying to conceive for the first time. I'd had a wonderful son, but not until I had taken an ART hormone therapy which I would have liked to have avoided. You enabled my husband and me to complete the perfect family we always dreamed of having.*

•
C
A
S
E

S
T
U
D
Y
•

---

## NUTRITION COUNSELLING

In 1971 Agnes Higgins described the Montreal Diet Dispensary Study: 'Twenty-three years ago, we were impressed by the research findings concerning the relation between maternal nutrition and birth weight, infant mortality and morbidity. Accordingly we decided to develop for disadvantaged pregnant women, a nutrition counselling method that would compensate for individual differences in income, nutrition, weight, and special conditions of stress, with a view to improving the weight and condition of the newborn'.[20] Why then, so many years later, are we still debating the same point and not putting it into action?

Foresight (The Charity for Preconceptual Care of Great Britain), has looked at research by Dr Weston Price, Dr Francis Pottenger and Sir Robert McCarrison into the influence of sound nutrition on health.[21, 22, 23] Their conclusions are that the quality of the food you eat confers good health. Healthy food emanates from healthy soil and good farming principles. Dr Roger Williams also points out that we are all biochemically different and that individuals' requirements for recommended daily amounts of nutrients may differ due to their unique body biochemistry.[24] A recent study noted that 'in pregnancy it is known that nutrient requirements alter. Women on good diets are seen to have healthier babies than those on poor diets'.[25]

In the UK Foresight (The Charity for Preconceptual Care) has reported pregnancy outcomes for 367 couples who, from 1990 to 1992, followed their suggested nutrition programme. The average ages were 34 for females (22–45 years) and 36 for males (25–59 years). Fifty-nine per cent of the couples had a previous history of reproductive problems; 37 per cent had suffered from infertility for between one and ten years; 38 per cent had had between one and five miscarriages; 3 per cent had given birth to a stillborn child. Of the children born, 40 were small for dates, 15 were low birth weight, and 7 were malformed. Forty-two per cent of the males had reduced sperm quality. After both partners followed the Foresight nutrition programme, an astounding 86 per cent of the women had become pregnant by 1993, and 327 children had been born (137 males and 190 females), all of them healthy at birth. Birth occurred at a mean of 38.5 weeks gestation and the average birth weight was 3,265gm (7lb 3oz). None was malformed and none had to go into special care baby units.[26] This shows what can be achieved by dietary changes and also by addressing genito-urinary infections (such as chlamydia) which may be preventing conception. This programme involves no drugs and no expense save that of buying good food, and requires minimal guidance.

## REPRODUCTIVE SYSTEM SUSCEPTIBILITY TO VITAMIN B COMPLEX

The hypothalamic–pituitary–gonadal axis is highly sensitive to the intake of the B vitamins (*see* figure 2.1). This axis is the main highway along which the hormones (chemical messengers) travel. The vital hormone messages which pass from one end of the highway to the other must be correct. As a recent study explains: 'Low intake of B vitamins depresses gonadotrophin releasing hormone (GnRH) secretion from the hypothalamus and thereby affects the development of the eggs and sperm in the gonads (ovary and testicles).'[27] Moreover, as another source elaborates: 'Low intake of B vitamins may also slow down the ripening of the egg before conception and be affecting fertility. The hypothalamus in other mammals reacts to a severe deficiency of any of these B vitamins (particularly riboflavin (B2)) by inhibiting GnRH secretion and so causing infertility.'[28]

Many people eat a diet of over-refined foods. Convenience foods are low in essential nutrients, such as magnesium, zinc, selenium and iodine, which are removed during the food-processing techniques. Fresh, unrefined foods are always the most nutritious.

## FEMALE ENDOCRINE HEALTH

The length and frequency of the menstrual cycle is an important biological marker when looking for toxic chemical effects on reproduction, but these effects are difficult to distinguish from the research paper effects of poor nutrient intake. As a research paper reporting findings explains, 'The highest susceptibility to nutrient deficiency in the female ovary is during ovulatory maturation and embryonic development; the first 30 days after conception are crucial'. The research indicates that 'a 70-fold increase in sensitivity in the ovary (to nutrient deficiency) occurs between 11.30 a.m. and 7 p.m. on the day preceding ovulation. It is therefore calculated that the period of highest susceptibility could be as long as 60 hours prior to ovulation'.[29] This research suggests that women should eat a healthy diet and reduce toxic overload at least one month before attempting to conceive, as should men. A recent study explains: 'Most of the defects in ova leading to miscarriage are already present in the embryo immediately after fertilization and they have their origin in male and female ova and sperm before fertilization.'[30]

This implies that the couple should both make sensible lifestyle changes for up to three months before trying to conceive to enhance their chances of achieving a successful pregnancy. The same study notes: 'The ova lie dormant from 15 to 45 years in a mother's ovaries until their turn comes to ripen and when the dormant chromosomes are tightly packed and apparently very resistant to any external influence.'[31] Keeping chemical exposure to a minimum would seem to be advisable. If you or your partner work with or near strong chemicals, take the recommended precautions. The one-month period of ripening in the follicle before ovulation is the susceptible time-frame.

The future reproductive potential of the developing fetus can also be affected by your nutrition, and exposure to harmful chemicals before and during pregnancy. So avoid exposure to anything harmful; it could affect the health of your children and grandchildren. The chemicals in some perfumes and powerful cleaning solutions may also have a detrimental effect on the immune system. Use more eco-friendly products or non-biological versions of these products.

The Dietary and Nutritional Survey of British Adults in 1990 used a category of persons – eating affected by being unwell, which involved 9.5 per cent of women in the survey, aged from 16 to 64 years. Calorie intake in this category was some 18 per cent below average, with nutrient intake similarly reduced. The survey concluded: 'Ten per cent of women may not be eating well enough to sustain a pregnancy.'[32]

When recovering from amenorrhoea (cessation of periods due to poor nutrient intake), there are menstrual cycles that are too long and luteal phases that are too short. Research at the University of Sydney suggested 'a recovery period of at least six months from amenorrhoea before attempting a conception.'[33] This allows all the body systems to recover sufficiently from the lack of nutrients. It takes the individual cells some time to regain their full capacity and be able to work at what is known as 'enzyme saturation level', i.e. all the enzymes are working at their optimum rate.

Research into restricted calorie intake has been done on monkeys at the University of Pittsburgh, and it was discovered that 'fasting for one day alone can change the hormone profile the following night;' moreover, 'missing a single meal could override the suppression of luteinizing hormone (LH)' … 'The implication for slimmers is that even short-term deficiency can have a profound effect on endocrine function.'[34] Other studies offer similar conclusions, suggesting that 'restrained eating may be a marker for metabolic and emotional disturbances, and may also be associated with biological consequences, as the LH should take a message from the pituitary to the ovary. If suppressed, no message would be sent. Women with abnormal menstrual cycles experienced ovulatory disturbances including low progesterone and short luteal cycles'.[35, 36, 37] If you are restricting nutrient intake in order to lose weight, you may be damaging your chances of becoming pregnant.

## BODY MASS INDEX

A body mass index (BMI) measure shows that women's weight:height ratio is a rough indicator of nutritional status. The body mass index chart has been designed as a result of feasibility testing. Low pre-pregnancy weight is a risk factor, with the risk increasing as the BMI falls below $24kg/m^2$. American data shows that 50 per cent of infertile women are below 20.7kg $m^2$. In a Hackney hospital study the mothers of the healthy weight babies had a BMI, on average, of $23.7kg/m^2$. A tool for determining BMI is based upon:

- Low BMI or underweight is   $<19.8kg/m^2$
- Normal BMI is                    $19.8–26.0kg/m^2$
- High BMI or overweight is     $26.1–29.0kg/m^2$
- Obese is                          $> 29.0kg/m^2$

The BMI is a good general guide to fertility. Indeed, nearly 80 per cent of infertile women have been judged to be underweight'.[38]

To work out your BMI:

BMI = weight in kilogrammes ÷ height in metres squared

e.g. if you weigh 52.5kg and are 1.52m tall, your BMI will be $22.7kg/m^2$ which is just below the optimum range.

BMI = $52.5 ÷ (1.52 × 1.52) = 22.7$

In animal husbandry, it is well known that animals conceive on a rising body weight, not when weight is falling. All animals have a fertility threshold and in farming there still exists the practice called 'flushing': 'The practice of giving ewes which are in fairly poor condition an improved diet for a few weeks before mating so that they are in a rapidly rising condition when they meet the ram.

Flushing is not fattening up; it means supplying all the essential nutrients to make the hypothalamus and pituitary gland (and ovaries) provide an excellent hormone profile'.[39] Dieting is a common cause of infertility.

## NUTRIENT NEEDS OF OVA

It can be seen from research that most nutrients are essential to ovarian function. A low protein diet causes fewer ova to ripen or be released, as does a very high protein intake. Therefore moderation is the key. Research suggests a protein intake of 75gm (3oz) per day. The endocrine system needs the coenzymes riboflavin (vitamin B2), pyridoxine (vitamin B6) and biotin to metabolize proteins efficiently. Studies show that 'a low protein intake depresses GnRH secretion'.[40] Deficiency of thiamin (vitamin B1) inhibits ovulation. Optimum production of ovarian hormones requires the vitamins pyridoxine (B6), riboflavin (B2), folic acid, thiamin (B1), and pantothenic acid (B5) and the minerals calcium and iron. B vitamins, magnesium and zinc are also important in the hypothalamus, the starting point for the process of reproduction. Other researchers suggest the ovaries are rich in vitamin C, iodine and selenium, as well as B vitamins, magnesium, essential fatty acids and zinc. A good nutrient intake in the months before conception should therefore ensure that the reproductive system is in tiptop condition.

'LUF (luteinizing unruptured follicle), where the follicle does not "pop" out an egg each month, has been reported in 79 per cent of women with endometriosis.'[41] One study on patients with endometriosis and infertility states that Riboflavin (B2) deficiency causes hormonal imbalances and [B2] is essential for the liver clearance of the steroid hormones oestrodial, which is a form of oestrogen, and progesterone (see chapter 7). Deficiency inhibits the LH secretion from the pituitary and GnRH from the hypothalamus. Riboflavin (B2) 'works closely with vitamin B5 and if levels of vitamin B2 and B5 fall below 80 per cent then the reproductive system fails.'[42]

### ZINC

A large percentage of couples who are referred to Foresight – the Charity for Preconceptual Care), are found to be zinc-deficient. High levels of copper and low levels of zinc, often with low magnesium and/or manganese levels, are the commonest finding, especially after using the pill or the coil.[43] Heavy metals, such as lead from petrol and cadmium from cigarettes, are antagonistic to zinc, as are high copper levels from excessive chocolate and tap water consumption. If the potential parents work in an industry where they may come into contact with heavy metals, or toxic chemicals, they should use the physical protection provided by the employer. If excess wheat is eaten, phytic acid present in wheat binds to zinc and prevents it from being absorbed by the body, so wheat-based foods should be eaten in moderation.

---

### Ann M of Lancashire

*I must admit that I found the diet extremely hard to follow and after three weeks I reintroduced dairy foods; fruit and bread more slowly. But I became far more sensible about the foods I was eating. Even now, almost five years on, I don't eat as much creamy food or add sauces even though I don't feel I have a problem with candida overgrowth any more. I feel that the pain I was associating with my endo was due to disruption of my gut flora which came from long-term Danazol treatments. I was utterly miserable before the candida was diagnosed and treated. I have since had two successful pregnancies and we are expecting our third baby.*

• C A S E   S T U D Y •

---

FERTILE WOMEN'S DIETS

Researchers have also investigated what happens in fertile women with different eating patterns. Research at Hackney Hospital looked at the birth weights of new babies, and investigated what their mothers had eaten prior to and during pregnancy: 'Mothers of low birth weight babies had been eating meat, meat products, white bread, refined sugars and soft drinks in greater amounts. Mothers of the healthy weight babies had been eating nutrient-rich foods – three regular daily meals (breakfast being the most important), with wholegrain cereals, muesli, oats, nuts and seeds daily, eggs, egg dishes, wholemeal bread, dairy foods, and lots of fresh fruits and vegetables.'[44] A developing embryo or fetus requires abundant nutrients via the placenta in order to become a healthy bouncing baby. High calorie, low nutrient, refined foods were obviously detrimental to the developing baby in the womb: 'The hypothesis of the Hackney study, that the diet of the mothers of low birth weight babies had too few nutrients in their diets, was supported.'[45]

The most insidious type of infertility is caused by the body's inability to maintain a pregnancy. Conception may take place but the embryo may be unable to plant itself in the womb lining if this is inadequate owing to the mother having a poor nutrient intake. A developing fetus with a proportionately higher nutrient requirement may also fail to thrive if the womb lining is inadequate by day 15 of the preceding menstrual cycle.

## FETAL NEEDS

The fetus needs to extract nutrients from its mother in order to grow, but the mother herself has nutrient requirements, and has to limit the amount of nutrients available to the fetus in order to protect her own health. If the fetus absorbs too many nutrients from its mother, she could become ill. A balance has to be struck. Somehow in the process of evolution the fetal actions are opposed by maternal countermeasures: 'The general impression is of a mysterious symbiotic relationship, in which the mother and fetus conspire to realise the outcome that is so clearly desirable for both – the birth of a normal healthy baby.'[46] It can be deduced that 'if the mother is nutrient-deficient the fetus will struggle to survive'.[47]

### ROLE OF THE PLACENTA

A mother's pre-pregnancy nutrition is crucial to a healthy baby because it determines whether or not the mother will be able to grow a healthy placenta. Nutrients reach the developing infant in the uterus through the placenta, which develops in the first month of pregnancy. The placenta plays an active role in supporting the pregnancy: 'Far from being passive in its transport of molecules, the placenta is a highly metabolic organ producing some 60 enzymes of its own. It uses energy to fuel its work. The placenta's work consists of actively gathering up maternally produced hormones, nutrients of all descriptions, and forcing them into the fetal bloodstream.'[48] It also produces an array of hormones and other chemicals itself, that maintain the pregnancy and prepare the mother's breasts for lactation. Therefore the health of the placenta is a central consideration: 'If the mother's nutrition stores are inadequate during the time when the placenta is developing, then the placenta will develop poorly. As a consequence, no matter how well she eats later, her unborn baby will not receive optimum nourishment.'[49] This results in a low birth weight baby, with a risk of adverse health consequences: 'After getting such a poor start in life, a girl or boy child may be ill-equipped, even as an adult, to store sufficient nutrients, and so may be unable to reach full developmental potential.'[50]

The mother's body has to be prepared for a pregnancy by being well nourished. If you restrict your calorie intake, you run the risk of damaging the tissue which will develop into the placenta and the fetus.

## NUTRIENT NEEDS

Vegetables make a major contribution to the intake of B vitamins important minerals, including magnesium, as studies suggest: 'Vegetables were indeed the most important contributor of magnesium, with dairy produce in second place, and were more important than dairy produce as a source of B vitamins.'[51]

Eating patterns have changed so much over the past 40 years, from the consumption of regular meals with fresh vegetables every day to the non-stop 'grazing' on wheat-based snack foods. This snack food has much of its original nutrient content removed during manufacture, and often has to be fortified with synthetic nutrients. This type of diet can lead to low blood sugar (hypoglycaemia) and problems such as fatigue, irritability, dizziness and mood swings. New research shows that fruits and vegetables contain fewer nutrients than before as soils become depleted from overfarming (*see* chapter 9).

Many mothers do not have access to prenatal care and receive very little advice on diet and nutrition. Midwives legally cannot give dietary advice, and very few women see a dietitian. This can lead to poor health outcomes. Research in America shows that prenatal care is cost-effective: 'Saved dollars amount to $3.38 (£2.11) saved in direct medical care expenditure for every dollar spent on prenatal care.'[52]

## Jackie H of Nottinghamshire

*When I discovered that I had endometriosis I embarked upon a series of quests which I hoped would lead me to the desired goal – another pregnancy. A visit to a Foresight clinician advocated an anti-candida diet – no tea, coffee, sugar, chocolate, fruit for one month, and no yeasty foods etc. This alongside dietary supplements of vitamins and minerals, zinc and vitamin C. For the first two weeks I felt tired and suffered dreadful headaches and then started to feel better. However, the endometriosis symptoms did not abate and the much longed for pregnancy did not happen.*

*My next visit was to a macrobiotic consultant. This time the diet was extremely strict and very narrow, unnaturally so. For a few months I lived off brown rice, oats, barley, organic vegetables, pulses, seaweeds, miso and very occasionally a small amount of fish. This regime stopped the pain and also my periods, but quite frankly was not a diet that I could stick to for any length of time. However, I did discover that organic vegetables tasted far nicer than ordinary vegetables and this is something that I have continued to include in my diet.*

*Vitamins, minerals and any other supplements were advised against. However, I did continue the Foresight vitamins and minerals as I considered the diet to be too restrictive – still no pregnancy.*

*In desperation I finally turned to you as my nutritionist to advise me in detail about foods and their effects on the body. I learned about the effects of gluten in susceptible people, the importance of cold-pressed oils and the link between animal fats and over-production of oestrogen in the body. For the first time somebody was actually taking time to explain the effects of food in detail. I modified my diet with the help of Dian and for the first time felt comfortable with how I was eating. She also prescribed vitamins and minerals, such as a multivitamin-mineral, zinc and vitamin B6, antioxidants, probiotics and a digestive enzyme, all tailored to my needs. I felt so much better and shortly afterwards became pregnant with my second child and surprise, surprise, two years later produced my third child! The gynaecologists had said that my endo was too bad for any pregnancy to take place. Throughout the various regimes I followed I learned something new about nutrition and these things I follow to this day, with the result that the endometriosis has completely cleared up and there has been absolutely no recurrence.*

There are three steps which will help to promote positive nutrition among women during pregnancy and lactation:

1  Increasing access to prenatal care.

2  Standard screening and intervention for poor nutrition, especially vital after the first miscarriage.

3  Delivering nutritional advice before pregnancy through school programmes in health and sex education classes.

It can be seen that it takes 12 months to make a baby, not just the 9 months it is resident within the body. The quality of your diet during those three months prior to conception may well be crucial in maintaining and achieving pregnancy and producing a healthy child as the end result. The effort of eating well for 12 months is worth while for the lifetime of pleasure which children can bring.

That the maternal diet can influence pregnancy outcome even when energy intake is adequate is also well established. Burke and his colleagues looked at mothers who had eaten good/excellent diets: they gave birth to babies judged to be in good/superior health in 94 per cent of the time. Contrasted with mothers whose diets were classified as poor, and whose infants had good health only 8 per cent of the time.'[53] Diet is a vital consideration if a baby is wanted and needed so very much; diet is crucial to a baby's health as it grows and develops.  Shouldn't we give our children a head start through correct nutrition? Every child has right to reach his or her full potential.

Margaret and Arthur Wynn, a social scientist and scientist respectively, working from Hackney Hospital in London, have dedicated themselves to researching the link between the diet and infertility. They speculate that if a woman is infertile as a result of a poor diet and wishes to be fertile, two questions have to be asked:

1  What type of diet will replenish a couple's reproductive systems?

2  Can a woman and her partner be persuaded to consume a wholesome diet which can replenish them sufficiently?[54]

One study at the University of Mississippi suggested counselling by a qualified 'therapeutic dietitian' to promote fertility: 'Fertility was restored in 19 out of 26 women, who conceived spontaneously in due course. All the women had been underweight at the outset but were encouraged to gain half a pound per week. No drugs were prescribed.'[54] There is hope and although the process takes effort, it is not arduous.

---

### Christine F of Sussex

*I feel on top of the world, joyful. I was devastated when told that my chances of pregnancy were nil even with Clomid or surgery, so now after the nutritional guidance I am over the moon, I am just so lucky. It has been a difficult pregnancy as it makes me feel not so well, but to me it is all worth while.*

CASE STUDY

---

Women in all social classes appear to eat very inadequate diets, to a point where the menstrual cycle is affected or suppressed. Illness may be one reason for poor diet, but often it is their wish to be slim and attractive, in keeping with socially accepted body image. This wish may be damaging to the fertility not just of this generation, but also of generations to follow.

The image of a healthy mother holding a healthy baby relies on the quality of life, hygiene, living conditions and sound nutrition surrounding them both. If eating well makes a difference, why not give it a try? There are no harmful side effects, just good health, as the evidence suggests: 'The Hutterites' (a Germanic organic farming community in the USA) fertility is used as an example of how high fertility can be when a population is healthy, stable and not using contraception ... producing 11 live births per married woman. Their infertility rate was only 2.4 per cent.'[56]

In a study '55 per cent of all women in their childbearing years reported taking vitamin–mineral supplements rarely or occasionally'.[57] This research showed that 'women considered at the highest risk for nutritional inadequacy had lower rates of supplement use'. So the question must remain: should all women be given a supplement as part of a preconceptual care programme? Many doctors feel that this may prevent women from eating a healthy diet as they would rely on the nutrients in the supplement. But all the data suggest that women already taking supplements eat more healthily anyway as they are giving more thought to their diet and nutrient intake. The design of appropriate individual supplement programmes should be considered, as many women self-prescribe and may not know the correct levels for supplementation. Healthy babies and healthy mothers would save thousands of pounds annually in health-care budgets, and would also lead to happier families in whom poor health was less of a problem.

## SPERM QUALITY

Male infertility, particularly low sperm counts, is an increasing problem. A partner with a low sperm count may also require nutritional aid. Research on the subject states: 'The deteriorating quality of men's sperm has linked the problem with chemicals found in food, household products and the environment. Scientists are trying to find out why sperm counts may be falling. They have concluded that the chemical pesticides, which mimic female hormones, may also have contributed to rises in testicular cancer. The link is regarded as "plausible" by the Department of the Environment.'[57]

The suspect chemicals include pesticides; phthalates (a group of compounds that 'migrate' from plastic PVC wrappings and leak into such foods as cheese, meats, cakes, sandwiches and confectionery); phyto-oestrogens (plant oestrogens) occurring naturally in soya beans, which are widely incorporated into infant milk formula; alkylphenol polyethoxylates, used in detergents, paints and cosmetics; and ubiquitous industrial pollutants such as polychlorinated biphenyls (PCBs) which accumulate in fatty tissue. Even strong electrical equipment emits strong magnetic fields which may be detrimental to sperm health. Moreover, women working at VDU terminals also appear to have problems with fertility.[59]

'One man in 20 is subfertile' concluded an international study published by the Danish Environment Ministry and reported in the *British Medical Journal*.[60] The maximum sperm count a man can have is determined by the number of Sertoli cells, which provide nutrients to the developing sperm. As Sertoli cells are produced very early in life, a reduced sperm count implies that sperm damage is being done very early in fetal development, possibly via the mother's food intake and the environment. Moreover, 'spermatogenesis in the human takes 120 days to recover if there have been mutagens around. If the sperm are being damaged by chemicals the man must take precautions for the next three months whilst a new supply is being made.'[61]

Professor Niels Skakkebaek of the University of Copenhagen,

Denmark, was the first scientist to observe toxic changes in human sperm. He says that exposure of the male fetus to high levels of oestrogenic chemicals in the first three months of pregnancy could be the vital trigger: 'It is quite clear from laboratory and clinical studies that pesticides of all categories may influence the immune system resulting in endocrine dysfunction.'[61, 62] However, much more research is needed to look at the effects of this pollution on hormone levels.

## SPERM NUTRIENT NEEDS

'Sperm counts of over 10 million/ml are classed as healthy, but 9 million or below can bring problems.'[63] Sperm have to be healthy to swim the long distances through the womb and Fallopian tubes. They encounter fluids on the way which may harm them so their outer skin needs to be strong. The head of the sperm is rich in zinc which helps to penetrate the ovum. This union of sperm and ovum triggers a cascade of calcium to flow all around the fertilized egg. Subclinical deficiencies of various nutrients can affect sperm formation. Vitamin C protects sperm against free-radical damage, and the level of vitamin C in seminal fluid is much higher than in other body fluids. Vitamin E enhances the ability of sperm to fertilize an egg in test tubes. Zinc is critical in male reproduction (zinc and vitamin E increase testosterone levels) and low zinc status may contribute to infertility.[64] Vitamin B12 also appears to improve both sperm count and motility, and deficiency is linked to sterility. Vitamin A deficiency causes abnormalities in sperm shape and, if the deficiency is prolonged, the spermatids and spermatozoa disintegrate. Selenium and iodine deficiencies are also associated with low sperm count. Magnesium deficiency is linked to mutagenic changes and infertility. Research suggests that 'manganese deficiency causes testicular degeneration'.[65] The amino acid L arginine is essential for sperm production and motility, and L caritnine levels appear to be high in the epididymis and sperm, which suggests that it too must play a role in male reproduction. These vitamins and minerals should therefore be supplemented in cases of male infertility but not in excess: 'Excesses may also cause mutagenic changes so levels should be moderate.'[66]

It is wise to avoid excess fatty foods to ensure that the intake of harmful pesticide residues is kept low: 'Pesticides bind to fats and are to be found more commonly in fatty food. Once inside the body pesticides react like oestrogens, female hormones, and can upset the normal hormonal balance.'[67] The diet should be low in saturated animal fats, but some good quality cis oils such as flax seed (edible food grade linseed oil) and olive oils can be included. Eating organic food when possible can also help to avoid some pesticides.[68] In chapter 9 we will look at which supplements can be taken safely.

## COPING WITH INFERTILITY

We all lose our fertility at some point in our lives. The poet Donald Justice says 'We must learn to close softly the doors to rooms we will not be coming back to'. Women with endometriosis may have to learn to close doors earlier.[69] However, the British Endometriosis Society's motto is 'Never Give Up'. Many women achieve pregnancy in the end.

Achieving pregnancy takes an average couple 18 months from the time they first start trying for a baby. There are many factors with endometriosis which can cause problems, but male infertility should always be investigated before female infertility, as it is less traumatic to treat. It responds well to zinc and vitamins C and E and evening primrose oils.

The trauma which some members of the medical profession can provoke by stating that endometriosis is a cause of infertility and that a woman 'can never get pregnant' can be too much to bear. The link between endometriosis and infertility is poorly understood. It is a hypothesis based on investigating the chemical secretions from endometriotic implants, which may well be correctable by diet. If one-fifth of the population have difficulty achieving pregnancy it may not be endometriosis alone that is causing the problem; it could be a combination of environmental factors. Ensure your lifestyle is giving your health the space, relaxation, exercise and nutrition you need to strengthen all your body systems.

*Vicki D of London*

*In late September I went to see a nutritionist in a desperate state. Over 3½ years I had undergone 4 IVF and ICSI procedures, countless inseminations with ovulation induction drugs and 2 major surgeries for endometriosis costing $100,000. My husband and I then moved from*

CASE
STUDY

*New York to London in July before undergoing a fifth IVF and ICSI procedure. Our NY doctor was by then also recommending donor eggs!*

*I felt very sick and run down and sought nutritional advice at the end of September. After three months on a healthy eating regime I started to feel much better than I had in years. On January 15th my period was quite late and I took an at-home pregnancy test. Much to my joy and disbelief it was positive. My husband and I had prayed for a natural conception and we cannot express our joy and gratitude. Nutrition does work! [My son] was born in October, at 9lbs, 1oz, and is thriving.*

When a woman wants to hold her baby in her arms and her partner wants to look into the eyes of his child, but they are unable to have children, an enormous cavern, a yawning gap permeates their lives. This can generate tremendous stress of monthly trauma, of frustrated longing and desire. A cycle of distress which continues as each menstruation begins and hope ends; this can create chaos with relationships. This can be doubly so with endometriosis, if painful or difficult intercourse (dyspareunia) is also involved; it can cause distress and despair in itself. It robs us of a joy and comfort in life, particularly if you are desperately trying to get pregnant. Disbelieving GPs and rushed consultants may not take the time to help, plus many GPs are too embarrassed to talk about painful sexual intercourse. Ask for counselling and referral to a sexual therapy clinic or a clinical psychologist if you feel the need. Talking through the problems and getting the right sort of help is very important, although, when desire is there and the pain is real, referral to a psychiatrist is not the answer. You and your partner lose all spontaneity for sex, as deep pain sets you on edge and you expect the worst before it happens. When internal organs that are meant to slip and slide are glued together firmly with adhesions, agony ensues. However, there is a great variety of alternative ways of sexual intercourse other than penetration and ways in which we can show our love for one another. Healing can make this all come right again.

## KEEP TALKING

Communication is the most important thing. If love is strong and friendship profound, then keep talking to one another. Don't brush your deep distress under the carpet or try to ignore the problem. Talk things through, cuddle and cry together. Being together is the important thing, and recognizing that this is no one person's fault. You will overcome this problem, there is hope.

### Two men's experience

'My partner was diagnosed as having a cyst on her ovary. As a result she had surgery, and the cyst and the ovary removed. I took the time to read up on endometriosis while my partner was in hospital. Needless to say it was a traumatic experience to see the effects major abdominal surgery and general anaesthetic had on someone I love and care for. What was worse than seeing her look ill were the mental images of her being virtually sliced in half. I so wanted to do something to stop the suffering, but I felt so totally helpless and useless. All I could do was be there for my partner, to offer her support and also gain as much information as I could on endometriosis.'

'Endometriosis does really test a relationship. It also shows how sexist the medical services are – seeing 'women's complaints' as some form of neurosis or hysteria. What can a partner do?

'1  Become informed – find out what endometriosis is, so you can offer a more understanding ear.
2  Support your partner in any way you can. I was fortunate in having understanding management and colleagues who allowed me to juggle my work shifts so that I was able to offer my partner the care she needed.
3  When your partner tells you about the various pains, etc., take her seriously. This is so important in a society which does not take women's health seriously.'

Women are more likely to talk this problem through with one another. Often it is the male partner who suffers in silence. At a psychosexual workshop for partners held in Brighton more than 40 couples found help by talking this through together. It was refreshing for so many people to be open about their sexual frustrations, and it removed the feelings of isolation which many had felt.

## A husband's advice

'My wife was diagnosed as suffering from a disease called endometriosis. It sounded so, well, diseased! By becoming informed it provided us both with answers to questions which I am sure many other couples have agonized over. 'Why can't you have normal periods? How can it hurt to make love?' Being naturally shy I have not found it particularly easy to make the first move in discussing what is, after all, a very personal subject dealing with period pains, painful intercourse and the like. However, what I have found is that it is absolutely vital for your relationship to put aside such traditional taboos and express your willingness to discuss such matters. It helps to show your partner just how much you care.'

Sharing stories and experiences in a group of people who are going through the same problems can help a great deal in coming to terms with how they affect one's life. A good book to read is *On Death and Dying* by Elizabeth Kübler-Ross. It explains how the pain we feel when someone dies can be comparable to the pain, depression and anger that infertile people go through. It is the mourning for a child who has never been born, but who lives in the soul, which hurts the most. Understanding this may help to put things in perspective for you; trying to appreciate life around you which may occur as a blur as the years pass while you try for a baby. Hold on to what you have around you, the love of family and friends.

One lady explained it this way: 'There were other things that we did to get over not having children. We started to make the choice our own rather than something that happened to us. We began to recognize that life was good when you are child-free. We took a few trips alone together and started to do the things we had put off just in case we had a baby. I finally returned to my artwork, something I stopped doing during my eleven years of infertility. I am now able to concentrate again and to paint for several months during the summer when the art school is on holidays. My husband started playing hockey and baseball, and we both started skiing and working out regularly. We began to focus our attention on each other and rejuvenated our relationship. Let's face it, when sex becomes a monitored chore during the infertile years, it takes a while to get your love life back on track. Now the focus is on each other rather than wondering if this will be the time that you get pregnant.'[70]

Part of feeling better has to do with giving up the anguish related to infertility and getting on with life. Setting new goals, perhaps making a career change or learning new things can open up a new world. Take the time and energy previously spent trying to have a baby and channel it into new adventures. Many couples struggle to survive the pain of infertility together, and because it has overwhelming negative influences, it tends to drive couples apart rather than bringing them closer together. Find time to return to the love that brought you together in the first place.

Believe it or not, there is life after infertility, and it can be an enriching experience. The biggest step is deciding when you have had enough and then taking your new life one day at a time. What is so difficult with infertility is living in limbo for years. Once the decision to stop treatment is made you will be amazed at how much better you will feel. Regaining control over your life is a wonderful thing. *Sweet Grapes: How to stop being infertile and start living again* by Jean and Michael Carter, published by Perspective Press, is another good book to read.

## INFERTILITY

The endocrine system appears to monitor nutrient intake. If we fall below a certain level, the reproductive system stalls. A rising body weight from a diet full of fresh foods is very important – three regular meals each day, beginning with a nutritious breakfast. A selection of the following supplements may be supportive while the diet is adjusted:

- Multivitamin/mineral
- B complex (non-yeast based)
- Magnesium malate
- Iodine (kelp)
- Selenium (non-yeast based)
- Zinc citrate or gluconate
- Vitamins A, C, E
- Amino acid complex
- Evening primrose and fish oils
- Bioacidophilus

**SUMMARY**

1  The infertility rate is high (15–20 per cent) in couples around the world, and endometriosis may be one contributory factor, causing infertility in some 30 per cent of all infertile couples.

2  Endometriosis-induced infertility can be due to adhesions, early miscarriage (and vice versa), endometriotic implant secretions and anovulation (no ovulation), or impaired fertilization.

3  Nutrition will help improve your fertility. Nutrients are required for a healthy reproductive system.
(Look up www.makingbabies.com for more information.)

4  The body matures the sperm and ova months before conception takes place. The health of your partner's sperm and your eggs and womb lining are dependent on your nutrient intake. Putting a sorry-looking sperm into a starving ova and implanting the resulting embryo into a sick womb is a recipe for disaster.

5  To sustain a pregnancy you need a healthy body weight:height ratio (body mass index). Fertility improves on a rising body weight, not when the weight is falling.

6  In order to improve your fertility you need to eat nutrient-rich foods – three regular meals daily (breakfast being the most important), with wholegrain cereals, muesli, oats, nuts, seeds, egg dishes, wholemeal bread, dairy foods and lots of fresh fruits and vegetables, especially green leafy ones.

7  A healthy placenta has to be made to house the fetus for nine months. The only way nutrients can reach the developing baby is through the placenta. To prepare the body to build a healthy placenta each month the diet must be nutrient-rich all the time that you are attempting pregnancy.

8  Fresh, unprocessed foods are always the most nutritious. Chapters 9 and 10 will explain the dietary changes necessary to improve the health of the reproductive system. Changes in your diet will help enhance fertility.

9  Never give up. Take time out for yourself and your partner. The pain and distress of infertility is damaging to the immune, nervous, digestive and reproductive systems. It is very important to give yourselves time and space, and keep talking to one another.

10  Do things for yourself that you enjoy. Set new goals and create new 'moments' one day at a time.

# 5 Many treatments, few cures?

> Remember the 15th century proverb that
> summarizes the purpose of medicine:
> 'To cure sometimes, to relieve often, to comfort
> always'.
> *Burch, W M, Endocrinology 3rd ed., 1988*
> *Williams & Wilkins*

The true enigma of endometriosis is that we do not have a definitive cure for the disease. However, we do have access to many therapies that can ease the pain and symptoms of endometriosis and, in some cases, help the infertile patient. Endometriotic implants may first have been described by Aristotle thousands of years ago. Ancient writings appear to describe the random appearance of the implants and their adhesions in the abdomen of women. Indeed, Egyptian papyrus scripts speak of 'the wandering womb', an apt description if ever there was one! Here we are, over 2,000 years later, and we still do not have a 'miracle drug' that will cause the selective destruction of the endometriotic implant. As discussed previously, the problem facing modern scientists who wish to develop a cure for endometriosis is that endometriotic implants grow, look and behave like the normal endometrium of the uterus. Any drug that would destroy the implant would also destroy the normal endometrium of the uterus. Finding a cure sounds like an impossible task, but recent research shows that there are very subtle ways in which the implants differ in their behaviour to the real endometrium, and it is possible that drugs that target endometrial implants only can be developed. The cure needs to be able to target the 'rogue' tissue and leave the normal endometrial tissue intact.

Before we look at the role of nutrition or some of the non-traditional therapies as an aid for coping with endometriosis, let us look at what is available from your gynaecologist. In modern orthodox medicine five main types of therapies are available:

1  Drug therapies
2  Surgical therapies
3  Pregnancy induction
4  Analgesics
5  Antihistamines

Any one or any combination of these therapies can be used to treat endometriosis, dependent upon whether the treatment is meant to reduce pain or assist conception, or both. The choice of treatment is also influenced by the wishes of the woman and her age. In the majority of cases endometriosis symptoms often diminish with the advent of menopause, so an older woman might not want an aggressive therapy like surgery, but may just want to decrease her pain symptoms with analgesics or through complementary therapy treatments. Likewise, a young woman in her teens would not want to subject herself to drastic surgery or use pregnancy as a possible 'cure', and she may prefer one of the drug therapies.

●
CASE STUDY
●

### Ann W of Sussex

*After being on different drugs on and off over the past 15 years it is difficult to remember what did what. But I can remember you did suggest cutting out cow's milk and trying goat's milk. Following the diet and supplements did overall make me feel better in myself.*

## DRUG THERAPIES

The drug treatments usually mimic the beneficial effects of either pregnancy (high levels of progesterone) or menopause (removal of ovarian steroids). During pregnancy and the menopause, it has been noted that endometriosis becomes less active and may 'die back'. Drug treatments therefore try to mimic these natural chemical reactions in the body, by altering hormone levels so that they are the same as they would be during pregnancy or menopause.

### PSEUDOPREGNANCY DRUGS

The word 'pseudopregnancy' means false pregnancy and, in this therapy, the hormones of pregnancy are administered in an attempt to mimic the beneficial effect of a natural pregnancy on endometriosis.

*Birth control pills*

Some success has resulted from women taking large concentrations of birth control pills containing synthetic oestrogen- and progesterone-like hormones. These combination pills are taken continuously over several months so no menstrual period occurs. The constant exposure of the endometriotic implant to progesterone and the lack of the cyclic pattern of the oestrogen hormones of the menstrual cycle cause the implants to thin out or 'die back'. Unfortunately, the implants do not disappear entirely; they lie dormant, like volcanoes, and they usually reappear after withdrawal of the treatment.

The drug treatments merely suppress but do not cure this problem. To elicit a cure, we have to find the real cause. However, these drugs can give respite from the symptoms of endometriosis and, for women seeking to have children, they may open up a window of opportunity in which they can try to conceive, whilst the endometriotic implants lie dormant.[1]

For some women this type of hormone therapy reduces, and sometimes removes, the pain of endometriosis. Shrinking the patches of 'rogue' tissue may stop the implant producing harmful chemicals which alter surrounding tissue, and cause inflammation. This treatment is popular with young women, especially teenagers, since they feel it is more socially acceptable to take birth control pills than to take a hormone drug treatment for reproductive problems. However, the high doses of hormones, especially the presence of oestrogen, have side effects that makes this treatment undesirable for some women, who becomes bloated from water retention, suffer from migraines, have breast tenderness, or unwanted weight gain. Some effects are less obvious: 'The contraceptive pill changes blood biochemistry, so that higher levels of vitamin A and copper begin to circulate, but the levels of B complex vitamins and zinc are lowered.'[2] Hormone preparations also disrupt the balance of our 'friendly' bifido gut bacteria, the very ones which protect the endocrine and immune systems.

A more direct way of mimicking pregnancy is to administer long-acting progesterone-like drugs, such as depo-provera acetate. This treatment requires hormone injections only once every three months. However, the difficulty with long-acting progesterones is that they accumulate in fat tissue, and in some women, especially obese women, it may take a year after stopping treatment for menstruation to reoccur. For this reason women who want to become pregnant may not want to be exposed to long-acting progesterone.[3] On the benefit side, long-acting progesterone treatments do not usually have the side effects attributed to birth control pills, although some weight gain and bloating can occur. As with the birth control pill, the long-acting progesterone can reduce the symptoms of endometriosis by suppressing the cyclic activity of the endometriotic implant and impairing its growth. The implants and symptoms can reoccur after therapy ceases. Short-acting progesterone (medroxyprogesterone acetate) has also been used successfully as a pseudopregnancy drug. In women who desire fertility these drugs are preferred over the long-acting progesterone treatments because reproductive cycles start more promptly after cessation of treatment.[4] The efficacy of taking birth control pills as a preventative measure against endometriosis has been questioned: 'Some 80 per cent of patients in the Brisbane research trial (looking at women with active endometriosis) had taken oral contraceptive pills. Fifty four per cent were pregnant and many had lactated, so prior pill use, pregnancy and lactation do not necessarily protect against the development of endometriosis.'[5]

*Progesterone cream*

Mexican wild yams (and mistletoe) contain a substance known as dios-genin. When the yam undergoes a technical process in the laboratory, diosgenin becomes the product sold as 'natural progesterone'. It is very important if you wish to try this type of treatment to read about the form of the cream, which is only available on prescription in the UK. Small amounts of the cream are to be applied to various sites on the body during the second half of the menstrual cycle.

Progesterone is a steroid hormone, produced naturally in the body by steroid synthesizing cells, that is required for pregnancy. It makes the uterus relax and inhibits the ability of oestrogen to cause cramps. The progesterone from yams is not natural to the body. The structure of progesterone is the same for all animals. The term progestogen refers to any substance that has the same biological activity as progesterone. A progesterone-like substance derived from a plant is technically defined as a progestogen.

Progesterone has many effects on the body. It alters the electrical activity in the brain and in large doses acts as a sedative. When progesterone was first discovered at the University of St Louis, USA, its effects were tested on rabbits. The first doses given were high as the researchers had no idea what normal levels were. Although there were no serious side effects, the rabbits actually fell asleep.

Progesterone also increases body temperature (i.e. it is thermogenic). Since progesterone increases naturally after ovulation, this thermogenic effect is sometimes used to determine if a woman is ovulating. Many women with endometriosis have reported a lower body temperature, of around 36°C, and normalized progesterone levels may assist them by helping to correct their temperature regulation.

The purveyors of 'natural progesterone' creams attribute cures for endometriosis, PMS, fibrocystic breast disease, uterine fibroids, ovarian cysts and osteoporosis to these products. Studies have been done on osteoporosis and they do show benefits. More research is needed, however, to see what exactly is happening to the endometriotic implants when these creams are used. We would all like a cure to be forthcoming.

Wild yam diosgenin which has not undergone processing has an oestrogenic action. It is very important to have your hormone profile taken before using any of these products to ensure you are in need of them. You will not ovulate and are not likely to conceive with this programme, using the creams, from Day 7 to Day 28.

PSEUDOMENOPAUSE DRUGS

'Pseudomenopause' means false menopause. Since the symptoms of endometriosis usually disappear once menopause begins, several drug treatments have been developed that mimic menopause. The hallmark of menopause is the absence of ovarian hormones and the absence of menstrual cycles. Natural menopause involves the gradual winding down over several years of hormone production from the ovaries. Pseudomenopause drugs rapidly shut down the ovary's ability to produce oestrogen and progesterone, but the effects are reversible. Without the cyclic exposure to these hormones, the endometriotic implants should shrink and die back. These treatments can be very effective in reducing pain symptoms and can help the infertile couple. However, pseudomenopausal drugs have some serious side effects that many women find unacceptable to live with on a day-to-day basis. The side effects of each drug are explained in the following sections.

*Danazol*

The major hormone used as a pseudomenopausal drug is Danazol, which has a chemical structure similar to the male hormone testosterone. It can be taken as a pill once or twice daily. Danazol causes a hypo-oestrogen (low oestrogen) condition. How Danazol causes this is complex and not clearly understood, but the drug appears to have several effects which lead to a decrease in size of the endometriotic implants. Danazol has the following actions:

1  It prevents the formation of some steroids by the adrenal gland and ovary, thus preventing the production of oestrogen.
2  It acts directly on the endometriotic implant to prevent growth.
3  It inhibits the production of LH and FSH by the pituitary gland, which removes the major endocrine stimulus to oestrogen production by the ovary.[6]

Furthermore, Danazol treatment usually stops the menstrual cycle in the majority of women who take it. The lack of cyclic oestrogen and progesterone production inhibits the regrowth of the implants.[7] In short, the low oestrogen and the testosterone-like action of Danazol set up a hostile environment for the growth and development of the implants.

## Jacky H of Nottinghamshire

*My diet helped me with the effects of Danazol. I started taking Danazol in August and had the normal side effects. I put on a stone in weight and suffered from severe muscle cramps and joint pains. Then I had a flare-up of thrush so decided to go onto a yeast-reducing diet. For three weeks I cut out all yeast-based foods and took garlic tablets. The thrush went and so did the muscle cramps and joint pains. After three weeks I re-introduced bread into my diet and back came the cramps as bad as before. I was on Danazol for nine months and now so long as I avoid yeasts I have no cramps or joint pains. I eat soda bread which is easily obtainable.*

CASE STUDY

Unfortunately Danazol is not heaven-sent, and some women may experience aggravating side effects. As a result of Danazol's testosterone-like structure, it has side effects that reflect the action of male hormones. Some women complain of muscle cramps, acne, bloating, decreased breast size and, in rare cases, voice changes, hair growth on the face, an enlargement of the clitoris, headaches and nasal congestion. With voice changes, migraines and clitoral enlargement the drug should be stopped immediately after consulting your doctor. Another rare complication from Danazol treatment is liver problems, including an elevation of liver enzyme levels that can lead to the patient turning yellow (jaundice). Change in the digestive enzymes in the liver may affect digestion in some sensitive people. When Danazol is taken for more than six months, liver enzyme function tests should be performed by the general practitioner.

---

### Lesley B of London

*As I refused to take Danazol when I was first diagnosed, I took the nutritional path to quell the pain and tiredness. After a few weeks it began to reduce symptoms which fluctuated according to stress levels mainly caused by work situations. I have continued to use supplements increasing the calcium, zinc and trying such things as Ginko Biloba, Echinacea. As I still smoke and the balance of my lifestyle is still lopsided (always was, always will be!) I am prone to low immune system whatever I swallow. But I believe that you definitely are what you eat. My message to endo sufferers would be to take whatever medical route you think is best for you, but in addition try nutrition and look at your lifestyle. The supplements need to be of good quality and the amounts taken should be correct for your needs, enough to be of value. Thank you for all your support.*

• C A S E  S T U D Y •

---

Although most women do not suffer many side effects from Danazol, those who do can be devastated. Young women especially are concerned with the masculinization effects of Danazol since the changes to facial hair, voice and clitoral growth are not easily reversible. Also the excessive weight gain causes many women to diet, thus reducing their nutrient intake even further. Up to 20 per cent of calcium can be lost from the bones, but this change is usually reversible. Pregnancy rates and pain relief after Danazol treatment appear to be reasonable, and because of this some women risk the side effects.

*GnRH analogues*

Another group of pseudomenopausal drugs are GnRH analogues. GnRH stands for 'gonadotrophin-releasing hormone'. This is the hormone from the hypothalamus in the brain that controls the release of the pituitary hormones, FSH and LH (*see* chapter 2). The coenzymes for its release are dependent upon zinc and vitamin B6. The GnRH analogues are synthetic compounds that look very similar to natural GnRH, but are chemically modified to make them more powerful and longer acting than natural GnRH. GnRH analogues inhibit the ability of the pituitary to secrete FSH and LH, thus switching off ovarian function.[8]

Since LH and FSH are the hormones that stimulate the ovary to produce oestrogen, withdrawal of LH and FSH analogues leads to a hypo-oestrogen condition. As stated before, oestrogen stimulates growth of the implant and low oestrogen levels lead to a decrease in the size of the endometriotic implant. There are two types of GnRH analogues, the GnRH agonists and the GnRH antagonists.

The analogues most commonly used today are GnRH agonists, which stimulate the pituitary to produce LH and FSH. However, for the treatment of endometriosis, excessive amounts of GnRH agonist are administered and the pituitary becomes overworked and exhausted by this sudden and rapid stimulation – and it eventually fails to respond to any signals. This lack of response by the pituitary leads to decreased production of LH and FSH.

The GnRH antagonists, on the other hand, directly inhibit the pituitary gland from producing LH and FSH. It seems that the GnRH antagonists are better suited for the treatment of endometriosis. Unfortunately GnRH antagonists have serious side effects, e.g. hives, which hamper their use as a therapy.

Although GnRH analogues do not have any male hormone-like effects, both Danazol and GnRH analogues induce the typical side effects associated with menopause. These side effects include headaches, hot flushes, sweating, vaginal dryness, painful intercourse, nervousness and moodiness. GnRH analogues may also trigger bone loss (osteoporosis), but this bone loss is usually reversible and bone density may return to normal after the treatment ends.

## SURGICAL THERAPIES

The surgical approach to endometriosis treatment involves either the selective removal of endometriotic implants or the complete removal of the reproductive organs. In both cases we are talking about invasive procedures that are potentially painful, possibly expensive and somewhat traumatic. However, surgery can be very effective for some women.

### LAPAROSCOPY

The selective removal of endometriotic implants is usually done through a laparoscope (figure 5.1). This is a fibre-optic device, containing a telescope and a fibre-optic light, that allows the surgeon to work directly on the reproductive organs through a small incision in the belly button (navel). In a laparoscopic procedure, the abdomen is filled with an inert gas, the pressure of which pushes the intestines out of view. This also enlarges the peritoneal cavity so that the surgeon can see the organs clearly and can move them around to find the patches of endometriosis.[9]

By making a second puncture in the abdomen, the surgeon can insert a grasping instrument that enables him to manipulate the organs. The laparoscope sometimes contains a laser or an electric probe that can be used to burn away the endometriotic implant. The laser is a high energy light source that is powerful enough to burn tissue; it is so fine it can cut sections from a single hair. The strength of an extremely fine laser can be more accurately controlled than that of an electric probe, and the physician has much better control of the depth of cellular destruction. The laser can also be used to remove endometriotic implants from areas which are not easily reached with an electric probe. This operation is less invasive than a laparotomy but it still carries the slight risk of some side effects: the use of anaesthetics always poses some risk and a careless operator could harm the bowel or one of the major blood vessels, but this is *very* rare.

It is a good idea to combine the laparoscopy with laser treatment or cauterization or excision, to avoid having a second operation at a later date, with all the additional trauma to the body that this entails. It also reduces the amount of anaesthetics absorbed by the body. If you are having a laparoscopy, check with the surgeon and let him know that if endometriosis is found, it can be lasered away,

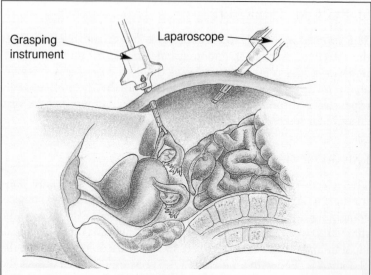

Grasping instrument

Laparoscope

Figure 5.1
Cross-sectional diagram of a woman's abdomen showing the placement of the surgical instruments used during a laparoscopic examination.

rather than having another operation later. Many doctors video this procedure so that a record can be kept for future reference. This can be useful when several doctors are involved with your case.

In addition to burning away or removing the implants, the surgeon can cut apart any adhesions that are present. As discussed before, adhesions are connective tissue bundles that attach the organs to each other. If the adhesions cover the Fallopian tube or twist the Fallopian tube away from the ovary, their removal may restore fertility. Adhesions may also stretch pain receptors in nerves and their removal can reduce pain. Some surgeons also cut the sensory nerves to the uterus to relieve pain; however, this may affect bladder function and ability to achieve orgasm. These various types of surgery can be very effective for some women.

In women with mild endometriosis pregnancy rates after surgery of 60 per cent have been reported, with a significant reduction in pain symptoms. Most women can return to a normal life two to three days after the procedure, which is a more rapid result than having to wait for the weeks involved in drug treatments. Most pregnancies that result after drug or surgical treatment occur 5 to 18 months after treatment. If pregnancy does not occur during that period then the chances of getting pregnant are reduced unless other methods of treatment are tried. This failure to conceive is primarily due to the regrowth of the endometriotic implants after treatment. Because of this, some physicians like to couple surgery with various drug treatments to extend and enhance the effects of therapy. Remember that drug and surgical treatments only suppress symptoms; only rarely do they cure the disease.

## HYSTERECTOMY AND OOPHORECTOMY

In desperation to alleviate the extreme pain, some women elect to have their ovaries (oophorectomy) and uterus (hysterectomy) removed. This can be very effective in removing pain symptoms, but is a drastic action that obviously cannot be undone. This type of surgery will overnight make a woman menopausal whatever her age, and she will have to contend with the rapid onset of the extreme symptoms of menopause. Natural menopause can take up to seven years, as the ovaries gradually cease their function. The hot flushes and mood changes associated with menopause can be aggravated after a complete hysterectomy since the procedure involves abrupt removal of the ovaries and hence ovarian hormones. This procedure should not be entered into lightly and trying the least harsh treatment method first (such as nutrients and diet) and working up can prevent this more drastic action.

Laparotomy, which may be used for hysterectomy or exploratory surgery, involves a 4–5 inch cut in the abdominal wall at the bikini line. Some hysterectomies can be done via the vagina or by laser laparoscopy.

The lack of ovarian steroids after a complete hysterectomy and oophorectomy can also lead to rapid bone loss (osteoporosis), especially in women with a family history of bone loss with ageing. The sudden loss of oestrogen slows calcium deposition into bone. Because of the menopausal and other side effects (i.e., sweating, vaginal dryness, painful intercourse), a woman who has had her uterus and ovaries removed should think about taking supplemental oestrogen therapy or hormonal replacement therapy (HRT). It is often recommended that women with endometriosis should wait at least 6–9 months after hysterectomy and oophorectomy before taking HRT, to allow any endometrial implants on the peritoneal cavity walls, bowel or bladder to die back. Immediate use of HRT gives the body access to more oestrogen which could trigger these endometriotic patches to become active again, causing the pain to reoccur.

In some cases women who have never previously had endometriosis or period pain symptoms, suddenly develop endometriosis after being given HRT patches. More research is necessary to discover exactly what is triggering this disease to take hold, but it is clear that oestrogen levels are the key factor.

In the USA 33 per cent of women have had hysterectomy by 60 years of age; in Australia 20 per cent of women have undergone the procedure by 50 and in Britain 20 per cent have a hysterectomy by 55.[10, 11, 12] Many doctors feel one-third of hysterectomies performed because of excessive bleeding are unnecessary. Hysterectomy as a panacea for endometriosis has come under considerable scrutiny in recent years. It is a complex procedure, and should not be entered into lightly. Take your time to make the decision, find out as much as you can about it, and discuss it in depth with your partner, doctor and other women sufferers. Recent information shows that pelvic damage can ensue.

## PREGNANCY INDUCTION

Having a child is a life choice, not a treatment for endometriosis. The high levels of pregnancy hormones seem to suppress endometriosis in most cases. Unfortunately, this represents a Catch-22 situation – endometriosis appears to impair fertility while pregnancy inhibits endometriosis. But pregnancy is not always desirable at a time when a woman's reproductive system appears to be very sick. Looking after a baby while in pain from endometriosis is not a life choice many women would want to make. The benefit of pregnancy in reducing endometriotic implants has been noted in many cases, but the duration of this benefit after the child is born is highly unpredictable. Some women go for years after a pregnancy with no symptoms of endometriosis, while others have endometriosis symptoms as soon as one month after the birth of their child. Discussion and information should be key factors in helping to make the right decision. There are many considerations: 'breastfeeding every 7 hours for 2 years has also been suggested to keep endometriosis at bay'.[13]

For women with endometriosis who want to have children, getting pregnant would have the double benefit of conception with remission of endometriosis symptoms. The two major treatments for enhancing the chances of getting pregnant are:

1  Ovarian superstimulation coupled with interuterine insemination (IUI) or normal intercourse.

2  In vitro fertilization.

These techniques are called Assisted Reproductive Technology (ART).

## ARTIFICIAL INSEMINATION OR INTERUTERINE INSEMINATION (IUI)

There are several drugs a gynaecologist can administer that stimulate the ovary to produce more and larger follicles, that will improve your chances of getting pregnant. The two major types of drugs used to stimulate the ovary are either drugs that 'fool' the pituitary gland into producing extra FSH and LH, or drugs that contain FSH and/or LH. Once the physician has stimulated the ovary to be more active then, at the anticipated time of ovulation, the patient can either have sexual intercourse or undergo interuterine insemination.

The benefit of the artificial insemination is that a larger number of sperm can be placed close to the area of fertilization and thus increase the chances of getting pregnant. The drugs used to stimulate the ovary can be quite expensive. However, the increased chances of pregnancy offered by interuterine insemination may be desired by many couples. One possible drawback to ovarian stimulation is that the high levels of steroids present during this procedure can also stimulate the endometriotic implants and increase the symptoms of endometriosis, as well as enlarge ovarian cysts. This is again a Catch-22 situation. Being informed is vital in order to make the right personal decision.

Dr Kamal Ahuja of the IVF fertility centre at Cromwell Hospital in London has cited 60 studies in the *Journal of Human Reproduction*, representing hundreds of cases of ovarian cancer reported worldwide that may be linked to fertility drugs.

ART treatments involve risks, as research has shown: 'Both the mothers who conceived multiple gestations by means of IVF and their neonates are at an increased risk of having multiple morbidities. The IVF infants had longer hospitalizations, respiratory distress and had to be given oxygen therapy. It is concluded that IVF couples are at increased risk of giving birth to low birth weight infants.'[14] It may be that couples wish to run these risks and try to become pregnant by artificial means. In any event, all the ethical dilemmas should be explained by the staff at each unit to couples thinking of undertaking these procedures. Other research has looked into the risk to mothers who have been exposed to the fertility drugs involved in IVF procedures, as there have been concerns that these procedures may be associated with breast and ovarian cancers. The suggestions are that long-term follow-up examinations of these women must be undertaken in order to analyse the risk statistically.[15]

The authors of this book would recommend that couples try the least harsh method first, which would involve healthy lifestyle changes to diet, patterns of exercise and relaxation – all of which cost very little – before embarking on costly IVF procedures. By taking the simple option first there is nothing to lose and everything to gain.

## IN VITRO FERTILIZATION (IVF)

In vitro fertilization (IVF) is a complicated and very expensive procedure. It can, however, be a means of getting pregnant. The reason that IVF is effective is related to the aggressive nature of the procedure. In IVF the ovary is superstimulated to produce an excess of eggs (rather than just one) and these eggs are removed from the ovary before ovulation by inserting a needle through the wall of the vagina and directly into the ovary, under ultrasound control.[16] The eggs are sucked from the ovary into a test tube, placed in a dish with the sperm and sometimes fertilization occurs. The resulting embryos are then transferred, by a long thin tube, through the cervix and into the uterus. These procedures can be physically, emotionally and financially stressful and have less than a 10 per cent success rate for women with endometriosis. (Remember, in the endometriosis patient, the peritoneal fluid contains the chemical secretions from the endometriotic implant which may damage the egg or sperm and prevent conception.)

Many scientists and physicians have debated whether or not IVF has any substantial benefit in getting the endometriosis patient pregnant.[17] Research has indicated that IVF has the same benefit as Danazol in increasing the pregnancy rate, i.e. 10 per cent. However, recent research also suggests that the older endometriosis patient (i.e., older than 35 years of age) has a better chance of getting pregnant with IVF than any other treatment.[18] Patients with auto-immune antibodies benefit more from IVF plus immunosuppressive drug treatment.[19]

Despite the cost of treatment, success cannot be guaranteed: 'Treatments cost several thousands of pounds or dollars so that only couples with sufficient disposable income can afford this path. Live births following IVF treatments range from 23.3 per cent to 4.8 per cent at clinics in Britain, the national average being only 14.2 per cent.'[20] This means that the top rate is 23.3 live births for every 100 treatment cycles. Almost 20,000 women in the UK had test-tube baby treatment in the year ending March 1995. Costs range from £3,000 to £5,000 per cycle but financial concerns are not the only consideration: 'Since the Human Fertilization and Embryology Act came into force in 1991, more than 500,000 human embryos have been created. Fewer than half are used in treatment and by March 1996 about 20,000 babies had been born.'[21] It is suggested that 'nutritional medicine should play a role in handicap prevention and medical treatment of infertility alongside IVF and GIFT'.[22] There are concerns that use of these techniques is increasing too rapidly. Researchers at a Dutch university in 1995 found that the fetuses of five out of twelve women who conceived through micro-assisted fertilization received the husbands male infertility genes.[23]

Speroff and Walsh (1987) quote health-care costs for infertility in the 1980s as $200 million (£125 million) per year; it must now be much more.[24] Combining orthodox fertility treatment with sound nutritional principles can only have beneficial consequences for both the health and the wallet. In England the highest success rate for IVF is 23.3 per cent. In combination with nutritional counselling, this rate could increase greatly. One only has to look at the Foresight success rate of 86 per cent when nutritional advice is given together with eradication of genito-urinary infections. Costs are much lower for nutrition consultations (£30–£50 per hour) than IVF treatment and for fresh foods and supplements for a few months.

## NUTRITIONAL IMPACT ON FERTILITY IN ASSISTED REPRODUCTIVE TECHNOLOGY

Vitamin C is vital to uterine health. In Japan it was found that 'when giving women who fail to ovulate vitamin C at 400mg per day combined with Clomid [ovarian stimulation] all the women ovulated. It potentiated the effect of the Clomid [ovarian stimulation]'.[25] It is also seen from research that 'vitamin E prevents miscarriage by allowing the embryo to attach firmly to the uterine wall and a normal placenta to develop around it'.[26]

Clomid has side effects, such as weight gain, breast tenderness, abdominal bloating and discomfort. Perganol likewise notes oedema as a side effect.[27] Zoladex and Danazol also list weight gain as a side effect.[28] These side effects can have far-reaching consequences: 'Women placed on these medications are often found to be uncomfortable with the amount of weight gained and put themselves on a reducing diet, thus cutting down the essential nutrients available to them.'[29] At a time when women are seeking to become pregnant, they are reducing their nutrient intake. This would appear to be the very worst time to try to diet. IVF treatment is expensive; in addition to the treatment the couple should concentrate on eating well in order to maximize the chance of a pregnancy. Remember that fertility increases on a rising body weight and decreases with a falling body weight.

## ANALGESICS

Painkilling drugs can be taken to reduce the pain of endometriosis, and coping with pain is dealt with in detail in chapter 3. The most common pain suppressants are antiprostaglandin drugs (e.g., aspirin, Motrin and Distalgesic. These antiprostaglandin drugs inhibit the production of prostaglandin E and prostaglandin F which are produced in large amounts by the endometriotic implant. Unfortunately, the disease itself is not affected by analgesics, so endometriosis will continue to develop unchecked but with a reduction (a dulling) of pain symptoms. Because of this, analgesics are usually used in conjunction with the other therapies. Analgesics may also contain caffeine: 'Caffeine is a weak stimulant that is often included in small doses in analgesic preparations. It is claimed that the addition of caffeine may enhance the analgesic effect, but the alerting effect, mild habit-forming effect and possible provocation of headache may not always be desirable.'[30]

## ANTIHISTAMINES

Antihistamines (which inhibit histamine production) can be short acting and in high doses have the disadvantage of causing drowsiness. As histamine release can be quite strong around endometriotic implants, antihistamines can sometimes be beneficial in pain reduction. Some antihistamines must never be taken with grapefruit juice. A substance in the juice called furanocoumarin attaches to an enzyme in the small intestine, which normally breaks down drugs. Prescription drug doses take account of that process, but because the furanocoumarin in the juice blocks this enzyme, it greatly increases the potency of the drug. Drugs taken for allergies, high blood pressure and heart disease can therefore be too strong.[31] (If you take antihistamines, ask your pharmacist for advice about the brand you use.) Vitamin C is also a powerful antihistamine and this may be why it appears to reduce endometriosis pain in many women, especially when combined with bioflavinoids.

## ETHICAL DECISIONS ABOUT TREATMENTS

With so many different and sometimes drastic treatments available it can be bewildering as to which way to turn and which direction to choose: 'Decisions can only be made on a basis of information and if a woman is not properly informed about the diagnosis or treatment of her condition, her chances of making a meaningful choice are diminished.'[32] Doctors often use highly technical language which makes it difficult sometimes to follow their gist. The doctor and consultant are in their roles to heal, and they can find it very difficult, even uncomfortable, when they are faced with a patient with a disease for which there is no cure: 'Doctors have been trained to be positive and helpful to patients and they do not like to send them away empty-handed.'[33] Knowing that with the placebo effect 30 per cent of people may get well even when given sugar tablets, many GPs are reluctant to be totally honest about drug side-effects.

There is at present no definitive medical cure for endometriosis but if you become informed and work with a nutritionist you might relieve the pain and the symptoms of infertility.

The shock of being diagnosed with a chronic condition brings its own anxiety and fear. Modern Western medicine conforms to our cultural myth that the body can be controlled; we always want to believe that someone can 'make it better'. In a clinical situation, lack of knowledge, lack of information, or lack of instruction, can provoke even more anguish.

Informed consent is extremely important, and there are ethical choices for both doctor and patient to make before choosing the treatment most appropriate to you as a unique individual. Building up a relationship of trust and confidence with your doctor is vital.[34] Providing information can itself lessen the pain, anxiety and tension. No doctor can do anything to a patient without his or her consent, and coercion should never be used. Each woman has a right to know how the drugs and surgery will affect her body, so information should be forthcoming from the health professional in each case. If a consultant expects you to comply to treatment without you being fully informed, you may need politely to question further about the efficacy (effectiveness) of the treatment.

The law ensures that your doctor should not have a hidden agenda when prescribing your treatment: 'Doctors, dentists and pharmacists who accept inducements to prescribe or supply medicines and other health products will also face fines of up to £5,000 or, in the most flagrant cases, a maximum of two years in jail. The move is in response to the increasingly lavish scale of gifts and other rewards being offered by some pharmaceutical companies and wholesalers, in an attempt to win orders. Offers which alarmed ministers include competitions with prizes of holidays or video cameras, and in one case bottles of wine simply for ordering a particular medicine. A government minister agrees that the public does not expect health-care professionals to be influenced in their decisions by incentives to prescribe or supply particular medicines.'[35] In America the American Medical Association has also clamped down on such practices.

Never assume that you are being given all information available, always dig a little deeper. Some charities are controlled by drug company interests and will only give one side of the story in order to boost sales. There are always two sides to a coin.

Health professionals should always work towards the good of the patient. Pellegrino, a medical ethics expert, gives his sense of the patient's good as 'the good most proper to being human', and that this 'involves the right to make choices, to plan for one's future and aim at goals, so that each individual is given the respect of patient dignity and human freedom'.[36] Whatever decision is made, it should come from the information given by the medical staff involved in a patient's case. Never be afraid to ask for more information if it is not clear.

The final decisions can only be guided with competent discussion between you and your consultant. 'They focus their (and our) attention on cures and imminent cures, on successful medical interventions, research funding and medical care and are more directed toward life-threatening conditions than toward nursing for chronic illness and disabilities'[37] is a criticism that has been levelled at the medical profession. Try to achieve a balanced exchange of information: 'The medical intervention should be modifying the disease using the craftsmanship of the physician or surgeon. Plus there is the sense of good as the patient's own concept for his or her own good, which takes into consideration what the patient feels is worth while and in their best interests.'[38] Most people know little or nothing about how to live with long-term or life-threatening illness; how to communicate with doctors and nurses about these matters; or how to live with uncertainty and pain when doctors cannot make them go away. Patient support groups have arisen to fill this gap for people suffering from every type of illness and disability. Some forward-thinking doctors even run doctor/patient forums to share information about how diseases impinge on life.

We need to to consider the ways in which we create new life. The practice of IVF means that thousands of embryos are created, some of which are implanted, others are used for research, others destroyed. With HFEA approval, embryologists decide which ones are to be screened out. At the extreme, IVF can be a bad science with unscrupulous multi-million pound pharmaceutical companies using children like commodities.[39] Yet, with nutritional guidance, eating well and using supplements for 3 months, women who have tried IVF without success have become pregnant. Try this simple, healthy route first before resorting to other treatments.

We need to aim for preventive medicine, to prevent the endometriosis and infertility from taking hold in the first place, but also to encourage all health professionals to listen and respect what the patient feels is right for her as an individual.

> Human destiny is bound to remain a gamble, because at some unpredictable time and in some unforeseeable manner nature will strike back.
>
> *Rene Dubos*, Mirage of Health, *1959*

Studies show that, in America, 'at present hysterectomy is the most performed major operation for American women between the ages of 15 and 45; the average age of elective surgery is 35 years. In 1985 one million women were given hysterectomy and over 35 million American women have had hysterectomies. Over half these women had their ovaries removed as well, even if the organs were not diseased. A half of all women in the USA have undergone hysterectomy by the age of 65 years.'[40] In the UK the situation is not dissimilar: '53 per cent of general practitioners believe that hysterectomy should be used only as a last resort in menorrhagia. 14 per cent of all UK women will have a hysterectomy before the age of 65 to solve this problem.'[41] The level of hysterectomy varies widely from country to country and from area to area: 'In California barely half of all women will carry their uterus to the grave, whereas a gynaecologist in Saudia Arabia may do no more than one hysterectomy per year. Perceived abnormal bleeding accounts for 70 per cent of all hysterectomies in premenopausal British women. About one woman in seven will decline a hysterectomy if she can be shown to have blood loss in the normal range.'[42] We all have to ensure that only essential hysterectomies are performed and that other treatment options are always offered. Informed choice is your key here. Ensure that you are always given sufficient information to make the right choice for your unique circumstances. Choose only that option that feels right to you. Always take the time to read your consent form completely and be sure that you agree fully with all the terms before any surgical procedure is undertaken.

All treatment decisions should be made on the basis of the knowledge as to how it may affect your future health. The outcome is important as it impinges on life. Try to become informed and make an informed decision.

## COMMUNICATING WITH YOUR DOCTOR

Making yourself understood during the few precious minutes you have with your doctor is vital. You will need to understand his or her point of view in order to communicate effectively. Express yourself articulately. You may need to take along a list with helpful reminders on points you wish to raise. You could also jot down any advice you are given. Then you will be in a position to discuss your treatment options and explain any anxieties you may have. Occasionally the doctor may record on cassette the advice which he gives, so that the implications can be fully understood when listened to again in the comfort of your home.

Many people are overawed by doctors' authority, since they are experts in their field and have so much knowledge. One often feels obliged to accept their suggestions without question. This only becomes a problem when we feel unhappy about a particular treatment. However, you have rights as an individual and as a patient, and there are many ways in which you can help yourself become more assertive in expressing your needs and desires.

Concrete steps you can take include making sure that you have the right doctor and becoming educated yourself about endometriosis. Local endometriosis groups usually know which doctors in their locale are the most sympathetic to the symptoms you experience. By understanding the symptoms and treatments available for endometriosis, you will be able to converse intelligently with your doctor. Analyse what your aims in treatment are – having a baby or eliminating endo-related pain. Explain these goals to your doctor and persist in finding a way to achieve them. Indicate any self-help methods you are using. In this way you should be taken more seriously.

Obtaining feedback from partners, close friends or those in a similar predicament can also be useful. It helps to put all the ideas and options into perspective. Other women with the condition may have been along the same route as you and can offer sympathy, as well as making practical suggestions. Talking through the options will help you to clarify your own position. As a unique individual your decision depends upon what you consider is right for you.

Finally, if after this much effort on your part, you are not receiving the kind of health care you require, you may consider asking for a second opinion. It is no sin to disagree with your doctor and should you be unhappy with any of the advice you are given, you are entitled to ask for an appointment with another doctor. The following checklist may help you:

- Is the doctor giving you respect as a person in your own right?

- Does the doctor believe that all the symptoms you describe are related to endometriosis or does he or she suggest that you are exaggerating the pain, or that other conditions may be complicating the diagnosis? Are you being taken seriously?

- Do you feel reassured that your doctor is listening with compassion to all the symptoms you are describing. Does he/she believe what you are trying to explain?

- What happens when your problem becomes urgent? Does the doctor see you quickly or do you have to make an appointment days ahead?

- When your GP responds to you, is he/she expressing things in ways you can understand or is he/she spouting jargon?

- Can you put your trust in this doctor?

- Does this doctor have your complete faith when it comes to operations? Has the doctor been open and informative about the surgical techniques and drug treatments beforehand (especially important if this is a new technique or part of a drug trial; medical ethics are involved here)?

- Do you feel confident that this doctor is open and honest with you about all the treatments which may be available?

When you are chronically ill, it can be difficult to appear self-assured, and doctors often misconstrue the distress of the condition as a woman being weak and emotional. Taking a friend along to the consultation for moral support can be helpful under these circumstances. Feeling drained is often a part of this disease pattern; the body is ill and trying to tell us that it needs nurturing back to health. Don't feel guilty about being ill. Just listen to your body. Perhaps it is asking for a rest.

## MEDICALLY TRAINED DOCTORS AND NUTRITIONAL ADVICE

Be aware that your doctor may not have received much training in nutrition: 'On average medically trained doctors only spend between 7 to 14 days during their 7-year training actually studying aspects of nutrition.'[43] However, most nutritionists have spent three to four years studying their subject, some many more. Nutrition is crucial to health and is the mainstay of preventive medicine. When the World Health Organization states that over one-third of all cancers develop as a result of poor diet, we wonder what other illnesses we could avoid if we all ate healthier diets.

A recent report indicated that only 20–25 per cent of medical schools run nutrition courses. Nutrition was perceived as a 'soft' topic and was not considered as a science amongst physicians. It was found that 'nutrition knowledge was low amongst physicians in practice and that this decreased with the number of years in practice. Lack of time was cited as a barrier to doctors discussing disease prevention with patients and many doctors had little confidence in their ability to change health behaviour in their patients.'[44] Dr Alan Levin, a doctor of environmental medicine in the USA, states that, 'Even today in the medical schools, preventive medicine and nutrition are very, very minor courses. Everybody laughs at them ... The important things are pharmacology, internal medicine, surgery, and how to deal with a disease once it happens. They are not concerned with altering people's diets or environments so that they don't develop a disease.'[45]

The World Health Organization stated in 1973 that all doctors should work alongside a nutritionist and yet, over a quarter of a century later, there is still no sign of this. Nutrition is complementary to orthodox medicine and the one can help the other. The main problem is that nutrients are natural, and drug companies cannot patent natural products like vitamins and minerals so they cannot make money from their sales. Only formulated chemical drugs invented by pharmaceutical companies and unique to their laboratories can be formally patented, enabling big profits to be made. Food is often seen by governments as a commodity, not as a health-giving substance. It is sold for profit, not for health, so food standards often fall short of what our bodies desire. Meldrum states that, 'nutritional therapies ... improve both health promotion/prevention and treatment/care services at no extra cost in the short term and with the prospect of a reduction of costs in the medium to long term'.[46]

Trained nutritionists work with their clients to assess biochemical individuality by looking at nutritional status, and using blood and tissue tests. They work on a one-to-one basis to correct any imbalances and resolve symptoms. They examine the root of the problem to elicit a cure, rather than just suppress symptoms, and will, for example, look at strengthening the immune and reproductive systems. They support the client through changes in eating patterns, encouraging the choice of foods which are nutrient-rich rather than high in empty calories, thus improving nutrient intake; and they may suggest nutritional supplements for three to four months to help correct imbalances.

Consultations with a nutritionist normally last for one hour and people are seen on average four times. In order to be effective, nutrition requires perseverance and skills in food choice, and this comes with encouragement. With face-to-face, one-to-one guidance and counselling clients feel the support and see the results of nutritional medicine. If doctors and nutritionists could work together towards improving health, great leaps in health care, and particularly fertility treatment, could be made.

Nutrition consultations should be part and parcel of all health care programmes. This is particularly important after stillbirth and miscarriages. Seek out a well-qualified nutritionist in your area and talk with him or her. Most practitioners offer a free 15-minute consultation first to consider the options open to you.

## SUMMARY

1  There is no known medical cure for endometriosis at present.

2  Traditional medicine can suppress endometriosis symptoms with a variety of strategies including: drug therapies which stimulate pseudopregnancy or menopause to suppress endometriotic implants; surgical therapies which remove the implants; pregnancy induction; analgesics or antihistamines to dull pain.

3  Become informed. Whatever decision is made should be based on the information that you have been given honestly by the medical staff involved in your case. Also read books, scan the internet (*see* www.makingbabies.com) and talk to other women.

4  A good line of communication must be established between the endometriosis patient and her physician in order for trust to develop.

5  Medical treatments can be beneficial if the patient has faith in her doctor's caring and knowledge. If you think your doctor requires more knowledge, you can ply them with the vast number of information leaflets provided by the endometriosis associations around the world. Their aim is to help educate health professionals in the immensity of the impact on life from this disease.

6  If you have seen more than four physicians, then nutrition is a possible answer. See a nutritionist for a full assessment of the underlying nutritional imbalances.

# 6 The holistic approach to endometriosis

> Edison's electric lamp is a completely
> idiotic idea
>
> *Sir William Preece, FRS,*
> *Post Office Chief Engineer, UK, 1876*

Truth is not known until it happens. Some holistic therapies work whether they appear to have a scientific reason behind them or not. There are things in heaven and on earth which our science does not yet understand ...

Your health is dependent upon fresh air, clean water, a variety of nutritious foods, your living conditions, cleanliness and good hygiene. We have a modicum of control over these things. We cannot change the genes that we have inherited. But it is suggested by some research that 'whilst nutrition (or specific nutrients) cannot negate one's ultimate genetic fate, it can modify the time frame during which the characteristics of this fate appear. Some nutrients turn on or turn off the expression of specific genes, and genes can affect the use of specific nutrients'.[1]

Your body is not just a set of disparate organs. Modern medicine has broken the body into compartments for treatment, but that is not how the body works. Each system is linked to the other by receptor cells which send chemical messengers to each other. It is like networking, or living in symbiosis – you scratch my back and I'll scratch yours. If one system begins to fail, the others will rally round and take the burden to allow healing to take place. The body works as a whole and we have to treat it as such.

How do you really feel? When we ask someone the question 'How are you?', the majority of people politely say, 'I'm okay, thank you', even when what is going on in their mind may be totally different. They could have a backache, headache, sore throat, or indeed any of a myriad of minor problems that often lurk behind our usual facade.

It is amazing that we tend to ignore what our bodies are trying to tell us. The headaches, bad period pains, constant infections and sore throats, stomach aches and that awful tired feeling (as though you are up to your knees in a tin of treacle) all happen for a reason. Why do we consistently ignore these warning signs? This is our body's way of letting us know something is going awry. In fact, sometimes the body positively shouts at us. But we ignore it as life rushes past at an alarming rate, and we have to keep up, so we push ourselves to the limit.

Life has far more stressors and strains than ever before. Worrying about where the next meal is coming from is not so much of a problem any more. We do not have to chase our prey or go out gathering and foraging; it is all neatly packaged in the supermarket. We go along and pick out the ready-made meals, place them in our home freezer and take them out when we need them. In the evenings when we return from work we are often too exhausted to cook anyway.

If we are ill and have to take time off work, it is the pits. We feel so guilty knowing our desk will be covered with mountains of outstanding work, so we rush back to the normal routine before we are properly cured. People often return to work too soon, before the immune system has restored itself to a strong position, ready for the next onslaught of bacteria and viruses to hit our systems. In the olden days there were convalescent homes where we were allowed to be ill, and where the staff nursed us back to health over several weeks. Good food was served and, as we began to heal, we worked in the gardens growing fresh vegetables for our meals. That brief respite from daily life with clean air and good food allowed the immune system to renew itself. That really was a holistic approach.

A holistic approach to illness can cover different angles. There is not much point in trying too many therapies at once. You need to choose one or two therapies with which you feel comfortable. We all have a sixth sense which many of us try to ignore. In order to be 'in tune' with our own bodies' needs we have to sense what is best for us. This is a part of being true to yourself – knowing what feels right and what feels wrong.

## Sheena M of Devon

*I decided to follow the 'complementary' path of treatment for my endometriosis and infertility which included acupuncture, homeopathy and nutrition. In addition I had the support and prayers of my husband, friends and family. I now have two extremely healthy, bright children – Verity, aged 3, and Henry, 8 months. I fed Verity till she was 18 months and intend to do the same with Henry. I have had no more pain despite my periods returning about 8–10 weeks after both births and, considering they were both by Caesarean section, I feel incredibly fit and healthy. Which therapy helped the most? I'm sure they were all just part of the whole but the results are wonderful and five years ago it was difficult to contemplate such a happy end to my story. Thank you.*

CASE STUDY

It helps to know that you are not alone with the pain of endometriosis, that while you are curled up with a pillow in bed, other women are in pain at that same moment. Some women find joining a support group helps to share the steps forward, or at least talking with the local group leader for support.

Endometriosis is like a game of snakes/shutes and ladders. One day you feel so ill and the next you feel 'normal'. It is so good to feel normal again, you can overdo it and relapse the following day. There is a trick in knowing when to rest. Giving in to pain can be distressing and many women tend to push themselves too hard. The immune system renews itself when the body is at rest, so quality time for yourself is valuable to the healing process.

Knowing how to help yourself heal is also important. A combination of orthodox and complementary medicine may be suitable for you. Sometimes a medicine will work for you and at other times it won't. One treatment style may be useful on its own, but occasionally two will enhance each other. Because we are each unique human beings, what works for one person will not always help another. But modern medicine tends to treat us all the same, even when it is so obvious that we are completely different, inside and out. You need to find the right path for you by a process of trial and error.

As Charles Duell (Director of US Patent Office, 1899) believed: 'Everything that can be invented has been invented!' But there is much we still have to learn about the workings of the human body. Even the workings of some of the drugs offered to you for endometriosis are not fully understood. There are many paths left unexplored, and one of them is the role of nutrients in the endocrine and immune systems. As drug companies can make no money from selling these nutrients, they see no point in doing the research.

The term 'biochemical individuality', coined by Dr Roger Williams, implies that each of us has a subtly different body biochemistry. Organs are slightly different shapes; enzymes work at different levels; drugs work in slightly different ways.[2] But finding the combination of therapies that is right for you is where your sixth sense comes into play – listen to what your body tells you feels right.

## Liz N of Yorkshire

*I have continued to eat a healthy diet based on the principles you outlined. I have also bought the books* Optimum Nutrition *and the* Fatburner Diet *by P Holford. This has helped my overall general well-being and I try to do regular exercise to keep fit, and get fresh air and natural light to help my psychological state. Overall this strategy (including the vitamin supplementation) has helped me to keep my endo under control. Certainly the other symptoms, such as PMS, mood swings, irritability and anxiety, have all decreased. I use homeopathy and reflexology, both of which improve my feeling of well-being to a limited extent but they did not affect the underlying endo.*

• C A S E   S T U D Y •

## RELAXATION

Every day you need to take 'time out' for 20 minutes and allow yourself space to just be. Relaxation time is very important when the rest of life is so stressed. Your body requires a period of rest each day to recharge the immune system. Research has shown the body heals much faster while we are asleep. At first it can be nigh on impossible to relax if you are used to doing everything for everybody. Choose something to help you relax. Lie in the bath with favourite music and candles; go for a walk; spend time on a hobby you really enjoy; or spend time with a valued friend – just sharing life can be very valuable. Let the world rush by you for a change, while you step into your own area of peace for your special moments. We stretch ourselves to the limit and those few minutes of relaxation, which you deserve, may help your body to begin to recover. Do not feel guilty, everyone is entitled to some time for themselves. Your body deserves a rest for healing purposes. Be kind to yourself, as you are unique in the universe.

## EXERCISE

If possible, take a short walk after your evening meal as this will aid your digestive processes as well as help you relax. You could take up an exercise (this does not have to be as hard as aerobics and jogging). A gentle walk or swim will help your muscles increase their mitochondria (cell organelles which produce energy, *see* chapter 2). The more mitochondria you have in your muscles, the more energy you can make.

Exercise not only tones the muscles and keeps the heart and lungs fit, it also stimulates your digestive tract to help you digest food effectively and excrete harmful substances more rapidly. You are also making the lymphatic system work by triggering movement of the lymph, so that the white blood cells of the immune army move around the body.

Exercise also raises the levels of endorphins (brain chemicals which act as natural painkillers) in the bloodstream, which also help to elevate your mood. Feeling positive can help to stimulate the immune system. Exercise also aids the proper excretion of oestrogen and cholesterol from the body. Research has shown that oestrogen and cholesterol when bound to fibre are excreted in greater amounts when exercise is undertaken (*see* pp 171,190, 218), which prevents them from re-circulating and causing health problems.

If you are in great pain from endometriosis you may not feel like aerobics or jogging, but gentle walks, swimming for pleasure or yoga may help to move stiff muscles. A short, brisk walk of 20 minutes, 3 times a week, also helps to put calcium into bones to prevent osteoporosis. If you exercise in daylight and eat sufficient zinc- and vitamin B6-rich foods, then your pituitary gland functions effectively to produce the hormone signals necessary for ovarian function.

Never stress the body with too much exercise, be moderate. Over-exercising is stressful and uses up the body intake of B vitamins, zinc and magnesium, the very nutrients the pituitary and ovary most require. (This is why athletes and ballerinas who train constantly and are underweight often have amenorrheoa (lack of periods). Their BMI is too low and they may become deficient in nutrients vital to the ovaries.)


## NATURAL DAYLIGHT

Research has revealed the importance of natural daylight for health: 'The retina of the eye and its zinc and vitamin B2 level are crucial in the formation of hormones. When the eye registers the presence of light, a signal is sent to the hypothalamus in the brain. The hypothalamus then begins to produce hormones which trigger the pituitary gland which instigates production of the sex hormones required by the ovaries. The pituitary produces gonadotrophic hormones which stimulate the ovaries or testes to produce the female and male sex hormones.'[3] We all require 20 minutes of natural daylight on the retina of the eye to begin this process. If you work in an office with fluorescent lights, it is important that you escape at lunchtime and have a walk, especially in the winter months when we travel to and from work in the dark: 'Fluorescent lights impair the function of the pituitary gland . . . in natural daylight the ovaries can produce their oestrogen and progesterone.'[4] Research would appear to confirm the connection between natural light and the good health of the reproductive system: 'There is a positive correlation between follicular fluid melatonin and oestradiol. This suggests that melatonin may be involved in the regulation of hormone production in the ovaries.'[5]

The connection between natural light and female reproductive health in particular was highlighted in a study of women undergoing IVF treatment: 'Follicular fluid samples were obtained from the largest pre-ovulatory follicle of 120 women undergoing in vitro fertilization, and were examined for melatonin levels. The concentration of melatonin and progesterone during the autumn and winter (dark) months were significantly higher than those of the spring and summer (light) months. By contrast, oestradiol concentrations were significantly lower during the dark months than during the light months. There was a positive correlation between follicular fluid melatonin and progesterone concentration, and a negative relationship between melatonin and oestradiol. This suggests that melatonin may be involved in the regulation of hormone production in the ovaries.'[6] We can conclude that natural light and zinc intake are very important to our fertility.

## HEALTH'S INTANGIBLES

Some researchers feel that there is a mind–body connection to health, and that the pineal gland in the brain may be the link. But whatever the link, the body has an amazing ability to heal itself if we allow it time and space and fill it with healthy air, food and water. Research scientists know that there is a 30 per cent recovery rate from the 'placebo' effect. (A placebo effect is a positive therapeutic effect claimed by a patient after receiving a dummy tablet believed by him to be an active drug.). This may be because they are taking part in a clinical trial and feel they are actually doing something positive to help themselves, or they feel someone is taking care to help them try to get better. Whatever this mystery factor, it would appear that the combination of trying to help yourself to get better and having someone care that you do get better has a profound effect on health outcomes.

## RELAXATION TECHNIQUES

Sleep can be elusive when you are in pain. Try going to bed and listening to some favourite music to lull you to sleep, or buy a relaxation, self-hypnosis or sleep tape to talk you through the relaxation techniques. Consider magnesium supplements – 'Magnesium might be of benefit both in calming you down and in helping you sleep at night, as it is a natural tranquillizer with no side effects and no possibility of addiction.'[7] One company (see p. 356) produces a pain tape which helps to calm pain down, and they also produce sleep/relaxation/health tapes. There are many ways in which you can try to help yourself and they are not difficult or expensive. Visualization therapy (see p 45) has helped many people with cancer and it may work for you. Prayer can be a powerful tool for some people, as can healing circles.

When you are extremely debilitated and life looks bleak, when friends are getting on with their lives but you are stopped in your tracks by intractable pain, then positive thinking is needed to lift you up. One helpful relaxation tape suggests very simply: 'Stop hating the part of the body that is letting you down. Rather look upon it as a sick little child and love it better.'[8] This has the immediate effect of softening your feelings towards yourself. Hating bits of your body for ruining your life is no help to recovery. What you need to do is accept yourself as being ill, and try to love yourself better. Pamper yourself, put yourself first for a change, get the environment right, reduce the stressors, and let go of the pain and terror and cast it away. By doing all the positive things you can to move forward, even if at first it is only inch by inch, the first steps on the road to health can be taken.

## COMPLEMENTARY THERAPIES

A variety of complementary therapies have become popular and may help you to control the symptoms of your endometriosis. (If you wish to further your knowledge in this area, please see the reading list provided at the end of this book.) This section will look briefly at therapies which have helped some women.

N. B. Always ensure that you are using a qualified practitioner who is insured to treat you. They should have a certificate displayed in their offices and belong to their governing or regulatory body.

---

### Lorraine W of Avon

*I was diagnosed with endo after a laparoscopy 18 months ago. After nine months of various hormone treatments and no improvement I went to see a herbalist. My symptoms were irregular cycles (36–72 days), heavy and painful periods (8–10 days), PMT for 2 weeks before the period began, weight gain but inability to lose weight, listlessness, distressing hair loss, and spots, irritability and sudden bursts of tears for no apparent reason. After initial herbal medicine and vitamins and minerals my condition started to improve. I began an anti-candida diet, i.e. no fruit for one month only, no refined sugars, yeasts and I excluded dairy products as I felt I had an intolerance to them. Five months since I began the diet I have noticed a large improvement in my condition. My last period was almost pain-free with no PMT. The cycle was 35 days only and the bleed lasted only 6 days. My hair is growing thicker and my skin is improving, and my energy level has increased so much*

• C A S E  S T U D Y •

---

*that I can now do a six-mile bike ride each night and keep fit with Callenetics twice a week. I am still taking some vitamins. I have no dairy products, no yeast products, and am trying to keep refined sugars and caffeine to as low a level as possible. My diet is mainly raw and steamed vegetables with stir fries. I try to follow the Hay system, i.e. not mixing starch and proteins, and my digestion has greatly improved and so has my temperature. I always felt cold before.*

•
C
A   S
S   T
E   U
    D
    Y
•

## ACUPUNCTURE

Many women with endometriosis have been helped by acupuncture. In this ancient Chinese therapy needles are stuck into certain known pressure points or invisible energy channels called 'meridians', which are believed to run between the organs of the body. The needle manipulation is said to unblock channels of energy in the body (called 'Qi'). The body is viewed as a balance between opposing forces, 'yin' and 'yang'. Yin is passive and tranquil, representing darkness, coldness, moisture and swelling. Yang is aggressive and stimulating, representing light, heat, dryness and contraction. Any imbalance is thought to be a cause of illness, for example, too much yin can cause dull aches, pains, chilliness, fluid retention, discharges and tiredness. Always consult a qualified practitioner. Letters after the name include MBAcA, FBAcA, MIROM, MRTCM, MTAS, BAAR, LicAc, BAC, DrAc.

## AROMATHERAPY

Aromatherapy involves treating illness with essential oils extracted from plants, which are believed to have medicinal qualities. Essential oils are produced by tiny glands in the plants, and these oils are distilled and dissolved in alcohol. In Britain the diluted oils are used mainly for massage treatments or are added to baths, cold compresses or used as inhalations. They are absorbed through the skin into the bloodstream and work internally. You should never swallow the oils. A trial using aromatherapy with sufferers of endometriosis was undertaken, using specific oils. Over half the women in the study experience a reduction in pain and depression, and had an improved sense of well-being.

## BACH REMEDIES

Bach remedies are a series of 38 preparations from wild flowers and plant extracts, first made by Dr E Bach in 1915, and they are available from most good health food stores and pharmacies. The remedies are used to treat the whole person, not just the illness from which they are suffering. Bach believed that the dew on the plants was impregnated with their medicinal qualities. He collected this dew, distilled it and dissolved it in alcohol to give to patients. The remedy is chosen according to the patient's psychological and emotional states. The remedies are sold in a concentrated form which needs diluting in spring water. Put four drops of the concentrate into a small amount of water or drop them directly onto the tongue. Bach's Rescue Remedy is popular with women with endometriosis as it seems to speed up recovery from stress, pain and exhaustion. There is no register of practitioners using Bach remedies, though some courses are offered.

## BIOCHEMICAL TISSUE SALTS

Biochemical tissue salts are natural mineral salts in tablet form which are essential for health. A lack of these salts or imbalance can cause disease. These salts provide a small, easily absorbed dose to help the body heal itself by restoring the correct balances. There are 12 tissue salts prepared in a homeopathic way. Combination N is for menstrual pain; combination B is for nervous exhaustion, edginess, general debility, and aids convalescence. The tablets are lactose-based, and so are unsuitable for anyone with a milk allergy. They are prescribed by naturopaths, herbalists and homeopaths.

## CHIROPRACTIC AND OSTEOPATHY

Using the hands to manipulate the body, chiropractors and osteopaths can correct disorders of the joints, muscles and spine. Spinal problems can cause referred pain in other areas of the body, e.g. the hip or leg. In some cases these problems can be the cause of period pains or constipation. Displacement of lumbars 4 and 5 (vertebrae in the small of the back) can be related to problems in the reproductive area as these hold the ligaments that support the uterus and Fallopian tubes. A twisted pelvis can lead to infertility, as the Fallopian tubes may be twisted away from the ovary, so correcting the tilt may be beneficial. The chiropractor makes greater use of X-rays and conventional methods like ultrasound than do osteopaths. Most chiropractors use the letters DC after their name, but from 1991 chiropractors trained at the Anglo-European College of Chiropractic at Bournemouth, UK, can use BSc Chiropractic. The letters MRO mean 'Member of the Register of Osteopaths' which is regulated by the General Council and Register of Osteopaths in Berkshire, England (*see* p. 358).

## HEALING

Some people have the gift of healing by the laying on of hands. This usually is done by someone with a deep faith in God, and who prays for healing power to flow from God through themselves into the individual seeking healing. Many healers can heal whether or not the person seeking healing is a believer. To find a genuine healer, work through a recognized church or try the addresses on p. 352. Many healings can hardly be called miracles, as they are understandable given the connection between the body and soul. Spontaneous remissions of disease can and do occur. To understand why, we might have to wait until until our understanding of physics improves. Our bodies comprise chemical, magnetic and electrical impulses which may or may not be involved in the healing process. True healing could never be a part of a money-making racket, so avoid all dubious institutions and seek those which feel full of reverence and peace. Search for sincerity, not charlatans.

## HERBAL MEDICINE

Herbal medicine treats the patient as an individual, with individual needs, and not just as another medical case history. Treatment is tailored to the specific requirements of the individual at that moment in time. Knowledge of the power of plants with healing properties has been passed from generation to generation. Indeed, it is the precursor of modern medicine – the use of digitalis (from foxgloves) for heart disease, willow (precursor of aspirin) for headaches, and blue cohosh (known as papoose root in the USA) for infertility. International scientific research not only confirms our knowledge of the healing powers of herbs but also enlarges it.

Trained herbalists have the letters MNIMH or FNIMH after their name, and can be found through the addresses on p. 352.

## HOMEOPATHY

Homeopathy first began in 1810 when Samuel Hahnemann discovered that fighting like with like seemed to help people heal. This was well understood by Hippocrates in the fifth century BC. He conjectured that illness symptoms were the body's way of fighting the illness. Hahnemann termed this new medicine 'allopathic', meaning against illness.

The homeopathic approach is based on the whole person, including their mental, spiritual, emotional and physical well-being. Therapists can be found through the Royal Homeopathic Hospital (see p. 353). There are five NHS homeopathic hospitals – in London, Bristol, Tunbridge Wells, Liverpool and Glasgow, and one private homeopathic clinic in Manchester. Each is staffed by medically qualified homeopathic staff.

## HYDROTHERAPY

Easing yourself into a comfortable hot bath can have a very soothing effect on aches and pains. Hydrotherapy (water treatment) is much more specific in its use of water's properties to cure ailments. At the root of this belief is the feeling that water is the essence of life. We are, after all, 70% water! In water's various forms (gas, liquid, solid, steam) it can be used to induce relaxation, to stimulate blood flow, to remove impurities, drugs or alcohol, to ease pain and stiffness, and to treat diseases. A list of accredited therapists can be obtained from the addresses on p. 353.

## HYPNOTHERAPY

Somewhere between sleep and wakefulness is the state of conscious-ness that hypnotherapists use to try to improve a person's health and relieve pain. Hypnotherapists induce a trance-like state and use it to bring about physical or mental changes in the patient, but treatment by an unqualified hypnotherapist can do more harm than good. For a list of well-trained therapists contact the addresses on p. 354.

## MASSAGE

Massage is one of the oldest therapies known to man, used since 3000 BC. Hippocrates wrote in 5 BC: 'The way to health is to have a scented bath and an oiled massage each day.' The use of massage helps to relax, stimulate and invigorate the mind and body. It also helps to improve the blood, lymphatic, muscular and nervous systems, helping to rid the body of waste products. Treatment by an unqualified masseur can do more harm than good, so contact the addresses on p. 357 to find a qualified practitioner.

## NATUROPATHY

Naturopathy helps the body to heal itself, for example, by fasting after an upset stomach, sweating out a fever, or submerging a sprained ankle into icy water. Naturopathy uses chiropractic, diets, exercise, massage, osteopathy, hydrotherapy, relaxation and breathing. It also encourages people to think positively about good health, and to live life as naturally as possible amid the pressures of everyday life. Naturopathy tries to identify the underlying cause of the illness and sets out to treat this, using diet and other therapies rather than just suppressing symptoms. Each case is treated as unique and naturopaths seek to complement and support conventional doctors. A list of qualified practitioners can be obtained from the General Council and Register of Naturopaths (*see* p. 357), and have the letters MRN and ND or DO after their name.

## REFLEXOLOGY

Reflexology involves massaging the reflex areas in the feet. These correspond to the 'energy channels' known to acupuncturists. Gentle massage can unblock these channels, allowing energy to flow again and heal damage to the body. It originated in China and is said to help people with pain, digestion problems, period pains and osteoporosis. Therapists use the letters MBRA after their name (*see* p. 359).

## SYSTEMIC KINESIOLOGY

Kinesis means motion, and kinesiology is the study of locomotion in relation to the structure and working of the muscles, for example, if leg muscles work properly then the knee will jerk when it is hit. This connection was recognized by a chiropractor in 1964. Systemic kinesiology works by correcting the motions of muscles and ligaments in the body.

Kinesiologists do not diagnose illness but look for imbalances or deficiencies in nutrition or energy, to locate physical problems. They give a light, fingertip massage to pressure points to stimulate the blood and lymphatic systems. This form of muscle testing gives a clear picture of a person's state of health. Practitioners can be found through the Academy of Systemic Kinesiology (*see* p. 359).

## YOGA

The postures and exercises which make up Indian hatha yoga are the best-known form in Britain. The philosophy stresses the influence of mind over body, and that mental and spiritual development are necessary to reinforce the benefits that physical exercises can bring. The movements are done slowly and never strained, creating an awareness of the body to allow a better relaxation of muscles. Conditions such as arthritis, backache, and period pains may be helped. Breathing plays an important part in the exercises. Skilled yoga teachers can be found through the Yoga Biomedical Trust and the American Yoga Association (*see* p. 360).

## CONCLUSION

There is a life out there to be led and if you suffer from endometriosis remember that this is only a phase in time when the body has succumbed to illness. The body needs a period of convalescence to heal; it needs looking after. Endometriosis is a jigsaw and you need to fit all the pieces together gradually, allowing each area time to heal. Everyone wants to be well very quickly, but when the body has taken a while to become ill, we have to be patient and work with it to achieve recovery.

### Angela A of London

*For my endometriosis I have taken Chinese herbs and vitamin and mineral supplements for about a year to help balance my hormones. Finding the correct balance to resolve the problem with hair loss is a challenge. Improving my diet, like stopping chocolates and coffee, cakes and biscuits and increasing good healthy foods, has been the key. However, if I follow a stricter regime I feel even better. Gone is the*

CASE STUDY

*horrible debilitating pain that put me in bed for a couple of days each period month. The terrible sharp drowning pain that went on and on is gone. All I have now is mild discomfort if I don't take some supplements such as the GLA.*

Try the various techniques we have discussed – relaxation, gentle exercise – and work with good friends and caring family members to help pull you through. Recovery doesn't happen overnight. Most people, when they are ill, expect to go to the doctor and take a tablet to put everything right. Endometriosis is not like that. It is far more complicated because it is systemic; it affects the whole person, not only the reproductive system. Begin to help yourself, and these positive actions may start to pull you out of the vicious circle that the pain of endometriosis can drag you into.

Your body does not want to be ill and it is constantly trying to heal itself. Endometriosis is nothing that we have done to make ourselves ill; it appears to be a combination of factors – environmental pollution, hereditary factors, poor diet, poor digestion, lack of exercise and relaxation in this mad world we inhabit. The body is out of balance and it needs rebalancing. You have the power to do that, and the time taken will be well worth it because it gives you your life back again. Go ahead, try it.

> If you do not take the time to be well, you WILL take the time to be sick!
>
> *Lindsey Duncan, Nutritionist*

## SUMMARY

There are a number of holistic therapies that appear to help with endometriosis, pain and infertility. We have looked at several, and they all are worthy of investigation if you feel that they may be of value. You must ensure that each practitioner holds recognized qualifications and seek advice from the organizations listed at the end of this book. Books on each speciality are available from local libraries.

1   Your health is dependent upon fresh air, clean water, cleanliness, nutritious food, good living conditions and hygiene. Assess your needs and do what you can.

2   Listen to what your sixth sense tells you. By becoming in tune with your body's needs, it helps you to judge what feels right and what feels wrong. You have the power to help your body heal – it is always striving to be well. Illness is not natural to it. Be gentle with yourself.

3   Every day allow yourself 20 minutes of 'me time'. When you can, just be.

4   Choose a treatment which feels right for your needs and try it for at least three months to give it a chance to work.

5   Ensure that you have 20 minutes each day in natural daylight to aid the function of your pituitary gland so that it can send the right messages to your ovaries.

6   Try going to bed and listening to some favourite music or a relaxation tape to lull you to sleep. Magnesium help you sleep at night, as it is a natural tranquillizer.

7   Feeling positive can help to stimulate the immune system. Try to take the positive step of recognizing that part of you is ill and sickly and needs looking after.

8   Exercise increases the excretion of oestrogen from the body. Research has shown that oestrogen bound to fibre is excreted in greater amounts when exercise is undertaken.

9   Be kind to yourself, look upon your ill body as you would a sick little child and love it better.

# 7 Strengthening the immune system

> The obscure we eventually see. The completely
> obvious, it seems, takes longer.
>
> *Edward R. Murrow*

Something major is going wrong with the immune system in endometriosis, and it may be that subclinical deficiencies of nutrients are not allowing the body to work at optimum efficiency.

## HOW THE IMMUNE SYSTEM WORKS

The immune system exists to protect us from danger. Outside our body are bacteria, viruses and parasites which can do us harm. The immune system consists of the liver, spleen, lymph glands (which filter cells), bone marrow and the thymus gland (which is located behind the breastbone). These are the chief organs which produce the white blood cell army (*see* figure 7.1). There are other tissues which are supportive of the immune system – the pituitary gland, adrenal glands, tonsils, adenoids, appendix and Peyer's patches in the lower part of the digestive tract.

The white blood cells behave like an army; they are the forces at the ready to do battle with an enemy invasion of the body. The lymphatic system is composed of the glands and lymph vessels, which are similar to the blood vessels, except the lymph is not pumped by the heart; it is moved by the body's movements. The vessels act as the main highway through the body on which the white blood cells can travel in the lymph (a yellow oil-based medium) to sites which are being threatened, the lymph glands. If the immune system begins fighting infections in the lymph glands, the glands enlarge (in the neck, groin and under the arms).

Research shows that 'over 2,000 immune cells per second are produced in our long (marrow) bones in the body'.[1] That figure, of course, presumes the body is healthy, fit and well fed. Such rapid

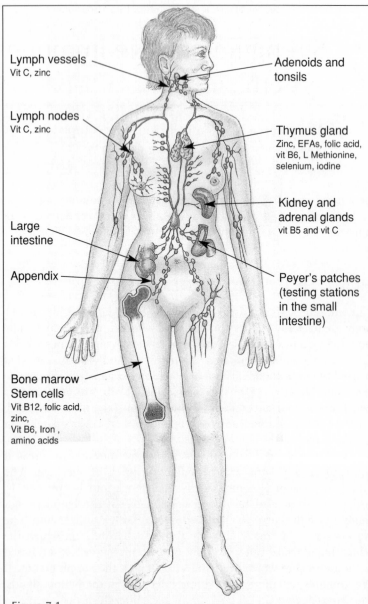

**Lymph vessels**
Vit C, zinc

**Lymph nodes**
Vit C, zinc

**Large intestine**

**Appendix**

**Bone marrow Stem cells**
Vit B12, folic acid, zinc,
Vit B6, Iron ,
amino acids

**Adenoids and tonsils**

**Thymus gland**
Zinc, EFAs, folic acid,
vit B6, L Methionine,
selenium, iodine

**Kidney and adrenal glands**
vit B5 and vit C

**Peyer's patches**
(testing stations in the small intestine)

Figure 7.1
The lymphatic system, showing the major tissues which are associated with the immune system.

growth and development deserves to be well supplied with the nutrients from your diet.

There are many different types of cell to suit all types of attack. They all originate from basic stem cells, primarily in bone marrow, which requires folic acid, vitamin B12, zinc, vitamin B6, iron and amino acids in abundance. If these are in short supply, the body cannot fight infections or remove cell debris (like endometriotic implants) efficiently. However, 80 per cent of the immunoglobulins (one of the major immune defence systems of the body) are made in the small intestine, therefore the gut membranes also need to be in the peak of health.[2] The gut as an area of immunity cannot be dismissed lightly. If your gut is ill, you will be ill.

Why are some people better endowed with stronger immune systems than others? Archibald Garrod in 1908 gave a lecture on inborn errors of metabolism at Yale University, USA, that is still pertinent today. He stated:

'The existence of chemical individuality follows of necessity from that of chemical specificity, but we should expect the differences between individuals to be still more subtle and difficult of detection. Indications of their existence are seen, even in man, in the various tints of skin, hair and eyes, and in the quantitative differences in those portions of the end-products of metabolism which are endogenous and are not affected by diet. Even those idiosyncrasies with regard to drugs and articles of food which are summed up in the proverbial saying that what is one man's meat is another man's poison, presumably have a chemical basis.'[3]

## Lynn S of Yorkshire

*Dietary changes as restrictive as the anti-candida diet are extremely difficult to adhere to if the therapy is started when the patient is at a low ebb. I could not cope with the withdrawal symptoms as I had recently had major surgery and felt too ill to start immediately. The dreadful aching in all my muscles as well as extreme fatigue meant that I was bedridden.*

*I tried again when I felt better able to cope. I feel building up the immune system by diet and good food and supplements is better used as a preventive measure, because once endometriosis is established, comfort eating comes into play.*

•
C
A
S
E

S
T
U
D
Y
•

## RECOGNIZING AN ALIEN INVASION

The immune system, as our first line of defence against infection and allergies, must be able to rapidly recognize 'alien' material like bacteria and viruses. In this way, as soon as our body is invaded, it can assemble the immune army of white blood cells and antibodies to rapidly destroy the 'alien' invaders. Inherent in this is the body's unique ability to recognize 'self' and 'non-self' material. As you may expect, this is accomplished very early on in our lives.

During our development as a fetus, the thymus gland in the chest and the other immunological tissues in the body compute and register all of the molecules that are present in the body as 'self tissue'. This stops our own immune system from attacking our own healthy cells.

However, there is a paradox with endometriosis. These cells are natural to the body, so they are not perceived as a threat. Or are they? Much of the pain from endometriotic implants could be from the release of strong chemicals as the macrophages try to remove these misplaced cells. There is only one other disease in the body where our own cells grow in the wrong places, and that is rare. This is splenosis and it only occurs when spleen cells are splattered after an accident. (The spleen is the only organ where endometriosis never appears to grow. It is the only part of the lymphatic system which filters blood.) All other body cells seem to behave themselves and stay where nature intended. If we can answer the question as to why endometrial cells roam, we may be halfway to finding the cure.

After birth any new molecules, like the molecules that make up the outer covering of a bacterium, are considered as 'non-self'. This is a miraculous system that is usually quite efficient at protecting us from 'alien' molecules which get into our bloodstream or lungs, or enter our bodies through breaks in the skin. However, there are some weaknesses in the system, one being that those tissues that are outside the body are not considered as part of the 'self' group. For instance, the sperm which are contained in tiny tubes within the testes are treated by the body as if they are outside the body, and are therefore recognized as 'non-self'. If you inject a man's sperm into himself, he will mount an immune attack against his own sperm! This may happen in women with endometriosis. The endometrium which lies in the centre of the uterus can actually be viewed as being on the outside of the body because it is open to the outside through the vagina, and the immune system may not consider it to be part of the 'self' group. When the endometriotic implants develop in the abdomen, the body responds with an immunological attack on the implants because it sees them as cells from outside the body – 'aliens'. Since the implants are the same as the normal endometrium, the antibodies we make then also begin to attack the endometrium within the uterus. When this happens, it may well interfere with conception and the reproductive process.

This immunological attack may actually be beneficial, in that women who do not have endometriosis may be devoid of the disease because their immune system constantly cleans up the endometriotic implants that form after each menstrual period. Women with an impaired immune system may not be able to clean up their abdomen of the endometriotic implants and thus they develop endometriosis.[4] How well we clean up inside the peritoneal cavity is dependent upon the nutrients which the white blood cells need for their function as 'rubbish disposal men'. If the white cells cannot do their job, then we fall ill.

Further research emphasizes the connection between endo-metriosis and an impaired immune system: 'Women with endometriosis have impaired ability of this disposal system, which is presumably mediated by either macrophages or peritoneal lymphocytes or both. Alternately, it is possible that there are differences in the capacity of endometrial tissues to be destroyed even in immunocompetent environments.'[5, 6]

It is possible that the endometriotic implants outside the womb behave in a different way to the endometrium inside the womb. The mystery deepens … it may be painful to us and cause a great deal of misery but the behaviour of this endometriosis tissue is very intriguing. If we can find out why it behaves in this way we can be closer to finding the cure.

It is felt that endometriosis may be an auto-immune disease (this is explained later on in this chapter). There is certainly immune dysfunction from many different perspectives (too many macrophages and too few natural killer cells) and whatever is happening also has a profound effect upon the reproductive system. The body tries to dispose of 'alien' endometriotic implant cells by phagocytosis (when white blood cells, the macrophages, come along and gobble up all invaders), but some mechanism goes wrong and some of the endometriosis is left behind. Women and researchers need to find out why. Then we will have the answer, the cure.

## THE IMMUNE ARMY

The white cells behave like an army, holding the forces ready for when they are called out to do battle with an enemy. Each part of this immune army has its own unique functions, but like any successful army they all have to work as a team. All the parts help each other and support what the others are trying to do. There are two main 'battalions', the cell-mediated and humoral systems. There are different levels of immunity; some happens inside cells, some occurs outside cells on receptors nearby. Plasma proteins act as another phase of immunity and circulating hormones give rise to a fourth level. It is useful for us to understand how our immune system works in order to help it improve its task of cleaning up endometriotic implant debris.

### CELL-MEDIATED IMMUNITY

Cell-mediated immunity involves many free-floating cells, both red and white, found in the blood. Zinc is very important in this system, and antibodies require B vitamins in order to produce T lymphocytes, which destroy 'alien' bacterial and viral infections. They 'eat up' all the 'aliens' captured by the immune army cells.

*Red blood cells*

Red blood cells deliver oxygen to all the tissues in the body, and they are always on the alert, watching for 'aliens'. If they find them, they arrest them and escort them to the white blood cells for destruction. Red blood cells require folic acid, iron, vitamins B12, B6, A and C, and zinc, calcium and magnesium, manganese, good quality oils and copper.

*White blood cells*

White blood cells are the main fighting force. They include:

1  Macrophages
2  Polymorphs
3  T lymphocytes
4  B lymphocytes
5  Mast cells

These all have different ways to attack 'alien cells' which threaten

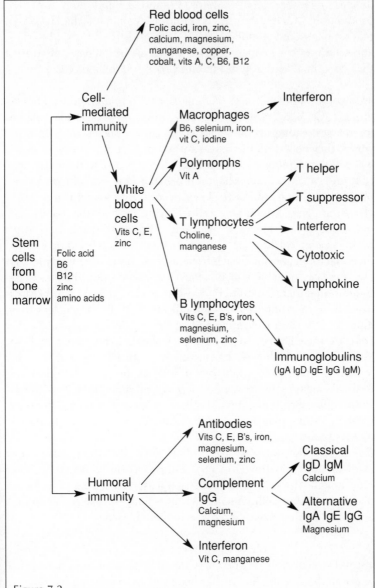

Figure 7.2
The immune system is separated into two main areas, the cell-mediated and the humoral. This diagram shows which nutrients each area relies on in order to work effectively.

danger. They require vitamins C and E and zinc for their production: 'One gram of vitamin C enhances the action of macrophages and stimulates the T cells and the B cells. (Aspirin is anti-vitamin C.) The macrophages which engulf 'aliens' only work if they contain at least 20μ of vitamin C per 100 million cells'.[7]

*Macrophages.* These are like 'Pac-men' in a computer game. They go around the body gobbling up cell debris or stay inside cells (as monocytes) eating up the garbage (phagocytic behaviour). In other words, they collect all the refuse and keep our internal organs clean. They have receptors on their surface which are able to recognize dead cells and 'aliens'. Macrophages also make enzymes which can clot blood and aid fat transport. They need ample calcium in order to absorb antigens, which are used to create lyzyme (the 'bleach' the macrophages use to digest the aliens). When we have a fever, we rapidly use up calcium supplies, so the diet needs to be complete, and then macrophages work much faster and are more effective. Selenium also increases the ability of phagocytes to clear away 'alien' cells and tumour material. Vitamin B also has a vital role: 'Vitamin B6 is needed by macrophages to work efficiently. If B6 is deficient these immune cells cannot clean up body debris inside the body cavity.'[8] By contrast, the effects of sugar have been shown to be detrimental: 'Dr Yudkin's research showed that sugar-rich foods interfere with the way in which phagocytic white blood cells clean up 'alien' invaders. Refined sugar was shown to depress immune function. Recent research has shown that this effect lasts for up to four hours after sugar is eaten.'[9] Macrophages also produce interferon and prostaglandins.

*Polymorphs.* Polymorphs are rather like *The Terminator* – they exterminate everything in sight. They work in kamikaze fashion; they engulf the 'aliens' and then release 'bleach-like bombs' at danger sites, thus killing themselves as well as the 'aliens'. Vitamin A is needed for the enzyme lysozyme in these bleaches.

*T lymphocytes.* T lymphocytes behave as homing missiles; they cruise around to survey areas and carry deadly chemicals on board ready to bomb the threat. Choline has been shown to increase lymphocyte production 3–4 times and helps the liver detoxify harmful chemicals. T lymphocytes lie in wait, watching for 'alien' invaders, and are ready to set off the alarm at any time if they are well nourished. They produce interferons.

There are four types of T lymphocytes, which watch out for viral infections:

1  *T helper cells* – look after all the other immune cells and try to safeguard the immune system from making mistakes. They have the power to stop or start the warfare, and are very powerful in switching the immune system off or on. They also protect us from both viral and fungal infections.

2  *T suppressor cells* – have the power to switch the immune system off only. They cannot switch it on. Once the threat of infection is over, they turn the attack off. There should be a ratio of 1.8 T helper cells to 1 T suppressor cell.

3  *Cytotoxic T cells* – behave like rockets and are very destructive. They seek out viruses hiding inside cells and hunt 'aliens'. They contain very powerful enzymes which are capable of breaking up and destroying infected cells.

4  *Lymphokine-producing T cells* carry 'killer missiles' to destroy aliens which travel between cells.

*B Lymphocytes.* B lymphocytes are very specific white blood cells which watch out for bacterial infections. They interrogate the 'alien' to discover its exact size and shape, and make a perfectly fitting straitjacket to hold it safe. B lymphocytes are able to form a production line making matching straitjackets to fit every 'alien' around. These are known as antibodies or immunoglobulins (Ig). Antibodies are able to arrest and hold the 'alien' until a macrophage can come along and gobble it up. B lymphocytes have memories, so if the same infection strikes again, they can go into production to make the right antibodies before the infection overtakes us. If we do get an infection twice, our immune system is functioning under par, and needs a boost. There are five antibodies in the blood all the time which are described in the section on 'humoral immunity'.

*Mast cells.* Mast cells are found all around the peritoneal cavity. They release histamines, serotonin and prostaglandins, which cause inflammation, increase blood flow, and may trigger acute food reactions. Prostaglandins can cause or dampen down inflammatory reactions and they modify one another's actions so they need to be in balance. They are constantly being made and destroyed.

## HUMORAL IMMUNITY

Humoral immunity involves immunoglobulins (Ig), produced by B lymphocytes, which form antibodies against 'alien' bacterial protein material.

### Antibodies

Antibodies are produced by B lymphocytes and they reinforce the humoral immune system response to danger. There are five types and they are labelled as IgA, IgD, IgE, IgG and IgM. Antibody production requires vitamin C, iron, magnesium, B vitamin complex, vitamin E, zinc and selenium. The different types of antibody have different roles: 'The IgE antibody, for example, is responsible for allergic reactions such as hay fever, asthma, eczema and arthritis. IgE is attracted to mast cells involved in allergic responses',[10] and 'IgG is required by cells active in destroying cancers and auto-immune diseases. It has the ability to activate the complement system of immunity.'[11] Research has shown that 'there was a trend to higher immunoglobulin IgG levels in women with endometriosis, than in controls. Women with endometriosis have significantly higher levels of antiglandular antibodies than cord blood or male controls.'[12] It has been suggested that 'IgG defends us against agents which invade tissues, which is why it is prevalent in endometriosis.'[13] IgG is involved in food intolerances.

IgA occurs in mucous membranes, and in all body orifices open to the atmosphere, e.g. the mouth, nose, ears, vagina, bladder, anus, etc. It appears to malfunction in people with food intolerances and allergies. IgD is present in only very small amounts and its function is presently unclear. It is found in semen and on the outside of lymphocytes. IgM is synthesized by immature B lymphocytes; it is the predominant type of immunoglobulin produced in blood plasma after initial contact with an 'alien' in food and bacteria. This is the largest mucus-like molecule found in the spaces between the blood vessels that line the throat, nose and vagina. It is also the first antibody produced in newborn babies.

### Interferon

Interferon affects both mind and body. Macrophages and T lymphocytes produce interferon, which is taken up by cells for their protection. Interferon shuts down the mitochondria (energy production powerhouse) in each cell to stop viruses using them for their replication. Interferon is dependent on manganese, choline and vitamin C. It has antiviral properties which prevent the virus from multiplying within the cells. As cells are damaged, they lose their ability to produce interferon. Damage can come from the external environment: 'There is a problem with the use of insecticides on crops as they inactivate choline-containing enzymes, which prevent the uptake of manganese by the plants. Overuse of insecticides can then lead to manganese deficiency in humans.'[14] Therefore our ability to produce interferon is reduced by pesticides. This implies that macrophages and T lymphocytes will not be as effective if the body has absorbed pesticides from foods.

*Complement*

Complement reinforces the humoral response and it acts in a cascade, rather like a tiered fountain. Once the cascade is set in motion, the complement cell dies. Complement production requires vitamin C. Complement works in two ways:

1 The classical pathway is activated by IgM and IgD and requires calcium.

2 The alternate pathway is activated by IgG, IgA and IgE and requires magnesium.

Complement destroys the 'aliens' by bursting cells using phagocytosis and inflammation, i.e. it 'blows up' dangerous 'alien' cells. Complement acts rather like the second unexpected, but spectacular, SAS-type assault on the battlefield. It provides specific immunity to complete the work begun by the T cells and B cells.

Antibiotics (which the body produces naturally) require vitamin C, as does the production of complement and macrophage ability to digest alien debris.

## Anon

*Although I have unfortunately never achieved a pregnancy, I feel it is very important to continue eating a healthy diet. My ME did improve but has never entirely gone away. However, the right supplements combined with a healthy diet went a long way to help improve my immune system and I have had better general health ever since.*

CASE STUDY

## AUTO-IMMUNE DISEASES

Auto-immune diseases involve a self-destructive element because 'in auto-immune disorders the immune cells make a big mistake and see their own "self tissue" cells as a danger.'[15] Auto-immunity is where the immune cells produced by the body begin to attack the body's own cells as well as 'alien' viruses, bacteria and parasites. This is, of course, bad news as healthy tissue can be harmed. Some researchers think that endometriosis is an auto-immune disease.

There is a strong connection between the immune system and nutrition, food allergies and intolerances, digestion and auto-immune diseases. Diseases such as type II adult onset diabetes, thyroiditis, systemic lupus and multiple sclerosis are thought to be auto-immune.

The three common features of auto-immune disorders can be described as follows:

1   The inside of cells becomes too acid.

2   The electron transport system malfunctions.

3   Nutrients which support the immune system are depleted.[16]

If we are subclinically nutritionally deficient because we do not eat well or because our digestive tract has been compromised in some way, then the uptake of vitamins and minerals will be low and this may have a knock-on effect on the immune system. Therefore, for a disease like endometriosis we need to eat a healthy, balanced diet full of nutrients, and ensure our digestive tracts are working at maximum capacity. Reducing our stress load, and allowing some time for ourselves (at least 20 minutes of relaxation each day) plus gentle exercise can benefit the immune system. The body heals faster when it is at rest. There are chemical dangers in the environment over which we have no control, and our bodies need to be strong in order to combat them, but other mechanisms could be at work.

## NUTRITION AND THE IMMUNE SYSTEM

If you are waiting for your ship to come in, start working days, nights and weekends building the dock.

*Paul Micall*

Trying to build up our immune system may be the best way for healing to occur. The connection between endometriosis and the immune system has been suggested by research: 'The hypothesis that the peritoneal "disposal system" may malfunction whilst trying to eliminate misplaced endometrial cells has been advanced to explain the development of endometriosis.'[17] The immune system is affected by the state of the reproductive system; they use many of the same nutrients. The rogue endometriotic implants should be removed and destroyed by the immune system's white blood cells before they take hold on the organs. But if the immune system has been compromised by poor diet, pollution or harmful drugs, it may be too weak to remove this rogue tissue.

Vitamin B6 is vital for the body macrophages so that body debris can be cleared away. If this is in short supply together with vitamin C, iron, magnesium, selenium, zinc and the antioxidants, trouble brews. Debris from old menstrual flow may accumulate but cannot be cleared away efficiently. As we have seen, 'a deficiency in vitamin B6 causes a decrease in the way the phagocytic cells hold the alien tissue captive so that we cannot clean up inside as efficiently as we should'.[18]

Vitamin B6 and folic acid together have beneficial effects on immune function. Research has shown that if there is a good supply of folic acid, zinc, methionine (an amino acid) and vitamin B6, the thymus gland in the chest is larger and able to produce more white blood cells. However, the size of the thymus changes naturally in the course of our lives: 'The thymus is a mysterious gland as it is large until puberty and then begins to shrink in adulthood, though is still recognizable.'[19] Research has shown that folic acid allows cells to divide therefore is essential for efficient immune system function, but folic acid has to be in balance with other B vitamins and zinc in order to work effectively. If women are zinc- and B vitamin-deficient, folic acid will not be effective.

## ENDOMETRIOSIS AND THE IMMUNE SYSTEM

The precise details of the relationship between endometriosis and the immune system need clarifying, as the following observations suggests: 'Endometriosis involves the implantation and survival of endometrial tissue on peritoneal surfaces in the pelvis. The process is stimulated by sex steroid hormones (oestrogen and progesterone);

other factors which determine the fate of endometrial tissue outside the uterus are unknown.'[20] Research shows that certain chemicals (cytokines, which may be produced by macrophages) are implicated in cell proliferation and inflammatory reactions: 'The volume of peritoneal fluid and its content of the inflammatory cells called macrophages have been shown to be significantly increased in patients with endometriosis, particularly in mild forms of the disease.'[21] This secretion of cytokines from macrophages may be the trigger for the cell proliferation seen in endometriosis, and may be responsible for the inflammatory response. Macrophages also produce interferons and prostaglandins, inducing inflammation and affecting the energy output of cells. Could this be why women with endometriosis feel tired all the time?

Menstrual debris is found in the peritoneal cavity of 90 per cent of women with endometriosis with open Fallopian tubes,[22] yet only 50 per cent of all women have active endometriosis. Therefore in 40 per cent of women their immune system is working effectively to clear away the menstrual debris and prevent it seeding itself onto other organs. It is suggested that the women with endometriosis do not have effective immune systems, possibly due to faulty nutrient uptake or an enzyme deficiency.

Research suggests that peritoneal fluid in patients with mild endometriosis supports cell proliferation owing to chemical signalling from the immune army as it attacks the site. Moreover, 'new research shows that endometrial tissue may be producing its own supply of oestrogen which would also trigger cell proliferation. Levels of interleukin-1 and tumour necrosis factor (types of cytokine) are increased in women with endometriosis'.[23] This points to inflammatory and hormone secretions from the endometriosis may be increasing the staying power of the rogue tissue. Normal endometrial tissue is natural to the body, so some immune signals try to maintain it within the womb. When endometriotic implants are outside the womb, other immune cells see it as growing in the wrong place and try to remove it. This is the dichotomy of endometriosis.

Johannes Evers, a prominent gynaecologist and researcher, suggests that one reason for the development of endometriosis may be that the endometrial deposits are so viable that the peritoneal macrophages do not recognize them as rubbish and do not try to remove them, allowing them to implant: 'Normal menstrual debris which enters the peritoneal cavity should be cleared away by the macrophages, but it appears that their capacity may be limited by some factor, either the quantity is too large or the disposal is inefficient and this leads to the cells staying around and implanting.'[24]

Is endometriosis growing where it should not owing to faulty macrophages? Are they deficient in vitamin B6, iron, calcium or selenium, so they can't work effectively? We need research to look at this question. It could be that more macrophages are in the peritoneal cavity as they are too ineffective in smaller numbers if these nutrients are poorly supplied. Both cell-mediated (T lymphocytes) and humoral (B lymphocytes) immunological defence mechanisms are involved in cleaning away debris from the peritoneal cavity. Antibodies to the endometrium, cell membranes and to the heart cells have been demonstrated in patients with endometriosis, indicating that the immune system is activated as a result of endometriosis.[25]

If there is some mechanism which prevents the white immune cell army from working at its optimum level, this may be due to a lack of nutrients, or it may be due to the effect of pesticides, such as dioxins, which are known immunotoxicants (poison to the immune system). This immune army needs feeding just like any other army. Without the necessary nutrients in plentiful supply, the cells will fail to complete their tasks efficiently. And if they are fed junk and pesticides, they will fail to protect you.

## ALTERNATIVE HYPOTHESIS

There are other immune interactions which could be going wrong. These problems may be similar to the auto-immune effects which cause endometriosis.

### MICRO-ORGANISMS AND VIRUSES

Let us look at the micro-organism that causes syphilis. An antigen (a substance that the body sees as 'alien' and therefore a potential danger) called cardiolipin on the surface of that micro-organism identifies it as the same as some of the heart muscle cells. When the immune system sees the syphilis micro-organism is causing damage it attacks it, but in doing so it also attacks the heart muscle (which has the same cardiolipin identity). Could a similar process be happening in endometriosis? Is some external micro-organism causing a problem? Some researchers wonder if endometriosis is caused by a type of virus, which triggers a cascade within the body cells.

Auto-immune ovarian disease is found in various endocrine syndromes. Several possible causes of immune activation are thought to occur as a result of tissue damage. 'Assessment of antibodies present in 40 patients with premature ovarian failure showed that, relative to controls, there was a significant increase in antibodies against thyroglobulin, nuclear antigens, heart disease and gluten, and increased levels of IgM. Decreased levels of complement were also described.'[26]

Gluten, the elastic protein in wheat, is also implicated in thyroid failure. Research at the ImmunoLaboratories in Florida is looking at the links between gluten and thyroid problems and it is thought that the gliadin portion of the gluten is the same as a protein in the thyroid: 'If the body builds up an intolerance to gluten then the immune cells will automatically begin to attack other similar tissue types, even though they are our own cells.'[27] It may be that both thyroid and ovarian cells come under fire. Much more research is needed in this area to show if it is of significance with endometriosis and infertility, but it is a very interesting hypothesis.

Research has shown that subclinical auto-immune disease may be involved with reproductive failure: 'Forty-four per cent of women who miscarried were seen to have antibodies implicated with anti-cardiolipin. It has also been speculated that two thyroid auto-antibodies are involved with reproductive failure. Thyroid auto-antibodies have been used as guides to point to women at risk from miscarriage.'[28] Research suggesting a link between coeliac disease (gluten intolerance) and auto-antibodies to the thyroid warrants further investigation, as 'adults tend to present with these problems in their 30s and 40s, tiredness, mouth ulcers, malaise, fertility problems and malabsorption being the main problems'.[29] All women with unexplained infertility should request very basic tests for auto-antibodies to the thyroid, coeliac disease (gluten sensitivity) and genito-urinary infections.

## EFFECTS OF STRESS ON THE IMMUNE SYSTEM

Prolonged or extreme stress can be very harmful to the immune army, sapping its strength when it most needs help.

The hormone cortisol (from the adrenal glands) is an

immunosuppressant which reduces the levels of T helper cells; increases the levels of T suppressor cells; inhibits production of natural killer cells and interferon; decreases secretion of interleukin 1 and interleukin 2; blocks the production of lymphocytes; shrinks the thymus gland; and reduces progesterone levels.

Studies show that 'cortisol secretion occurs usually for 6 hours around waking time, it prepares the body for action and in doing so suppresses sleep, growth, reproduction and libido. It also reduces production of GnRH, LH from the pituitary gland, oestradiol and testosterone from the gonads'.[30] Corticosteroids are stress hormones which are released from the adrenal gland when toxins, infections, emotions, pain and disease strike. Stress raises cortisol levels in the adrenals, and this hormone competes with progesterone production and lowers it, which in turn alters oestrogen levels. Ongoing stress is very damaging in any illness, but particularly in endometriosis as oestrogen levels must be balanced with progesterone. If the stress 'fight or flight' reaction is continuous, the adrenal glands would always be on red alert, constantly producing high levels of adrenaline and cortisol. This would have a knock-on effect on all the other endocrine glands, e.g. the pituitary, ovaries and testes. The pituitary gland in the brain co-ordinates immune activity in the head and neck areas, so stress also depletes the immune system, and it also causes blood to thicken in case of injury so that it will clot easily. Adrenal stress triggers an aching neck and shoulders.

Stress affects the reproductive system in many ways. Insulin, progesterone, testosterone and oestrogens decrease at times of stress, whereas corticosteroids, catecholamines, thyroxine and growth hormone output is increased when the body is under stress. Because the corticosteroids inhibit release of GnRH from the hypothalamus and LH from the pituitary, this has an effect on the reproductive, digestive and immune systems. Corticosteroids increase sympathetic nervous system activity which is implicated in a decrease in natural killer cell function. They also decrease the secretion of gastric juices and halt gastrointestinal mobility, i.e. peristalsis shuts down and the bowel begins to malfunction.

Try to understand how these three systems (reproduction, digestion and immunity) are interlinked and entwined. Nutrients and stress reduction are parts of our jigsaw, parts of the key to keep systems strong. Even the nervous system will be affected because neurons have receptors for luteinizing hormone. So stress damages the reproductive, nervous, immune and the digestive systems in one fell swoop. Stress reduction techniques described in chapter 6 can help to minimize the damage.

## OTHER DANGERS FOR THE IMMUNE SYSTEM

*Fluoride*

Fluoride breaks off a portion of the 'Y'-shaped antibody, breaking the antibody into two and making it ineffective; 'fluoride causes immune system weakness and reproductive problems'.[31] Perhaps women with endometriosis should avoid products containing fluorides in order to help strengthen their immune systems. This includes certain toothpastes, mouth rinses, medications, aerosols, pesticides, herbicides, foods processed with fluoridated water, shampoo, deodorants, etc. Look for those which are fluoride-free.

## IMMUNE SYSTEM SUPPLEMENTS

The immune system is our battleground against disease. We usually expect it to protect us against outside agents which try to do us harm, such as viruses, bacteria and gut parasites. When it starts attacking 'self-tissue', something drastic is going wrong. As many of the white blood cells rely on nutrients to supply their needs, what we eat is important in helping us to maintain the immune system's function. We should take in adequate amounts of:

- Selenium (yeast-free)
- Vitamins A, C, E
- Echinaecia (take in 3-week blocks only)
- Coenzyme Q 10
- Zinc
- Magnesium
- B complex vitamins
- Vitamin C

## STRESS

Once stress takes hold and the adrenal glands begin to work overtime producing adrenaline, we use up supplies of magnesium, zinc and B vitamins at an alarming rate. The adrenal glands require a constant supply of vitamin C, vitamin B5 and essential cis oils. The nervous system becomes involved and calcium, magnesium and B vitamins are required. We are thrown into the 'fight or flight' syndrome. Our bodies are preparing us for action. The blood thickens so that it will clot quickly if we are attacked; the digestive system shuts off to allow us to use the energy elsewhere and run faster. The liver throws more sugar into the blood to ensure we have enough fuel to get us away from the danger fast. The body is only meant to be in this state for a short period of time, so when the stress is prolonged, everything begins to go wrong. Being nutritionally sound helps to bolster us against this effect.

- Vitamin C
- Magnesium malate
- Zinc citrate
- B complex vitamins
- Lime blossom tea
- Probiotics (acidophilus)
- Manganese

- Pantothenic acid (vitamin B5)
- Calcium gluconate
- Chromium polynicotinate
- Bach Flower Rescue Remedy
- Multivitamin/mineral
- Digestive enzymes
- Choline and inositol

## SUMMARY

The immune system controls the ways in which the body copes with attacks from bacteria, viruses, cell debris and infiltrating tissue such as endometriosis. You can help to support your immune system to function by eating foods which are nutrient-rich. This gives the immune cells a fighting chance at eradicating misplaced tissue such as endometriotic implants.

1  Endometriosis may be due to immune dysfunction. Women who have endometriosis may have impaired immune systems which may not be able to clean up debris in the abdominal cavity.

2  A strong immune system is dependent upon a varied nutrient and phytochemical intake.

3  Make sure that your foods are rich in the antioxidant nutrients as they are protective – the mineral selenium and vitamins A, C and E.

4  Sugar-rich foods interfere with the way in which white blood cells clean up cell debris.

5  If you have unexplained infertility or if your endometriosis seems to be blocking your fertility, request tests for auto-antibodies to the thyroid, coeliac disease (gluten sensitivity) and genito-urinary infections, as well as for steroid hormone levels.

6  Reduce your stress levels wherever possible. Make a list of all the things which stress you and think hard about ways in which some of them could be eliminated.

7  Avoid products containing fluoride, such as toothpastes, shampoos and deodorants, as they can inhibit antibody function.

# 8 How digestion affects the reproductive system

> Throughout prehistoric times and historic times, supplies of food and resultant eating patterns have been powerful factors influencing human development and the human condition.
>
> *Stamler, 1994*

> Such is the idea that poor nutritional standards may be blocking humankind's path to future health.
>
> *Dian Mills, 1996*

You are what you eat. Rather – you are what your body can digest. That is far more important. You could be eating an amazing diet and yet not digest and absorb the nutrients effectively.

Does the food you eat really make that much difference to your health? Does your digestive system obtain the maximum amount of nutrients from the foods you eat every day? Are the foods you eat rich in nutrients? Many processed foods are high in calories but lack essential nutrients, therefore it is vital that you eat fresh foods daily. It is very important to have an efficient digestive tract, removing nutrients from foods, processing them and sending them into the bloodstream. These nutrients affect the way each cell functions, trigger production of hormones and enzymes and keep the body healthy.

A key to the whole reproductive system working normally is the regular supply of nutrients, and that is dependent upon the health of your intestines. Without absorption of nutrients, fertility begins to fail. Hormone production becomes erratic, affecting the function of the hypothalamus, pituitary gland, ovary and womb lining. Ensuring that your digestion is working at its best should be your number one concern.

Table 8.1
A comparison of foods 1939 and 1991[1]

| Food | Potassium 1939 | Potassium 1991 | % change | Calcium 1939 | Calcium 1991 | % char |
|---|---|---|---|---|---|---|
| Old raw carrots | 225 | 170 | -24% | 48 | 25 | -48 |
| Boiled cauliflower | 152 | 120 | -21% | 22 | 17 | -23 |
| Celery | 279 | 320 | 15% | 52 | 41 | -21 |
| Old potatoes | 568 | 360 | -37% | 8 | 5 | -38 |
| Swede | 138 | 170 | 23% | 56 | 53 | -5 |
| Lettuce | 208 | 220 | 6% | 26 | 28 | 8 |
| Onions | 137 | 160 | 17% | 31 | 25 | -19 |
| Tomatoes | 288 | 250 | -13% | 13 | 6 | -54 |
| Mushrooms | 467 | 320 | -31% | 3 | 6 | 100 |
| Cucumber | 141 | 140 | -1% | 23 | 18 | -22 |
| Chicory | 182 | 170 | -7% | 18 | 21 | 17 |
| Kellogg's All Bran | 955 | 1000 | 5% | 82 | 69 | -16 |
| Hovis | 243 | 200 | -18% | 28 | 120 | 329 |
| Kellogg's Cornflakes | 114 | 100 | -12% | 7 | 15 | 114 |
| Cheddar | 116 | 77 | -34% | 810 | 720 | -1 |
| Whole milk | 160 | 140 | -12% | 120 | 115 | -4 |
| Butter | 15 | - | - | 15 | - | |
| Eggs (chicken) | 138 | 130 | -6% | 56 | 57 | |
| Boiled chicken | 381 | 300 | -21% | 11 | 11 | |
| Beef roast/lean | 337 | 350 | 4% | 6 | 6 | |

In this chapter we are going to look at factors that help and factors that hinder the digestive system's ability to absorb nutrients from even the most superb of diets. Your digestive tract health is vital to the state of your hormone profile; it really is the body's first line of defence against disease.

**Nutrition is not an alternative approach like herbal medicine and homeopathy, it is essential to life. Eating is something we all do every day, it sustains us, it can keep us healthy – or it can make us unhealthy.**

We all try our best to eat the mythical 'well-balanced diet'. A new

| nesium 939 | Magnesium 1991 | % change | Iron 1939 | Iron 1991 | % change | Phosphorus 1939 | Phosphorus 1991 | % change |
|---|---|---|---|---|---|---|---|---|
| 2 | 3 | -75% | 0.6 | 0.3 | -50% | 21 | 15 | -29% |
| 7 | 12 | 71% | 0.5 | 0.4 | -20% | 33 | 52 | 58% |
| 0 | 5 | -50% | 0.6 | 0.4 | -33% | 31 | 21 | -32% |
| 5 | 17 | -32% | 0.7 | 0.4 | -43% | 40 | 37 | -8% |
| 1 | 9 | -18% | 0.4 | 0.1 | -75% | 19 | 40 | 111% |
| 0 | 6 | -40% | 0.7 | 0.7 | 0% | 30 | 28 | -7% |
| 3 | 4 | -50% | 0.3 | 0.3 | 0% | 30 | 30 | 0% |
| 4 | 7 | -36% | 0.4 | 0.5 | 25% | 21 | 24 | 14% |
| 3 | 9 | -31% | 1 | 0.6 | -40% | 136 | 80 | -41% |
| 9 | 8 | -11% | 0.3 | 0.3 | 0% | 24 | 49 | 104% |
| 3 | 6 | -54% | 0.7 | 0.4 | -43% | 21 | 27 | 29% |
| 0 | 210 | -50% | 10 | 12 | 20% |  |  |  |
| 0 | 56 | -30% | 3 | 3.7 | 23% | 257 | 190 | -26% |
| 0 | 14 | -18% | 2.8 | 6.7 | 139% | 58 | 50 | -14% |
| 0 | 25 | -47% | 0.6 | 0.3 | -50% | 545 | 490 | -10% |
| 0 | 11 | -21% | 0.08 | 0.06 | -25% | 95 | 92 | -3% |
| ' | - | - | 0.16 | - | - | 24 | - | - |
|  | 12 | 0% | 2.5 | 1.9 | -24% | 218 | 200 | -8% |
|  | 25 | -4% | 2.1 | 1.2 | -43% | 270 | 190 | -30% |
|  | 23 | -8% | 4.4 | 2.6 | -41% | 264 | 200 | -24% |

assessment of the mineral content of fruits and vegetables shows that vital minerals can be 30–40 per cent lower in 1991, compared with 1931. So even if we eat as well as people did in 1931, we still cannot take in the same amounts of mineral without eating more, and unfortunately most people eat far less fruit and vegetables today than was consumed in the early twentieth century.

Thomas McKeown has argued that 'the major changes in health status in the twentieth century have been due to improved personal hygiene, better housing and healthier diets rather than to curative medicine'.[2] This is real preventive medicine.

## LIFESTYLE AND THE PSYCHOLOGY OF EATING

We all want to enjoy the food we eat. That is a part of the pleasure of eating. The whole world over, people invite others into their homes and offer them a meal. Friendships are made, deals are struck, and families come together over the meal table. Mediterranean cultures are especially skilled at creating relaxing and enjoyable mealtimes. Preparing and sharing of food is a statement of caring for our fellow friends. Cooking is creative and people gain great pleasure in the giving of good food. We should all learn to take time out to enjoy the food we eat and share it with friends.

The following guidelines may help to improve your digestion.

1  Relax for ten minutes before you eat in order for the digestive enzymes to begin working.

2  Sit down while you eat; never stand or rush around with a sandwich in your hand.

3  Chew slowly in order to mix salivary amylase, the carbohydrate-digesting enzyme in the mouth, into the food.

4  Avoid too many distractions during mealtimes. Talking with friends is one thing, but if you are watching TV and trying to read the newspaper as well, you will not get the best enjoyment from your meals.

5  Take time to enjoy what you are eating, savour the flavours, and try to avoid 'snatch and grab'-type meals.

6  Prepare food just before you are going to eat it, and cook it as quickly as possible in order to preserve the maximum vitamin content. Steaming, grilling or stir-frying are the best ways to preserve nutrients.

To understand the quantities of foods required for mealtimes, the following old adage is still useful: eat like a king for breakfast, a prince for lunch and a pauper for dinner. This will allow the body to absorb the maximum nutrients needed at the beginning of the day to sustain energy in the hours to come.

## PATTERNS OF HEALTHY EATING

Man has drastically altered his diet over the past 50 years, and our digestive systems have not yet fully adapted to these changes. At first man was a scavenger, eating whatever came his way each day, and because he was nomadic; no stores of food were kept save those he could carry. Food (nuts, seeds, berries, fruits, wild vegetables, wild grass seeds, meat and fish, and occasionally honey) was eaten fresh when it was available, and in times of famine only the strong survived. Then around 6000 BC man learned to cultivate crops and herd animals, so the diet changed. More cereal grains were eaten and as hamlets were established, food was stored. Nowadays few of us grow our own food. Instead we rely on farmers and multinational organizations to produce the food for our meals. Apparently, '44 per cent of people rarely cook; they merely rely on processed foods, developed to have a long shelf-life'.[3] Studies show that '35 per cent of household food bills are spent on ready-cooked meals'.[4] The idea of eating really fresh, 'just picked', vibrant food has diminished.

We are thought to have been omnivores, implying that we ate a wide variety of foods in our recent past, and this is what our digestive systems still expect. Nowadays, however, we tend to have a very restricted diet and most people do not eat a wide variety of foods. The gut and liver have to deal with many new chemicals that are added to our foods in order to 'enhance' their taste and to give them a longer 'shelf-life': 'the average person eats an alarming 3–12 pounds of additives each year'.[5] If the liver is overtaxed with chemicals, it will need detoxifying before you can heal. Many cultures follow detox measures – Swedes have their saunas; American Indians have their sweat lodges; Arabs have Turkish baths; Eastern Europeans have mud baths, and Muslims their cleansing Ramadan fasts. All these activities draw toxins from the body to help it to remain healthy.

We need to look at the foods we eat and make sure that we choose well, as that will help our ailing digestion. The shops are full of foods which look tempting, but do they contain the nutrients our bodies require in order to keep us healthy? Wholemeal flour contains 22 nutrients. White flour has had 98 per cent of its vitamin B6, 91 per cent of the manganese, 84 per cent of magnesium and 87 per cent of its fibre, and most of its chromium removed by processing. Refined foods have a lot of nutrients removed by processing, and unfortunately many foods have additives, pesticides, antibiotics and hormones within them. Our digestive enzymes and body cells are not designed to deal with such a cocktail of these compounds, and some sensitive people can have extreme reactions over time as their livers, digestive and immune systems weaken in the face of chemical onslaught.

## THE DIGESTIVE TRACT BARRIER

Remember that your digestive tract is a 26-foot-long (780cm) tube, open at each end, so its contents are not really internal but are external to the rest of the body. It consists of the mouth, oesophagus, stomach, liver, pancreas, gall bladder and small intestine and large intestine (see figures 8.1 and 8.2). All these organs have a strong mucous membrane which acts as a barrier between the outside world and the bloodstream. This membrane protects us from harmful substances in the outside world. Only the nutrients, amino acids, glucose, fatty acids, glycerol, and phytochemicals should cross this mucosal barrier into the bloodstream. Larger molecules pass through, from the mouth to the anus, and are expelled as waste without causing harm; therefore 'this mucosal barrier has to be extremely resilient. Its surface is 300m$^2$ (almost the size of a tennis court), which makes it the largest surface area in the body which is in contact with external substances'.[6]

## THE DIGESTION AND IMMUNE SYSTEM LINK

Tissue called 'Peyer's patches' on our gut wall, sample and test all the substances we pour into our body. If they sense a dangerous 'alien' they call up the immune army by secreting IgA antibodies. IgA antibodies are part of the lymphatic system, the immune system. They are on watch all the time (like sheepdogs) for any dangers: 'The IgA binds to the antigen (alien bug) and makes it much bigger so it is more difficult for it to pass through the gut wall.'[7] The dimensions of the gastrointestinal tract reflect the importance of its role: 'Gut association lymphoid tissue (GALT) is distributed throughout the GI tract. GALT consists mainly of Peyer's patches and the total mucosal surface area of the adult human GI tract is up to 300m$^2$, making it the largest body area to interact with the environment, i.e. tennis-court size! This huge surface area has to be very effective at absorption and yet exclude all infectious agents, allergenic material and toxic substances from entering the bloodstream via the villi. The GALT makes the gastrointestinal tract the largest lymphoid or immune organ in the human body. It has been estimated that there are approximately $10^{10}$ immunoglobulin-producing cells per metre of small bowel – accounting for approximately 80 per cent of all immunoglobulin-producing cells in the body'.[8] This vitally important membrane is our first line of immune defence and needs looking after, and 'adhesion of the good bifido bacteria, the lactobacilli, to this mucosal lining may be a critical factor in stimulating the immune system'.[9]

We all have four pounds of gut flora living in the intestines of each one of us and by keeping this healthy and balanced we may improve our general health. The health of the digestive system can profoundly affect your immune and reproductive system, your fertility and perception of pain. It is in your interest to keep both systems in tiptop health.


FOOD INTOLERANCES

Some normal foods, such as wheat and milk, may suddenly begin to be a problem if they have not been digested correctly. The body becomes intolerant if large molecules pass through the mucosal barrier. Some of our white blood cells are thought to have a memory of three months, so avoiding a problem food for three months may solve the problem. You can then start to re-introduce the food gradually.

Why do food intolerance problems arise?

1  If the gut membrane becomes compromised in susceptible people by such irritants as excess gluten from wheat, food additives, pesticides, drugs or filaments from yeast overgrowth, etc., the protective mucous membrane can be breached.

2  If the gut flora become imbalanced by an onslaught of antibiotics or hormonal preparations (such as the contraceptive pill and HRT). Even severe prolonged stress can upset the balance of gut flora.

3  If the liver and pancreas enzymes are not fully functional.

4  If the stomach's hydrochloric acid supply is too low.

5  If gut parasites or food-poisoning bacteria or yeasts invade this space.
6  If the small villi (projections in the gut wall) are damaged by wheat bran or gluten, absorption of nutrients may fail.

Once large molecules get through damaged gut membranes into the blood, the body's immune army will react, as it perceives danger. You may begin to feel 'sick all over' from the toxins released into the body via the blood; this is known as auto-intoxication. It can also happen if the ileocaecal valve between the small and large intestine becomes faulty and allows backward flow of bacteria into the small intestine. Systemic kinesiology treatment (*see* p. 131) may help to correct this.

## *Ailish P of London*

*I have suffered from the debilitating condition of endometriosis since the age of 14. Over the years the pains and symptoms became worse until eventually the condition was diagnosed when I was 24. By the age of 31, now 31 years old and several hormone treatments and operations later, the disease was still affecting my life.*

*I suffered from lack of energy, poor concentration, bloating, bad skin and gums, and, of course, several days of every month severe abdominal and back pain. Throughout the month I had severe pain on defecation and alternated between having diarrhoea and constipation.*

*I realised that medical treatment was not really working and decided to try an alternative approach. Nutritional supplements and a healthy diet which excluded wheat seems to be the answer to my problems. I am now pain-free, have normal bowel habits, have much more energy and feel so much better – less anxious and depressed about the whole condition. It is hard to exclude wheat from one's diet as it is contained in so many foods. However, the benefits I have gained from this diet far outweigh the fact that I cannot have a hot buttery slice of toast in the mornings! It is far better to feel so well and switch to alternative foods – now toast does not seem very attractive any more.*

# FACTORS WHICH INFLUENCE NUTRIENT INTAKE

## DIGESTION AND ABSORPTION

Eating fresh and healthy food is not much help if the digestive tract is not working efficiently. Even if we eat organic food all the time, a damaged digestive system does not effectively break down the foods into nutrients, and, if there is any damage to the mucous membranes or liver, or if the pancreatic enzymes are poorly secreted, our absorption of nutrients will be impaired. According to one study, 69 per cent of the population studied showed signs of at least one gastrointestinal disorder over the previous three months. In the USA alone it is a common reason for people to seek medical advice and annual costs are $41 million (£25.6 million). Surveys show that 'constipation affects four million Americans each year. Physicians write more than a million prescriptions for constipation annually, and we [Americans] spend $725 million a year on laxatives.'[10]

Any disorder of the gut and its membrane (stomach upsets, indigestion, bad breath, abdominal pain, irritable bowel syndrome, diarrhoea, constipation, piles, anal irritation) implies that some degree of malabsorption may be present. This leads to poor uptake of nutrients no matter how healthy a diet is eaten.

> Every tissue in the body is fed by the bloodstream which is supplied by the bowel. When the bowel is dirty, the blood is dirty and so are the organs and tissues. It is the bowel that must be cared for first.
>
> *Lindsey Duncan, CN*

Illness is not always recognized as a subclinical nutrient deficiency; often treatment entails suppressing symptoms by drug treatments instead of addressing shortfalls in the diet. Doctors who take an interest in nutrients and foods which promote health are a rare breed. However, good nutrition is central to our well-being. The Office of Population and Census Statistics (OPCS) in 1991 reported that 'there were 28 deaths in 1989 and 32 deaths in 1990 due to avitaminosis (vitamin deficiency)'.[11] But many more people fall ill due to long-term subclinical deficiencies which deplete the

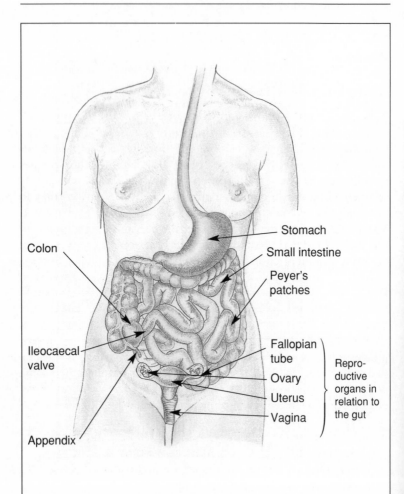

Figure 8.1 The digestive system is open to the outside at either end and therefore has to form a strong barrier internally to protect us from harmful bacteria etc. It does this through the good gut flora and the integrity of its mucous membrane. The GI tract consists of the mouth, oesophagus, stomach, liver, pancreas, gall bladder, small intestine and large intestine. The gut mucosal barrier requires zinc, beta carotene, biotin, butyric acid, pantothenic acid, vitamins A, C and E, and essential fatty acids and L glutamine for its health. Herbs like slippery elm can help protect it when it becomes inflamed.

effective way the body should be working. Low nutrient intake or poor absorption can reduce our ability to fight diseases, virus and bacteria. The link between many of the diseases of Western civilization and poor digestion is not yet fully recognized in orthodox medicine. The health of the digestive tract and the integrity of the mucous membranes which line the tract are vital to your health. This has to be the first line of your defence against endometriosis.

## FACTORS IMPORTANT FOR A HEALTHY DIGESTION

For the digestive tract to work efficiently and support the immune and reproductive systems, four factors have to come together:

1  Transit time is the time it takes for food to be processed in the digestive tract and to pass through the body.

2  Liver function tests; can look at how efficient the liver is at producing the enzymes required for good digestion and for degrading oestrogens so that they can be passed harmlessly from the body.

3  Healthy gut flora are vital to our general health as the intestinal flora  provide us with B vitamins and vitamin K and provide immune protection.

4  Fibre if regularly eaten, is vital for excretion of toxins and waste products from normal metabolism (*see* pp.171, 188, 218).

### TRANSIT TIME

Transit time is the time in which the food you eat is digested, absorbed and then excreted from the body. This is very important to your state of health. You can easily check your transit time by eating some sweetcorn kernels and watching how long it takes for them to reappear in your stools. Transit time for a healthy gut is 12–24 hours. Faster than that and the body will not have time to obtain sufficient nutrients from your food. Much slower than that and the waste fermenting inside your body can begin to putrefy the food and cause build-up of chemical compounds (some of which are carcinogenic).

If you have ever been constipated you may remember feeling

toxic and bloated, until the laxatives did their job. Fibre holds water and this keeps the stools soft. If the waste is kept for too long inside the bowel, the water is reabsorbed and constipation results. Both vitamin C and magnesium can soften stools and they can be used to help alleviate constipation. But if constipation is due to a food intolerance, the culprit food needs to be found and eliminated. Constipation is triggered in some people by wheat, eggs, bananas or dairy foods. Drink at least three glasses of water each day and take three brisk 20-minute walks each week to help stimulate peristalsis waves along the intestinal walls. This helps you expel waste and prevents the build-up of harmful toxins. Exercise in general helps to stimulate peristalsis in the gut and also endorphin production in the brain (which helps reduce pain levels). Diarrhoea, on the other hand, is saying 'get this stuff out of here fast'. Something is irritating the gut membranes and it needs to be expelled as it is bad for the body. Listen to what your body is trying to tell you.

## LIVER FUNCTION

The liver is a vast chemical factory which deals with everything the body takes in, and renders it safe. Liver enzymes have the ability to biotransform dangerous substances and make them harmless. The liver enzymes need a constant supply of B vitamins (found in green leafy vegetables), as well as vitamin A; L taurine, L methionine, L carnitine and L glycine (amino acids); vitamin E; vitamin B6; and lecithin (choline and inositol).

The foods which contain nutrients and phytochemicals beneficial to the liver are lemons, carrots, beetroot, cucumber, tomatoes, artichokes, chicory, celery, radishes, leeks, onions, cabbage, spring dandelion leaves, parsley, cold-pressed olive oil, apricots and grapefruit. For one day every three months you could eat a liver-cleansing diet of these foods in a salad. A glass of weak tea with lemon, hot water with lemon or organic carrot juice helps the liver work efficiently at detoxifying chemicals. You can also use lemon juice and olive oil as a salad dressing. Herb teas, such as thyme, rosemary, chamomile and meadowsweet, also aid liver function.

Foods which congest the liver are dairy foods, eggs, alcohol, meat, manufactured hydrogenated vegetable trans oils, sugar and tobacco. Obviously chemical food additives should be avoided wherever possible. Coffee and tea are best avoided in a liver-cleansing diet. Detoxifying the liver must be done gradually. As we detoxify, the toxic substances enter the bloodstream and they may make you feel unwell for a few days as 'die-off' symptoms (flu-like symptoms or headaches) may occur as the body begins to cleanse itself, but that means that you are getting on top of the problem. Drinking a lot of fresh water helps to flush out the system.

The road to wellness can sometimes seem like two steps back for every one step forward, but if you understand what is happening and why, it is easier to cope. As these are only the symptoms of a passing phase, they should be an encouraging sign that the right track is being followed. So whenever you undertake a detox diet, always take your time. The body does not need any more shocks to its system, endometriosis has been enough. If we have been ill for a long time it would be nice to take a 'magic bullet' tablet and get well overnight. Nutrition is not like that; it requires some perseverance to allow the body to heal in its own time. If it has taken several years for the body to become ill, be patient as healing may take 3–6 months. Reading the many comments from women who have followed this path of liver cleansing, you can see that it can be a fast or more gradual process, due to our inherent uniqueness and our biochemical individuality. We all react differently to different treatments.


## GOOD GUT FLORA

> Surely no man can live without friends
>
> *Aristotle*

About 2kg/4lb of friendly bacteria live in our intestines. We provide them with food and warmth and, in return, they help us digest foods, and they support immunoglobulin production. The good bifido bacteria make vitamins B and K. This is symbiosis – you scratch my back and I'll scratch yours. Drawing upon research findings, it is estimated that there are '100 trillion organisms in our intestinal tract – 400–500 different species with an active metabolic action equivalent to the liver'.[12] There is so much vibrant life inside us, which acts to protect us from harm if you look after it carefully.

The gastrointestinal tract acts as a strong barrier between us and the outside world. Think of the good gut flora as our protective atmosphere. Just as the atmosphere around planet Earth helps to protect it from radiation and meteorites, all these good bacteria are shielding and screening us from the dangers of parasites, viruses and bacteria lurking in food and water.

Three pounds of bifido bacteria and one pound of bacteriodes bacteria live inside us. The bifido bacteria are the 'good' guys who produce B complex vitamins and vitamin K. The bacteriodes bacteria are required to break down protein foods; in doing so they produce gases. Drugs such as antibiotics upset this balance. Antibiotics are 'anti-life' and kill off all bacteria whether good or bad, whereas probiotics, such as acidophilus, are 'for-life' and help to restore the levels of bifido bacteria to normal. It is very important to keep the ratio of three bifido bacteria to one bacteriodes bacterium in balance, by eating live yogurt or acidophilus after antibiotic or hormonal drug treatments, or if you are suffering from severe stress. If there is an excess of bacteriodes, too much gas will be produced; if there is too little bifido bacteria, insufficient levels of vitamin B complex will be produced to keep the gut membranes healthy.

We have often been taught that bacteria are all bad, but here within us we have some of the best bacteria one could ever wish for; they keep us in the peak of health if we look after them. The use of drugs (e.g. overuse of antibiotics, the oral contraceptive pill, hormone replacement therapy or hormone drugs, indigestion tablets, non-steroidal anti-inflammatories), sensitivity to gluten in wheat, even severe ongoing stress, take their toll. If you bloat a lot and experience abdominal pain, you probably need to take some digestive enzymes and acidophilus to replace the flora which are out of balance and to improve your digestion and speed up your healing process. This bloated condition is known as dysbiosis and it may also arise when the diet is high in animal fat and low in fibre.

The digestive enzymes help to rest the liver for a short time and they aid the breakdown of foods into nutrients. A nutritionist can guide you as to which supplements may speed up the healing of the gut membranes, for example, slippery elm, N acetyl glucosamine, L glutamine, essential fatty acids, butyric acid, vitamin A or zinc.

*Digestive enzymes*

A healthy liver and pancreas produce enzymes which help break down foods into nutrients ready for digestion. In fact, we begin producing enzymes even before we start eating. The thought of a tasty meal starts enzyme production, so that our digestive system is ready to receive food by the time we begin to eat, although American-style grazing and fast food has altered this pattern, and snacks often arrive in the stomach before it is ready to begin digestion. Stress also upsets enzyme secretion so that we cannot digest food when we are upset. Poorly digested food can cause a build-up of gas in the intestines. Flatulence is a sign that you are either not producing sufficient digestive enzymes or that the gut flora is unbalanced, leading to malabsorption. The worst foods for producing gas are beans, onions, eggs, meat, cabbage and sprouts. Drinking one small glass of fluid with a meal may help. Vitamins C and B6 can improve absorption of nutrients from the gut into the bloodstream, as they act as carrier molecules to take nutrients from the gut and into the bloodstream.

Digestive enzyme tablets (available from health food stores or by mail order) are made from animal and/or vegetable sources and can be taken with meals to aid digestion and absorption if you have liver or pancreas problems. They consist of:

1  Amylase to digest carbohydrates.
2  Lipase to digest fats.
3  Protease to digest proteins.

| Organ | Enzyme | Food | Digested particle |
|---|---|---|---|
| Mouth | Salivary amylase | Carbohydrate | Simple sugars Glucose, fructose, galactose |
| Small intestine | Pancreatic amylase | Carbohydrate | Glucose, fructose, galactose |
| Stomach | Pepsinogen | Proteins | Amino acids |
| Small intestine Pancreas | Trypsin | Proteins | Amino acids |
| Pancreas | Chymotrypsin | Proteins | Amino acids |
| Pancreas | Carboxypeptidase | Proteins | Amino acids |
| Intestinal membranes | Aminopetidase | Proteins | Amino acids |
| Pancreas | Lipase | Fats and oils | 40+ fatty acids Glycerol |

Table 8.2 Taking digestive enzymes for a short time if the digestive system is malfunctioning may enhance the body's digestion of these vital nutrients while the body is trying to heal.

If you are unable to digest fats, this upsets their potential to manufacture steroid hormones, the good anti-inflammatory prostaglandins which aid the body to heal wounds, reduce pain, increase immune potential and enhance fertility. Blurred vision and left-hand-side rib pain are signs of pancreatic insufficiency. A sluggish liver can produce various symptoms such as fibrocystic breasts, food intolerance, acne, fatigue, nausea, greasy fatty stools, intolerance of fatty foods, itchy skin, rashes, a bitter taste in the mouth and PMS. Choose reputable digestive enzyme tablets containing lipase, amylase, protease, bromalin (a digestive enzyme found in pineapples) and papain (found in papaya), and avoid those enzymes derived from animal glands and especially from a bovine source.

## Probiotics

Probiotics may be required if the body's natural bacteria have been compromised in some way. Probiotics are live microbial supplements, taken in either capsule or food form (e.g. live yogurt, kefir etc.), which help to replenish the bifido bacteria and increase the number of naturally resident bacteria in order to benefit the host's health. Research shows that 'the main positive effects associated with probiotics include cholesterol and/or triglyceride reduction, anti-tumour properties, increased vitamin production and stimulation of the immune system'.[13]

Research also suggests that improving the gut flora is critical to improving health. It is suggested 'that the adhesion of lactobacilli to mucosal epithelial cells may be a critical factor in immune stimulation'.[14] Choice of a good probiotic is very important, as some of the cheaper ones are less effective. Look for dairy-free formulations which contain lactobacillus acidophilus and bifidobacterium bifidum, where each capsule delivers 4 million live bacteria. These products must be pure and must persist when in the GI tract. A nutritionist will guide you as to the best products available.

## Fructo-oligosaccharides (FOS) or Prebiotics

Fructo-oligosaccharides (FOS) are comprised of sugars linked together in a way which stops the body digesting them, and the bifidobacteria use FOS for their own growth. The Japanese regularly use FOS in over 500 of their foods. Research revealed that feeding 15mg of FOS per day to healthy volunteers caused bifido bacteria to become more predominant in faeces, showing that their intestinal environment was healthy. Ninety-five per cent FOS encourages the growth of beneficial bacteria and reduces the growth of unfriendly bacteria, and they may also help relieve constipation. FOS are found naturally in honey, barley, rye, garlic, asparagus, onions, bananas and artichokes, but in insufficient quantities to be of benefit. Studies show that 'chlorine in the water supply has a damaging effect on our good bacteria, so FOS are of help in maintaining the correct environment in our gut'.[15] Water filters could be used to remove chlorine.

*Fibre*

Fibre is a cellulose form of carbohydrate which the body cannot break down and it therefore passes through the GI tract more or less unchanged; however, in doing so it absorbs toxins, cholesterols and oestrogens, holds water to keep the stools soft, and stimulates peristalsis contractions.

Fibre also delays the absorption of glucose and improves glucose tolerance, thereby keeping blood levels normal and preventing mood swings, and the presence of fibre promotes 'good' bifido bacteria in the intestines. It improves faeces transit time and reduces the muscle strain that can lead to piles. Fibre keeps us 'regular'; a healthy stool should be brown and float because it is high in fibre. If stools sink this is a sign that not enough fibre is being eaten.

There are different types of fibre, some of which are insoluble, e.g. bran, and some which are soluble, e.g. pectins in fruits and gums and alginates from seaweeds. Other sources of fibre include cereal grains, fruits, vegetables, nuts and seeds. However, many people experience digestive problems with cereal grains, and may be better off consuming fruits and vegetables. Wheat bran can make some people constipated, so choose oat bran products instead.

Importantly, as fibre absorbs degraded oestrogens and helps to eliminate them from the body, it prevents them from stimulating more endometriosis to grow. Therefore eat lots of good sources of fibre, such as fruits and vegetables, nuts, seeds and cereals to help to protect yourself against high oestrogen levels which could trigger endometriotic implants. The role of fibre will be discussed in greater detail later in this chapter (p188). We should all eat around 30mg of fibre per day.

## Lisa C of Sussex

*My menstrual cycle has always been a cause for concern to the extent that I had gone for periods of 12 months without menstruating. In early 1994 my symptoms peaked, after 3 months' antibiotic treatment for a throat infection. I suffered months of recurrent thrush, cystitis and bacterial vaginosis. My periods became extremely heavy and very painful. I either suffered from constipation or diarrhoea, especially before menstruating. I felt cold all the time, my hair thinned and I had all the classic PMT symptoms and developed a rash on my upper body. Finally I began to experience acid indigestion after each meal.*

*After numerous exploratory operations it was established that I had endometriosis, irritable bowel syndrome and hiatus hernia. The nutritionist advised me to change my diet and exclude many foods that could be aggravating my condition. I excluded all foods containing the following: sugar / honey, salt, preservatives / additives, chocolate, coffee, tea, alcohol, dairy foods and yeasts. I adopted what is known as a wholefood diet, eating all foods from fresh to help the healing process. A daily salad, green leafy vegetables, red / orange-coloured vegetables, 1–2 pieces of fruit (not citrus), wholegrains (rice, oats, rye, corn, etc.), 3 organic eggs a week, 10 almonds per day, some live soya yogurt, chicken, fresh fish, seeds, pineapple juice and plenty of fresh water.*

*In addition to those dietary changes I began to take some supplements daily: an acidophilus, a multivitamin / mineral, digestive enzymes, vitamin C, magnesium, vitamin A drops, and I followed a gentle colon cleanse with herbs.*

*Slowly my symptoms began to ease. My periods became lighter and considerably less painful. My hair began to thicken and look healthier. My skin rash completely disappeared and I now very rarely suffer vaginal infections. Although there are a few foods I still cannot tolerate when I try to reintroduce them, I am now able to reintroduce many into my daily diet. I still have a few bowel and indigestion problems but I would say they have improved by over 50 per cent. Fourteen months after beginning this programme I am expecting my first child in 20 weeks' time. I believe that this would not have been possible so soon if I had not adopted this wholefood diet and supplement programme.*

# FACTORS HARMFUL TO DIGESTION AND ABSORPTION

Having looked at three areas which support the health of the digestive tract, we will now turn our attention to the five areas which are detrimental and can cause great harm to our health. These are a leaky gut, chronic candidiasis, malabsorption, food intolerances, and the harm caused by environmental oestrogens (as well as the build-up of natural oestrogens if the diet is low in fibre and high in fat).

## LEAKY GUT DYSFUNCTION SYNDROME

### Julie A of Kent

*The one important factor I learned was to listen to your body. It soon tells you what it needs and what it does not want. How you feel after drinking or eating certain foods tells you a lot. The worst part was excluding dairy foods and wheat for three months. That was really hard, but it does open your eyes to the effects of food on your body, and I felt much better for it and am now able to eat normally again with no problems. I certainly learned a lot. Healthy eating is a great way to achieve normal weight.*

• C A S E   S T U D Y •

In leaky gut dysfunction syndrome, damaged mucous membrane wall in the intestine allows food particles to be absorbed into the bloodstream before their digestion is completed. The gut wall can become leaky through damage to the membrane by drugs, gluten or *Candida albicans* overgrowth. Unfortunately the immune cells in the blood think that the undigested food particle leaked through is 'alien' and dangerous, and therefore they attack it. Often the particles are the protein parts of foods, small chains of five amino acids joined together like popper beads. Normal food molecules are recognized by the immune system cells as normal and are left alone, but larger, partially digested molecules (exorphins) are seen as 'alien' and may be attacked. If this happens, susceptible people develop food intolerances to quite normal foods. Metabolites enter the bloodstream leaving you feeling sick all over. The liver can become overloaded and digestive enzyme production may be affected.

Once we have antibodies to foods they can attach themselves to a lung space or in a joint and cause inflammation reactions. This is how auto-immune diseases begin.

These exorphins (exogenous morphine-like molecules) are very similar to endorphins, the natural pain killers produced by the brain: 'If they manage to get through the liver, experiments suggest they may affect mood, inducing a sense of comfort and craving for yet more of that food.'[16] This would explain why we crave the foods which are doing us the most harm. Deficiencies of protein-digesting enzymes would affect the way in which the body deals with exorphins.

It is reported that 'research at the National Institute for Health in the USA has shown that these larger food particles may get into the bloodstream where they are able to bind to receptors for endorphins'.[17] Yet more research is needed in this area to see how this affects body chemistry.

An article on research into the intestinal absorption of macro-molecules reports: 'Normally proteins would be broken down by digestion into amino acids but if they are still large peptide (protein) molecules, an attack can be mounted. Generally the mucosal barrier allows substances less than 0.4mm in diameter to be absorbed into the body, while preventing larger molecules from entering.'[18] Beads of amino acid chains will get across the barrier if the mucosa has been breached by candidiasis. *Candida albicans* hyphae (long thin filaments) could penetrate the membrane and cause the gut to 'leak' large molecules into the bloodstream to which the immune system reacts.

It has been found that 'increased permeability is a highly sensitive measure of disruption of the normal mucosal barrier function of the small intestine and it is therefore not surprising that many potential toxic agents cause increased permeability – NSAIDs, alcohol, cytotoxic drugs, bile salts, detergents, gold compounds, chelators, ischaemia and dietary idiosyncrasies'.[19] Stress and hormonal preparations can have similar effects.

Mary Lou Ballweg, of the International Endometriosis Association, reports: 'Rarely lumps of endometriosis implants grow inside the bowel, causing obstructions (lumps the size of a grapefruit have been removed having the texture of black rubber). Out of five thousand endometriosis patients ten per cent have significant bowel involvement.'[20]

## CHRONIC CANDIDIASIS

An overgrowth of the single-cell yeast *Candida albicans* in the gut flora has also been associated with endometriosis and leaky gut syndrome. Candidiasis is very difficult to diagnose, as the yeast occurs naturally in all of us.

---

### Liz R of Croydon

*I followed an anti-candida-style diet from September to December 1993. Before following the diet my symptoms were hypoglycaemia, tingling and numbness in my arms and legs and anxiety attacks. I was taking the drug Fluanxol for these symptoms which my doctor felt were stress related. I had read a lot about candida and my symptoms were much worse after eating sweet foods and refined carbohydrates. I thought that was the problem so gave the diet a try. On the diet the symptoms initially got worse but then when I stopped the Fluanxol I had no symptoms. I assume the diet cured me.*

•
C
A
S
E

S
T
U
D
Y
•

---

How can a tiny organism cause health problems? *Candida albicans* is a one-celled yeast. We all have this yeast within our digestive tract, normally living in harmony with us. Only when it grows out of proportion can it become a problem.

Symptoms from disrupted intestinal flora can include constipation and diarrhoea, or both; headaches; chronic fatigue; depression; dizziness; bloating; poor concentration; vaginal irritation; sugar and bread cravings; mood swings; PMS; digestive problems; and blurred vision. You know best how you feel. If you are experiencing these symptoms this may be an area to explore.

### *The harmonious relationship between yeast and gut flora*

Three things can play havoc with the delicate balance of intestinal flora, weakening the immune system so that it is less able to cope with yeast overgrowth:

1  A diet high in saturated and trans fats and refined sugars.

2  Prolonged use of antibiotics, the contraceptive pill and HRT, or exposure to toxic substances.

3  Prolonged stress.

*Candida albicans* is a very aggressive yeast and if it sees a space for growth, it will proliferate. It can change from a one-celled yeast into a 'hyphal' form, spreading long filaments (hyphae) which may puncture minute holes in the intestine wall, causing a 'leaky gut' (*see* p. 173).

## Carol B of Suffolk

*The anti-candida diet has brought about a remarkable improvement in my condition. I am 42 and suffered from distressing symptoms (including anaemia) for at least 5 years before being referred to a gynaecologist 15 months ago. A laparoscopy revealed really quite bad endometriosis. But hormone treatments (Danazol, Provera, Primolut) were unsuccessful. I was attempting to come to terms with the prospect of radical surgery when a lessening of symptoms occurred during a weight-reducing diet. I subsequently purchased the* Candida albicans *book by Leon Chaitow, and felt that prolonged stress could have been responsible for the manifestation of yeasts. I embarked upon the recommended diet, taking supplements. The first change was the absence of pain, which had been very severe and accompanied by nausea and diarrhoea, and I was able to abandon the six-hourly use of Ponstan. After several months the flow has also lessened, and I now have no flooding or large clots, and the most recent improvement would seem to be the absence of mid-cycle bleeding.*

• C A S E   S T U D Y •

Candida also has the potential to upset the hormone balance: 'Candida has receptor sites in its cell membranes which accept hormones; if progesterone binds to candida it fails to reach its destination.'[21] Acetaldehyde (breakdown product of alcohol produced by candida from sugar) reacts with the neurotransmitter dopamine to cause emotional disturbances like anxiety, spaced-out feelings and depression. Aldehydes cause suppression of T cell function, increased susceptibility to infection and inability of the immune system to respond efficiently to infections or allergens.[22, 23] *Candida albicans* yeast needs to be contained at a low rate in the gut, but overgrowth upsets your well-being.

## Penelope S of London

*My diet includes omitting as much yeast as possible (i.e. bread, cakes, pickles, etc.), limiting refined sugar intake, no coffee, only Earl Grey tea or herbal teas. I have a list of 'mould' foods to avoid, e.g. mushrooms, and I eat no milk or milk products, except live yogurt and cottage cheeses or feta cheese. I follow this as much as possible and have found that lapses, such as coffee, cause the niggley pains to restart. I sometimes live on the threshold of cystitis which is kept under control with Cynoloen and feel that my endometriosis is closely related to candidiasis.*

### Redressing the balance

Treatments are best undertaken with a nutritionist's guidance, and some environmental medicine practitioners may be able to offer advice. The first area of attack is to reduce the *Candida albicans* yeast to normal proportions via the following four steps:

*Diet.* It is important to reduce the foods which are 'feeding' the yeast. *Candida albicans* thrives on sugars (sucrose, glucose, fructose, dextrose, maltose, honey, molasses). Therefore refined sugars, yeasts, fermented foods, dried fruits, dairy foods (other than *live* yogurts) should be removed from the diet for 2 or 3 months. This diet can seem daunting but with the right guidance it is easy to find a vast range of alternative foods to provide the nutrient intake you require. Some diets recommend no fruit for the first two to four weeks to cut out the fruit sugar, fructose. After that you eat one piece of fruit a day.

For the first month you can eat plenty of fresh vegetables, pulses (legumes), wholegrain cereals, meat and fish, nuts and seeds, which provide substantial meals. Avoiding snack-type foods is important. The body craves nutrients from fresh meals; it needs solid wholefood meals but many people replace wholesome dinners with sugar- and wheat-based snacks which are nutritionally unsound. The following foods have anti-yeast properties and should be used frequently: garlic, onions, cabbage, broccoli, Brussels sprouts, kale, watercress, mustard cress, cauliflower, turnips, cinnamon, olive oil, and aloe vera juice. Pau d'Arco tea from South America also has an anti-candida effect.

*Antifungal treatment.* If the overgrowth is chronic and allergies abound with intolerances to ordinary foods, then diet alone cannot help. You will need antifungal agents to help reduce the candidiasis. These are available from the doctor as Nystatin, Diflucan or Betacanzale, or from health food shops as caprylic acid. Garlic is also excellent at reducing yeast overgrowth, with the aid of Pau d'Arco tea and aloe vera juice. Occasionally chronic candidiasis can produce headache and flu-like symptoms. This is because toxins are released into the bloodstream as it dies off. If this happens, reduce the antifungal treatment and drink lots of water for two days to help cleanse the system. Then you can add the antifungal agents back into your regime. Two to three months' treatment may bring vast improvements to your health.

*Beneficial probiotic bacteria.* In order to replenish and repopulate the intestinal flora, lactobaccillus acidophilus and bifido bacteria can be taken. Two very good forms (bioacidophilus and acidophilus plus) are acid-stable and capable of surviving the gastric secretions of the stomach. The repopulation of the digestive tract with these good bacteria is important so that B vitamin production can be maintained, especially after taking antibiotics, oral contraceptives and HRT. Take a B-complex supplement whilst on such drugs.

*Nutritional supplements.* While the diet is being adjusted and food exclusions are undertaken, a short-term supplementation with vitamin and mineral tablets, and digestive enzymes and acidophilus will help to ensure that all essential nutrients are being absorbed. The supplement must be yeast-, sugar-, dairy- and gluten-free.

## Sally G of Tyne and Wear

*You had been advising me for quite a while to go onto a candida-style diet to help my endo. To be honest, at the time (about 4 years ago) I had just turned 18, been diagnosed with endo and didn't believe that nutrition would help. I first cut out wheat and yeast products and much to my surprise there was a huge improvement in pain. I've then gradually eliminated foods from my diet such as processed foods and refined white sugar and have increased my nutritional supplements and fresh foods. I wish I had done it earlier.*

*I find that out of all the supplements I benefit the most from*

CASE STUDY

•
C
A
S
E

S
T
U
D
Y
•

*Efamol Marine which helps to decrease inflammation, hence reducing pain (plus the added bonus that it is great for the skin!!). I've had three laparoscopies and on my second and third my surgeon expressed how surprised she was that there was such little inflammation present (although the endo had spread). It is hard for most people to stick to a 'nutritional path' but when it works, you know it's been worth it. You have to listen to your body, take regular exercise (even just gentle) and eat well. I am a great fan of complementary therapy. My favourite is reflexology which I just love. It is relaxing and alleviates digestive and menstrual problems.*

*Everyone is different, and different things work for different people. I've had three colonics very close together and in my experience it was a bad move. A year later I still suffer a lot of pain in my colon. I would think very carefully before using such aggressive therapy again.*

## MALABSORPTION

By now we have established that 'you are really only what your body can digest and absorb'. What you eat is vital to your health, but if the digestive tract is on the blink then it does not matter if we live on organic wholefoods as those nutrients will not be effectively absorbed and the body may still become subclinically deficient.

If you suffer from bloating, stomach upsets, abdominal pain, poor digestion of fats, diarrhoea or constipation, anal irritation or bad breath, these need sorting out before you can get better. Consider reducing your sugar intake as 'even excess sugar can cause proliferation of E. coli bacteria which trigger infections in the intestines'.[24] Refined sugars can disrupt the balance of gut flora. If you take indigestion tablets, diuretics or laxatives, this will reduce absorption of vital minerals even further.

Many long-term steroid treatments may disable the gut flora which would normally produce B vitamins which aid in oestrogen degradation. Maintaining vitamin B production is crucial for all women with endometriosis. Malabsorption may be improved by following a healing programme. The use of the herb slippery elm, probiotics and digestive enzymes during drug treatments may help to correct some of the symptoms.

## FOOD ALLERGY AND INTOLERANCES

'A little of what you fancy does you good' is a saying which food-intolerant people should be wary of. To believe that ordinary foods can make you ill is sometimes hard to swallow! A true allergy is an immune response to a foreign substance (antigen). It is usually an IgE over-reaction which, at the extreme, can prove fatal. A food intolerance to 'normal' foods may be 'masked', as a weakened immune system tries to defend us from attack but reacts with ailments/distress signals – often an IgG response.

Studies suggest a link between food intolerances and endometriosis: 'American research points to a higher incidence of allergic-related symptoms in endometriosis sufferers.'[25] Many women with endometriosis often appear to have food allergy or intolerance problems to very ordinary foods and chemicals. To relieve the pain from endometriosis and to try and get pregnant, women have taken many different drugs, which may have affected the bifido factor bacteria which inhabit the small intestine. In some cases drugs and foodstuffs can also damage the mucous membrane lining of the intestines.

More and more people are becoming sensitive to ordinary foods: 'Food sensitivity or intolerance is more common than true food allergies, around 24 million American adults are affected by the foods they consume.'[26, 27] This may be due to environmental pollutants, chemicals within food, changes brought about by genetic engineering, poor gut mucosa or a weakness inherited from the family. But the result is usually the same – damaged intestinal lining and reactions within the immune system which trigger reactions in other body systems.

Some families are 'atopic' – that is, they have a history of illnesses such as asthma, eczema, hay fever and arthritis: 'The risk of being predisposed to an allergen is 50 per cent if one parent has an allergy. It rises to 75 per cent where both parents are involved. However, a third of atopic people are born into families where no intolerances have been recognized. The most usual symptoms are recurrent headaches, regular bouts of indigestion or persistent fatigue.'[28]

Which foods make you feel drained of energy and which foods revitalize you? The most common food intolerances are to cow's milk products (cheese, butter, yogurt, cream), food preservatives and colourings, wheat (cakes, biscuits, pastries, pastas), chocolate, eggs, citrus fruits, and foods containing salicylates (e.g. apples, cherries, grapes, peaches, aubergine, broccoli, tea and coffee).

*Wheat intolerance*

Most British foods use wheat as their staple base. In America it may be corn, in Japan soya, in India rice, etc. It can be easy to eat an excess of wheat over one day, with wheat bran and toast for breakfast, sandwiches for lunch, pizza or pasta for dinner, and various cakes and cookies throughout the day. Wheat, barley, rye, oats and spelt are known as gluten grains because they contain a stretchy protein called gluten, which can inflame the lining of the gut membrane in sensitive people. The non-gluten grains (rice, corn, buckwheat, quinoa, sago, tapioca, arrowroot and millet) can be used instead, although millet, corn and rice may also affect extremely sensitive people. Health food shops, nutrition cooperatives, Lifestyle, Gluten-free Bakery and the Allergycare Company (*see* p. 354) have lots of wonderful alternatives (*see* the Useful addresses section).

Sometimes eating one type of food too often can cause intolerance. If you feel you are wheat intolerant, avoid wheat for 30 days and use the alternatives, such as rye crispbreads, oatcakes, ricecakes, corn pasta, corn tortilla and tacos, buckwheat pasta, millet flakes, quinoa, potato-based pizza, and pastry made from ground almonds and brown rice flour. Many women with endometriosis have found that excluding wheat helps to reduce much of the bowel pain they experienced.

---

## Barbara H of Cheshire

• C A S E   S T U D Y •

*During the nutrition trial it was pointed out that I was eating a lot of wheat products. This probably stemmed from earlier attempts to lose weight via the F-Plan Diet, and a general belief that large quantities of fibre via bran and brown-bread products was beneficial. Actually I think now that the wheat products were doing me harm.*

*Some years after the nutrition trial I had a period of very bad health following some surgery for other health problems (and was taking antibiotics for flu). [Excess use of antibiotics can adversely affect health as antibiotics may damage the protective gut flora, which can lead to the onset of many diseases.] I had now developed what was recognised as food intolerance, mainly to wheat-based products and dairy foods. With nutritional advice I was able to cut out the foods that were making me ill. I also lost a stone in weight.*

*The supporting nutritional supplements helped me at a time when I was suffering from a lot of pain from endometriosis and very low energy levels. I therefore continued to take nutritional supplements for five years on and off. However, I have improved all the endometriosis symptoms. I now take a low dose multivitamin/mineral every day.*

### Dairy intolerance

Dairy foods are mucus-forming and may affect people who come from an atopic family (a family with a history of asthma, eczema, psoriasis, hay fever or arthritis). By excluding dairy foods for one month you can see whether your symptoms improve. A generation ago, the average dairy cow yielded eight quarts of milk per day, ate mainly grass and produced only one part per hundred million of antibiotics to a pint. Today a typical cow yields fifty quarts per day, may be fed meal made from bone and blood (from cattle, pig and chicken carcasses) and produces on average fifty-two different residues of antibiotics, plus blood and pus, in milk.[29] Alternatives to dairy foods include soya milk substitutes, rice dream or oat milk, tofu, soft soya cheeses, hummus, avocado pâté, fish pâté and nut butters (*see* p. 250 for a list of calcium-rich foods other than dairy products).

### Lisa C of London

*In the past 2½–3 years I have been suffering from a whole range of symptoms including dysmenorrhoea, amenorrhoea, digestive and bowel complaints, skin rashes and depression and so the list goes on. After numerous examinations and operations it was established that I have acute irritable bowel syndrome, endometriosis and hiatus hernia. I was virtually told that there was no permanent cure and the various drugs I had been prescribed had only worsened my symptoms. I have been seeing a nutritionist for seven months and following a strict dairy exclusion diet supported by supplements. However, I have been eating more wholefoods than ever before. My symptoms have improved by about 70 per cent and with a little more help, one day I hope to have the old me back again.*

CASE STUDY

*Food exclusion diets*

To show intolerance to particular foods, nutritionists may ask their clients to remove that food from the normal diet for one month; then to reintroduce it, and watch for any symptoms which may arise over a 24-hour period. When the excluded food is reintroduced there may be reactions such as headaches, flu-like symptoms, extreme fatigue or blurred vision, or a sense of mental grogginess. If there is a reaction, that food is best avoided for three months then reintroduced into the diet very slowly.

---

### Natalie C of London

*I eliminated cheese and caffeine. At laparoscopy nothing was detected and I am expecting a baby at Easter.*

CASE STUDY

---

Some people comply with the exclusion, but many do not. This can be due to such factors as cost, availability of alternatives, or being 'conservative' about food and therefore unwilling to change even if it means better health. Or they may not understand the full implication of the damage that is being inflicted on their gut membranes and immune cells when that food is eaten.

While on an exclusion diet, you can eat alternatives to provide nutrients and take a multivitamin/mineral supplement. If necessary, foods not in your normal diet can be eaten to increase the nutrient intake. There is less likelihood of an allergy to foods you have not eaten before, such as, for example, starfruit, kumquats, salsify, kale or celeriac.

Understanding why you need an exclusion diet is half the battle. Food molecules to which we are allergic can weaken the immune system. The white blood cells react to large molecules, the 'exorphins'. An over- or under-reactive immune system can affect the reproductive system (*see* chapter 7).

Leading health writer Leon Chaitow reports: 'Alterations in gut flora are felt to be linked to auto-immune disorders. Research at King's College London has looked at the body's way of ridding itself of undesirable bacteria by attacking its own tissues instead.'[30] If you feel that a certain food does not agree with you, see how you feel when you remove it from your diet.

The important thing to recognize is that if a food has become a problem, then something has to be done. It may mean avoiding that food for a few months and, if that is all it takes to get well and feel healthy, then surely it is worth a try.

*Immune responses to food intolerances*

The body struggles to deal with what it sees as 'alien' molecules. Once they have been 'captured', they are generally devoured or occasionally they are sent along to the joints (often used as a dumping ground for waste), which can cause aching joints. Orthopaedic surgeons know this dumped material as 'plica'. The incidence and amount of plica has increased over the past 10 years.

## FOOD ALLERGY AND INFERTILITY – COELIAC DISEASE, HYPOTHYROID AND INFERTILITY

Coeliac disease is a condition where the small intestine fails to digest and absorb food due to a sensitivity to wheat gluten (gliadin). Hypothyroidism occurs when the thyroid gland in the neck becomes sluggish. In adults the symptoms are sensitivity to cold, constipation, coarse skin, slow pulse, mental and physical slowing, and the outer third of the eyebrows can be lost. Infertility is a condition where both male and female can find it difficult to achieve conception (*see* chapter 4). In this section we will look at the links between these three conditions.

Research has linked coeliac disease and thyroid disease with possible thyroid auto-antibodies and infertility: 'Fourteen per cent of women with coeliac disease were found to have thyroid disorders.'[31] Recent research has estimated the numbers of women affected by hypothyroidism in the UK: 'Hypothyroidism is prevalent in 1.4 per cent of women. The commonest cause is auto-immune failure and the measurement of thyroid auto-antibodies confirms the diagnosis.'[32] These figures lead to the suggestion that 'testing for thyroid disease seems to be warranted in all women and men with unexplained infertility'.[33] This suggestion would appear to be supported by tests that are already in place: 'Autoimmune diseases such as those involving the thyroid, are thought to be involved in infertility. Indeed thyroid auto-antibodies are used to predict women at risk for miscarriage.'[34] As two-thirds of all pregnancy loss occur before the pregnancy is recognized, testing for thyroid auto-antibodies would help to catch those women in need of support. The human placenta produces the hormones human chorionic gonadotrophin (hCG) and human chorionic thyrotrophin which may interact with thyroid auto-antibodies. More research is needed in this important area. How many women with fertility problems are screened for thyroid auto-antibodies as a matter of course?

When symptoms of coeliac disease were removed by excluding wheat gluten from the diet, many infertile patients became pregnant. It is very important for doctors to check for coeliac disease in patients presenting with unexplained infertility and endometriosis. Many of the painful abdominal symptoms experienced in endometriosis could also be caused by gluten intolerance. The incidence of coeliac disease in Europe has been estimated as follows: 'The prevalence of coeliac disease varies from one person in every 2,500 in the UK, to one in 3,000 in the USA, one in 10,000 in Denmark and one in 300 in the West of Ireland.'[35] However, new research suggests these figures may be an underestimate.

Other research suggests that the longer women with coeliac disease are left untreated, the greater the risk of developing auto-immune thyroid disease and infertility. Tests for both conditions should be done automatically when infertility is present. Studies show that 'in males gliadin (the active portion of gluten) reduces semen quality in susceptible people. Deficiencies in zinc, folic acid, B12 and iron have been implicated in coeliac disease. Successful conception was reported after gluten exclusion in patients with infertility.'[36] It is thought this is a subclinical disease which subtly alters immune system function, and also causes malabsorption of vitamins and minerals from the digestive tract due to the damage inflicted on villi by the gluten.

It has been found that 'untreated hypothyroidism and hyper-thyroidism can both give rise to very similar changes in the gut mucosal damage, as can coeliac disease, which makes diagnosis difficult'.[37] Research from the seventies highlights the connection between the health of the digestive system and general well-being: 'All those tested had IgA antigliaden antibodies, showing that they were wheat intolerant. Failure to recognize either of these conditions, the researchers felt, could lead to a lack of response to treatment. Oral gliadin has been shown by research to affect neurotransmitters, dopamine and noradrenaline, in the brain.'[38] Get your doctor to check for both hypothyroid and coeliac disease as a matter of course. Coeliac disease can also lead to short-term lactose intolerance (intolerance to dairy foods). This should also be assessed.

---

### Barbara W of London

*After three years of trying for a baby, and with four failed IVF attempts behind me and a diagnosis of endometriosis, I had almost given up hope of ever becoming a mother. My marriage was in tatters, I was badly depressed and couldn't bear to look at a baby in the street, let alone the babies of my friends. I was desperate. I decided half-heartedly to have what was probably a final attempt at IVF, but at the last minute it was called off as my hormone levels were too high. The news devastated me and I came to the conclusion that I couldn't stand the IVF emotional treadmill any more. With one last heave of my depleted energy I decided to work on my diet and I visited Dian. She told me about the possible link between wheat gluten and infertility and told me about a client with endometriosis who had phoned in pregnant after following a gluten-free diet. I took that story away with me and it inspired me to begin a strict wheat- and dairy-free diet, making sure I used all the alternatives. A few weeks later I discovered to my shock and amazement that I was pregnant – naturally! I am still struggling to believe that after all this time such a miracle could have happened and I still have months ahead before I can be sure that this pregnancy will work out. But I hope that this story gives others the hope I needed to keep going.*

• C A S E   S T U D Y •

---

Coeliac disease would appear to be affecting greater numbers of people: 'During the 1980s and 1990s it has become apparent that coeliac disease is under-diagnosed and that the clinical features have changed in both children and adults. The shift has been towards milder symptoms, such as indigestion in adults and recurrent abdominal pain in children. The prevalence of coeliac disease from recent screening studies has been found to be as high as one in 100 to one in 300. Infertility or miscarriages have been described in women and reversible infertility in men.'[39] This change in prevalence may be due to wheat being genetically engineered or diets containing excess hidden wheat: 'In Ireland the highest reported figure (of coeliac disease) in a random sample of the general population has been found to be one in 122 people.'[40] Research shows a definite link between coeliac disease and infertility which the medical profession and IVF units seem to ignore and never test for when infertility is unexplained. However, the evidence for a connection is powerful: 'Coeliac disease is associated with infertility in both men and women. Subclinical coeliac disease in women may be an unexpected cause of delayed menarche, amenorrhoea, premature menopause, recurrent abortions and low pregnancy rate. Many individuals without apparent symptoms who are found to have coeliac disease remark on a new-founded vitality and sense of well-being when started on a gluten-free diet.'[41]

Removing as many problems as possible from an ailing immune system will enhance its strength and improve fertility, as health begins to be renewed. In susceptible people, the gliadin in wheat causes tremendous damage to the gut mucosa and is seen to be toxic to human tissue cells in culture. We need to encourage more testing and research in this area of infertility.

Under-nutrition has always been suspected when fertility is impaired. During wars and in famine areas, it has been noted that fertility was reduced at times when the food supply was cut off. This is due to atrophy of the reproductive organs. If the gut mucosa are badly damaged, then nutrients will not be absorbed.

## NUTRIENTS WHICH STRENGTHEN THE GUT MUCOSA

To improve the function of the gut mucosa the nutrients zinc, beta-carotene, biotin, butyric acid, pantothenic acid (vitamin B5), vitamins A, C and E, essential fatty acids and L glutamine are known to be important. Slippery elm can have a soothing effect as it builds up a protective layer of mucus on the membrane, allowing healing to take place. Often the mucosa may be inflamed from the substances which irritate it. The body then acts in one of two ways: it either rushes to expel the offending food, causing diarrhoea; or it seizes up altogether and we experience constipation. Either way we are left with a malabsorption problem.

# NATURAL AND ENVIRONMENTAL OESTROGENS

## NATURAL OESTROGENS OF BODY ORIGIN

Natural oestrogens are made from cholesterol in the ovaries, testes and the adrenal glands in response to signals from the pituitary. They can also be made by every fat cell in the body. From these sites they are secreted into the blood and are carried to the cells of the breasts and reproductive organs. Oestrogens send chemical signals or messages to help other cells respond to the body's internal environment, and oestrogens are responsible for cell growth in the breast, uterus, bone, liver and cardiovascular system. However, some environmental synthetic chemicals, such as pesticides, insecticides and herbicides, appear to mimic the role of oestrogens in the body.

Natural oestrogens come in many types and vary greatly from one another, for example, 'oestradiol is 12 times more potent than oestrone and 80 times more potent than oestriol'.[42] Carlton Fredericks states that 'control of natural oestrogen is a nutritional process which is disturbed by too much sugar, too little protein and is incapacitated almost completely by lack of vitamin B complex'.[43] Indeed, it is our digestive system, in particular the bile from the gall bladder and the liver, which aids the excretion of oestrogen from the body. This is very important to all women who have endometriosis. You can help control oestrogen in your body through your diet and gentle exercise.

## FIBRE AND OESTROGEN EXCRETION

Excretion of oestrogens bound to fibre is another key to our management of endometriosis: 'Dietary fibre increases excretion of excess oestrogens from the body.'[44] The Western diet rich in animal and trans fats elevates the levels of sex hormones produced in the body. Fats and fat cells store oestrogenic pesticides and cause a build-up of free radicals which can damage cell membranes, so a low-fat diet is advisable. Avoiding the bad saturated animal fats and trans oils, and eating mainly the good cold-pressed cis oils is vital to health as we saw in chapter 3.

You can take action to aid excretion of oestrogens:

1  The best fibre to eat is found in unrefined wholegrain cereals, nuts,

seeds, berries and the pulse/legume vegetables (peas, beans and lentils), although the cellulose in soluble vegetable fibres are more effective in triggering the normal processes of breakdown in the colon than fibre from grains/cereals e.g. oats. Fibre also binds the oestrogens and inhibits their reabsorption: 'Some fibres such as the lignins found in rye, other grains and seeds are changed by gut flora to form anti-oestrogen compounds, enterolactone and enterodiol, which are protective against cancers.'[45] There is a direct effect of the quality of plant fibre consumed: 'Good quality fibre encourages a hormone known as serum hormone-binding globulin (SHBG) which can be used as a marker for steroid hormone abnormalities. SHBG is a unique transport system for oestrogen, because while the oestrogen is bound to the SHBG it cannot exert any biological effect within the body.'[46] If the diet is low in fibre, then the oestrogens can have a biological effect. The other soluble fibre we referred to earlier as FOS also aids oestrogen clearance.

2  The bifido bacteria also encourage oestrogen clearance by inhibiting an enzyme known as beta glucoronidase. This hormone normally encourages the deactivated safe oestrogen to become reactivated, so that it can be sent back into circulation (not a good idea with endometriosis).

3  At least four vegetables, two fruits and a handful of nuts and seeds should be eaten each day with some wholegrain cereal. These will also speed up the transit time of food through the digestive tract. The best vegetables to eat are those from the cruciferous family, all rich in B complex vitamins and magnesium: cabbage, Brussels sprouts, broccoli, cauliflower, kale, turnip, swede, radish, horseradish, mustard and cress: 'These contain three unique compounds – indoles, dithiolthiones and isothiocynates, which influence certain enzymes that rev up the body's degradation system [...] oestrogen is "metabolized" and ultimately excreted from the body.'[47]

4  'Other protective factors may be the phyto-oestrogens from soya [see p. 197] and a high natural level of selenium in foods';[48] for those suffering with endometriosis it is in our own interest to keep circulating oestrogen levels moderate. Therefore by eating green leafy vegetables, a little soya protein and selenium-rich seafoods we are helping our body to protect itself. So granny was right when she told us to eat up our greens!

5   The clearance system for oestrogens, cholesterol and toxins is the liver. The steroid hormones are metabolized (broken down) in the liver. The bile from the gall bladder stores these inactive hormones and excretes them bound to fibre in the stools. Choline and inositol make up lecithin which helps the liver deal with fats. The herb silymarin and zinc methionine may also assist in liver cleansing (*see* p. 166).

As other scientists have demonstrated, 'we know from research that the form of oestrogen known as oestradiol causes tissue proliferation'[49] and that 'uncontrolled levels of oestrogen, if the body goes into oestrogen dominance, have been indicated for contributing to the serious problem of endometriosis and breast cancers'.[50] When this oestradiol form of oestrogen reaches the liver, enzymes which use B vitamins as co-factors, change this sex hormone into the less harmful oestriol. A healthy liver with a plentiful supply of B vitamins can degrade oestradiol into oestriol which is important for optimum well-being: 'If the sum of oestrone and the oestradiol is greater than the oestriol in a 24hr urine sample, women may be at greater risk of illness related to oestrogen excess.'[51, 52] Your doctor can check your oestrogen levels with a simple blood or saliva test.

Oestriol is the form in which oestrogen can be bound to fibre and excreted. Therefore the diet needs to have sufficient fibre and B vitamins to help the body deal with the constant breakdown of circulating oestrogen. If the diet is high in animal and trans fatty acids and low in fibre, the gut flora in the bowel behave differently and change the way they break down oestrogen. If the gut flora in the small intestine and the liver enzymes are in a poor state, the levels of oestradiol and oestrone in the blood may become higher than they should and this can unbalance reproductive hormones.

Research shows that 'dietary fat may influence oestrogen metabolism due to the stimulation of animal fats upon the growth of colonic bacteria which are capable of synthesizing oestrogen as well as breaking the oestrogen–glucoronide linkages'.[53] Eating fish can be beneficial: 'A diet rich in fish oils (herring, mackerel, sardines, pilchards, salmon, trout, tuna) has been shown to help women suffering from high circulating oestrogen levels and also help those with PMS who are oversensitive to the hormone prolactin.'[54] Though women must make sure that the fish they choose is from a clean source low in pesticides. Deficiency of B complex vitamins may impair the liver enzymes function in inactivating oestrogens.

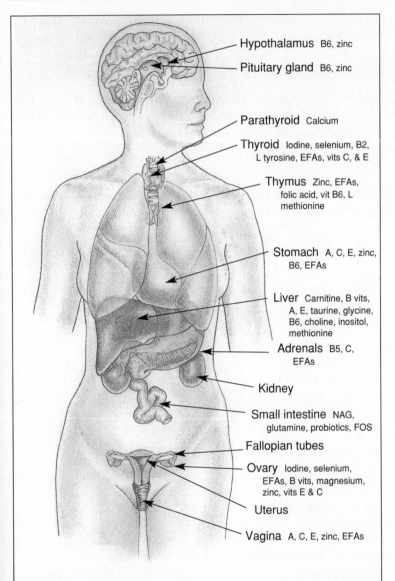

Figure 8.2
The endocrine system is responsible for balancing all hormones in the body (*see also* figure 2.1). Here we can see the main nutrients known to be involved for each organ. These are all dependent upon the nutrients eaten and absorbed by a healthy digestive tract.

How the environmental synthetic oestrogens behave when reaching the liver requires far more research.

## UNNATURAL OESTROGENS

Unfortunately natural oestrogens made in the body have mimics, some naturally occuring in foods and others man-made, which confuse the normal hormonal messages.

1  Exogenous oestrogens or xeno-oestrogens which our bodies metabolize from pesticides are thought to be dangerous.

2  Phyto-oestrogens naturally ocurring in foods such as soya are felt to be helpful during menopause.

3  Endometriotic implants are thought to produce their own oestrogens directly into the abdominal cavity (*see* pp. 69, 282).

*Xeno-oestrogens*

Unfortunately some of the food we eat contains pesticides which have an oestrogenic effect (xeno-oestrogens).

Dioxins, PCBs and nonylphenols have an oestrogenic effect in body cells, i.e. they produce chemicals which act exactly as oestrogen does in the body. These are false oestrogens and they are bad news: 'Suspect chemicals include pesticides and phthalates (nonylphenols), a group of compounds which migrate from plastic wrappings and leak into the foods we eat, such as cheese, meats, cakes, sandwiches and confectionery.'[55] Research from around the world has shown that these compounds have a detrimental effect upon the reproductive systems of both humans and animals: 'USA production alone of synthetic organic chemicals (including pesticides) amount to 197.5 billion kilogrammes in 1992, with similar production in other countries. They ignore geographical boundaries and are found in rainwater, lakes, oceans and in the fat cells within our bodies.'[56] The effects of xeno-oestrogens are insidious: 'Biologists feel that these xeno-oestrogens can mimic the actions of natural signalling molecules such as oestrogens and also growth factors, i.e. a "natural" signal may be being sent by an "unnatural" signalling molecule. They do not alter genes themselves but may alter the way they (genes) are expressed.'[57]

In 1979 it was realized that diethylstilboestrol (DES), a synthetic man-made oestrogen used to prevent spontaneous abortion in pregnancy, caused a specific vaginal cancer in the daughters of women who had taken DES while pregnant. DES acts as a transplacental carcinogen, i.e. when given to the mother it causes cancer in her daughter; it also causes testicular problems in sons. Therefore, worries about other synthetic oestrogen mimics which are awash in our environment are well-founded. We need to know what the long-term effects will be, and whether or not the increase in endometriosis and other reproductive disorders are linked to the use of pesticides.

Naturally occurring oestrogens are important in normal growth of organs. But these 'mimic' and synthetic xeno-oestrogens are soluble in all fats and oils, so they can cross cell membranes into the nucleus and can activate or repress gene expression; that is, they can change the cells' programming (even though they bind in a much weaker fashion than natural oestrogens). It is also known that the body's own metabolism can alter these chemicals, possibly to even more potent forms in the body: 'Metabolism can convert non-oestrogenic substances into ones with hormonal activity or they may just disrupt normal hormone levels. When one research group tested a combination of chemicals their oestrogenicity jumped by 160 to 1,600 times their individual potency, probably due to synergy. So together they may be more potent than when alone.'[58] We need more research to look at exactly what these chemicals do to our oestrogen balance.

The International Endometriosis Association, headquartered in the USA, discovered a group of monkeys in the University of Wisconsin Primate Center who had been treated with dioxins and had developed spontaneous endometriosis: 'The disease pattern found in the monkeys was in direct correlation with the amount of dioxin they had been given. The 15-year study indicated that latent female reproductive abnormalities may be associated with dioxin exposure in rhesus monkeys.'[59]

*Dioxins in foods.* Unfortunately dioxins come to us from plants and animals through our foods. The higher up the food chain, the greater the contamination with dioxins.

1   Eating from lower down the food chain may have a lesser effect, e.g. for a fish-eating vegetarian or lacto-vegetarian. The fats in

    meat and dairy foods may contain the highest levels of dioxins, so
keep intake very low.

2  Fish should also be from a relatively clean source, not a polluted
lake or river.

3  Trying to avoid fruits and vegetables which have been sprayed is
very difficult. Buying organic vegetables can be neither easy nor
cheap for most people and anyway dioxins are everywhere, even
on the skins of organic vegetables. However, it is extremely
important that all fruits and vegetables should be peeled in order
to remove the chemicals. Just washing them will not work.

4  Processed foods, such as cakes and biscuits, may contain
contaminated fats, so they should be kept to a bare minimum. If
cooking is done at home, there can be more control over the use
of pure ingredients.

We have to be aware but not anxious. Just do your best to avoid an
excess intake of these harmful chemicals.

    Dioxins build up in our fat cells. Internationally, there is some
debate as to the acceptable levels of these: 'The World Health
Organization and the UK authorities accept a tolerance of 10 units
of dioxin per day as acceptable. While USA authorities set the
minimum risk at 0.0064 units per day, stating that dioxins have a
cancer risk.'[60] For instance, a pint of milk contains five times the
quantity of PCBs contained in a single cod liver oil capsule; a pat of
butter contains three times the amount. Water should also be chosen
from purified sources. The way in which our liver enzymes deal with
these man-made oestrogenic chemicals requires more research.

**Weight loss and dioxins**. If you are trying to lose weight then do
it slowly, 1kg/2lb per week only. This is very important as a sudden
change in diet can result in too fast a release of dioxins from fat
cells, causing other symptoms such as feeling toxic and exhausted.
This fast release also greatly stresses the liver. The use of the herb
silymarin can gently cleanse the liver. One often finds a weight loss
of 2kg/5lb happens naturally over one month if on an exclusion
diet, as intolerance often causes fluid retention in soft tissue
(oedema). Researchers at the University of Los Angeles, USA, took
60 people off wheat for three months. At the end of this time they
were given one slice of bread. Twelve people put on 3.5kg/8lb in

weight overnight with fluid retention. Once the food is excluded again, the cells lose this fluid, the bloating sensation disappears and body weight normalizes. The use of good quality cis oils can also help weight loss when used wisely: 'Researchers have observed that the more linoleic acid in the fat tissue, the less obese the person.'[61]

If you are pregnant or breastfeeding, take care as some dioxins stored in body fat cells can transfer from mother to child.

## EFFECTS OF HIGH OESTROGEN LEVELS

A condition known as oestrogen dominance (i.e. oestrogen out of balance with progesterone) is under review by researchers. This may be due to the effects of the exogenous oestrogens or hormone disrupters from the pesticides which surround us. Also, a very low fibre and high fat diet can compound these problems. We do not know what subtle effects an excess of phyto-oestrogens or xeno-oestrogens may be having on us.

1  High oestrogen levels can be an abortive and can cause uterine cramping.

2  They may also cause an imbalance in brain chemicals, with too many excitatory neurotransmitters and too few inhibitory ones, thus causing mood swings.

3  High oestrogen causes high copper levels, and low zinc and low prostaglandin series 1 levels. High copper levels have been implicated as a nervous stimulant, triggering mood swings and can also inhibit essential enzymes which produce energy. High copper levels also compete with iron, lowering it and causing heavy blood loss during menstruation. High copper has been linked in research to ovarian cysts.

4  High oestrogen levels stimulate serotonin, a neurotransmitter, to release aldosterone, a hormone, from the adrenal glands. These glands control the kidneys' water and salt retention. Excessive amounts of aldosterone cause bloating. It is therefore important to eat a low salt, low refined sugar and low refined carbohydrate diet (white rice and white flours). The use of diuretics if you bloat just throws zinc and magnesium out of the body too rapidly and this will worsen all the other PMS symptoms. (Vitamin B6, zinc and magnesium are natural diuretics and will expel retained fluids.)

5   High oestrogen levels also correlate with low thyroxine levels as
    these two hormones are antagonistic to each other (i.e. act against
    each other). Hypothyroid symptoms can result – coarse skin,
    fatigue, constipation, feeling cold, weight gain, and hair loss
    (especially the outer third of the eyebrows).

6   Stress raises cortisol levels in the adrenals and this hormone
    competes with progesterone production and lowers it, which in
    turn raises oestrogen levels. Lowered progesterone reduces
    immune function and makes miscarriages more likely. Stress
    reduces the amount of B vitamins available to the body, so trying
    to reduce stress levels is a good idea. Taking a yeast-free B
    vitamin complex can be a good idea at such times, especially as
    vitamin B6 is the precursor to progesterone.

7   Women who take an excess of antibiotics (amicillin, penicillin,
    neomycin, etc.) change the amounts of oestrogen being recycled:
    'The quantity of oestrogen found in the faeces is increased up to
    60 times the normal levels. Looking at research, levels of aerobic
    and anaerobic bacteria drop to between 20–25 per cent of
    original levels during antibiotic treatment. In patients going for
    operations only 9 per cent contracted infections when taking
    antibiotics compared to 35 per cent of those not receiving
    antibiotics.'[62] So the benefit of taking antibiotics is important, but
    the gut flora must be replenished within three weeks of the
    operation.

8   With oestrogen dominance, several symptoms may occur:

•   weight gain (extra fat may be deposited on the waist, hips and
    legs)
•   heavy and irregular periods
•   fibroids on the uterus
•   swollen breasts and formation of cysts
•   water retention (soft-tissue oedema)
•   more pronounced PMS symptoms
•   cravings for sweet foods
•   lack of sex drive

If you have many of these symptoms, then this book should help
you find a way to correct the problem by normalizing hormone
levels.

To repeat what we have said, B vitamins are vital to the way the liver is able to break down oestrogens circulating in the blood (oestradiol which is known to cause cell proliferation is linked to endometriosis): 'Being able to break down oestradiol to oestriol, a hormone which is benign, is dependent upon the B vitamin levels in the liver.'[63] Therefore your diet is very important in controlling oestrogen levels. Oestriol can be bound to fibre from the diet and excreted from the body, so your fibre intake is very important. Only 30g of fibre per day are needed. Healthy eating therefore helps to control the processes which may lead to endometriosis. Choline and inositol (B complex vitamins) are very important in liver enzyme function and fat metabolism, so the diet should be rich in these B vitamins. Excess folic acid can increase oestrogen production, so care must be taken to keep it in balance with the other B vitamins.

## NATURAL OESTROGENS OF PLANT ORIGIN (PHYTO-OESTROGENS)

Phyto-oestrogens are naturally occurring oestrogens in plants, such as soya, wheat, alfalfa, red clover, citrus fruits, tofu, tempeh, miso, liquorice, rye, rhubarb, anise, bean sprouts, sunflower and linseed seeds, etc. (*see* table 8.3) Some research suggests that these natural plant oestrogens (known as isoflavinoids and lignans) are protective and may help to lower or balance the oestrogens produced by the body cells: 'They are very similar to oestradiol but are not the same as oestrogen produced in women. It is felt from research that they act like weak oestrogens or may have an anti-oestrogenic effect to block excess uptake of natural body cell oestrogens. One isoflavinoid (genistein) does three amazing things in the bodies of post-menopausal women: it delays bone loss, it reduces blood cholesterol levels and it helps to keep oestrogen levels high in them.'[64]

More research is necessary to see what effect phyto-oestrogens have on the levels of oestrogens in endometriosis. If it acts as an anti-oestrogen and helps to normalize levels, it could be very helpful; whereas if it raises oestrogen levels it may be detrimental. When phyto-oestrogens act as anti-oestrogens they can lock into the body's oestrogen receptor sites, rather like the US Space Shuttle Atlantis is able to dock with the Russian Space Station Mir. It is thought that they may therefore prevent the oestradiol (known to cause cell proliferation) from growing out of control, thus reducing the more potent oestrogens in the body from triggering other disease states.

Research done in America suggests that phyto-oestrogens may be protective against cancers of the breast, uterus and cervix. Indeed, 'in Japan breast cancer is low where the diet is high in soya products and fresh fish. Such a diet, which is higher in soya protein than in the West, indicates that Japanese women have lower oestrogen levels. Isoflavins present on soya beans have been seen to inhibit the growth of cancer cells.'[65] It is known that in cultures such as Japan where women eat an average of 100mg of indoles daily, there is a very low risk of breast cancer. In the West our average daily intake of indoles is a mere 20mg, far too low.

Endometriosis may respond to the use of 'good' oestrogens in the diet in some women. Moderation may be the key. However, in Japan the incidence of endometriosis is high, so it is unclear what is really happening with respect to phyto-oestrogens: how can they be protective against breast cancer in older Japanese women, but do not appear to lessen the levels of endometriosis in younger women? It is a mystery.

However, it is felt that a combination of phytochemicals is the most beneficial, so that by eating a variety of natural fruits and vegetables we take in beneficial combinations of foods. For instance, the allylic sulphides found in garlic and onions and the limonene in citrus fruits work as enzyme activators and strengthen the body's immune system. Many phytochemicals have antioxidant properties, so they disarm the free radical molecules which rush around inside the body causing damage to cell membranes and cell DNA.

To obtain extra lignans eat 1–3 spoonfuls of ground food grade linseeds every day with breakfast.

To obtain isoflavinoids, eat soya beans. The Japanese eat 100mg of soya beans per day; other Asians take in only 45mg per day from soya flour, tempeh, tofu or vegetable protein. Roasted soya beans contain 162mg isoflavinoid per 75g/3oz and tofu contains 62mg per 75gm3oz.

| | | |
|---|---|---|
| Carrots | Soya beans | Wheat + bran + germ |
| Rice + bran + polish | Oats | Barley |
| Potatoes | Apples | Cherries |
| Plums | Red clover | Mouldy corn |
| Citrus fruits | Ginseng | Alfalfa |

Table 8.3
Foods containing oestrogenic factors

Meat and dairy foods raise fat levels in the body and therefore contribute to oestrogen production. A low fibre diet with high animal fat can exaggerate oestrogen levels, so you should eat a selection of high fibre foods. A balanced diet is essential; never eat too much of any one substance in a day and always ensure that the diet is rich in a variety of different foods.

| | |
|---|---|
| Cottonseed | Safflower |
| Wheatgerm | Corn |
| Linseed | Peanut *(best avoided because of the afflotoxins)* |
| Olive | Soya bean |
| Coconut | Linseed oil + glutamic acid = anti-pyridoxine (need extra vitamin B6) |

Table 8.4
Oils which are oestrogenic. Use only one tablespoon per day of these good cis fatty acids. Buy only the cold-pressed, unrefined, un-hydrogenated versions (linseed, olive, safflower and corn oils).

*Diana G of Shropshire*

*I put my improvement in health and endo symptoms down to a non-dairy diet, drinking bottled water, no coffee and keeping more or less to a candida-style diet. i.e. no grapes, mushrooms or yeast-based foods. I also find that not eating brown bread helps me (I'm all right with white). A positive state of mind and not to give up is essential.*

CASE STUDY

A recent report from the UK Medical Research Council's Institute for Environment and Health concludes that 'though some epidemiological studies suggest that the consumption of foods containing phtyo-oestrogens may have beneficial effects, almost no evidence exists to link these effects directly to oestrogens'.[66] Recent American research has shown that low doses of phyto-oestrogens at dietary levels can cause breast cancer cells to proliferate. While all this debate is on-going about the true effects of phyto-oestrogens in normal healthy people, women with health problems related to imbalances of oestrogen need to be cautious in their use. Apply the rules of moderation and never eat in excess – try to avoid snacking or comfort eating.

## THE ROLE OF THE THYROID

The thyroid gland and its hormonal products play a vital role in our overall well-being. The major hormone produced by the thyroid is thyroxine which is the hormone that controls the basal metabolic activity of the body. Thyroxine speeds up most of the metabolic (chemical) reactions that take place in the cells of the body. Thyroxine acts like the thermostat that controls the heating of a house. When the house needs to be warmed up, the thermostat goes up and the furnace burns more fuel and heats up the house. Thyroxine causes an increase in the use of our dietary carbohydrate, proteins and fats by the body. Thyroxine also works with the other hormones of the body to enhance their biological actions.

When a person has low levels of thyroxine (i.e. hypothyroidism), the body slows up. An individual with hypothyroidism feels cold and becomes sluggish. But more important to our discussions in this book, hypothyroidism leads to infertility. Women with hypothyroidism may not menstruate. The absence of the menstrual cycle is technically called amenorrhoea. A normal menstrual cycle is dependent upon the presence of a properly functioning thyroid. Oestrogen is an antagonistic hormone to thyroxine, so if we have oestrogen dominance, then thyroxine levels may be low.

Thyroid hormone synthesis depends in large part on having an appropriate amount of iodine in the diet. Iodine is absorbed through the small intestine and transported directly to the thyroid where it is used in the synthesis of the thyroid hormones. Without iodine, the thyroid desperately tries to produce thyroid hormone with no success and the thyroid enlarges (goitre). A goitre can easily be seen as a lump in the region of the neck. Selenium is vital for the uptake of iodine so both should be taken together.

In addition to iodine, a healthy thyroid requires cis fatty acids, proteins, vitamins and minerals. The thyroid gland also produces T3 (triidothyrine) and T4 (thyroxine). These hormones have to be finely balanced as imbalances can lead to abnormal heartbeats, hyperactivity and irritability. Very high levels of these hormones cause hyperthyroid weight loss; low levels can lead to hypothyroid weight gain. The pituitary gland produces thyroid-stimulating hormone (TSH). If the level of TSH is found to be normal when tested, the patient will not be suffering from hypothyroidism. The level of TSH will change before thyroid hormone levels fall and is therefore an extremely sensitive index for hypothyroidism. If you suspect you suffer from a sluggish thyroid, check with your GP and ask for tests on T3, T4, TSH and auto-antibodies to the thyroid. It is very important for women with endometriosis that all four tests are done, not just the first two. Other findings from the USA National Center for Toxicological Research 'indicates that isoflavinoids could inhibit thyroid hormone synthesis, inducing goitre and even thyroid cancer'.[67]

| | | |
|---|---|---|
| Cabbage | Broccoli | Cauliflower |
| Fool's parsley | Mint | Brussels sprouts |
| Mustard | Turnip | Cress |
| Radish | Horseradish | Spinach |
| Carrot | Peach | Pear |

Table 8.5
Goitergens: foods which suppress thyroid function

Use the vegetables listed in table 8.5 freely but do not eat them in excess. The B vitamins and magnesium in them are necessary to your health. Cooking usually reduces the goitergenic effect; eaten raw they are effective at reducing thyroxine levels.

## ACHIEVING HORMONE BALANCE

It is in the interest of every woman with endometriosis to keep her hormones well balanced, and this is governed by the foods which you choose to eat and the state of your digestive tract. Correcting the digestive tract function with specialist supplements and by eating healthily will be of benefit. Foods containing both phyto-oestrogens and goitergens need to be balanced, and most of us do that instinctively by not eating the same food all the time. We are meant to eat some foods from each food group every day, but at the same time we need to try to avoid or keep to a bare minimum those which may contain dioxins and other oestrogenic substances (such as chocolate, which may contain the pesticide lindane). By being sensible in our choice of foods we ingest a wide variety of different nutrients each day (in Japan they recommend eating 100 different foods each day). We can try to do our own best, to choose and buy wisely, for our enjoyment of food must not be stilted. It is very important that we enjoy the foods we eat, so a balance has to be struck.

If you are extremely ill and one or two foods appear to be upsetting you, remove them from your diet, but ensure that they are replaced by similar foods in order to maintain the nutrient level you need. It may be beneficial to try an exclusion or a rotation diet. We must all take care to listen to what our bodies are telling us by using our sixth sense. Become aware of exactly how different foods affect your health. The judicious use of supplements may help to speed up the healing process and heal the gut membrane.

## THE MORAL OF THE STORY

You are what you eat only if your digestive system is able to obtain nutrients from the foods which you consume. You are only what you can absorb.

### DIGESTIVE SYSTEM HEALTH

The first step is to heal the digestive tract.

*Noel H of London*

*I would like to say to all the women out there who might read this book that diet is such an important factor in contributing to one's health. I eliminated dairy products, wheat, sugar, chocolate and anything with preservatives, colourings, tinned and packet microwaved junk foods. I now include fresh fruits and vegetables, organic when possible, have cut down on red meat, substituting chicken and fish. I found it strange at first, because I hadn't realized what ingredients were in most foods as I hadn't looked before. I was amazed to see all the unnatural constituents. It was difficult the first week, but gradually I enjoyed the change and now have a much healthier lifestyle. My bloating feeling had disappeared and my stomach cramps are almost non-existent*

CASE STUDY

*except when I am stressed or eat the wrong thing. I do think that the new healthier diet is an acquired taste; with most things it takes time to find the right alternative foods. Instead of chocolate I have carob bars and nuts. Instead of dairy products I enjoy goat's yogurt and soya milk and cheeses. It has made such a dramatic difference in my life. It was a week before I noticed any change. It was hard at first but I wouldn't go back to the way I was, because now I feel a totally new person. I know and feel that without this diet I would never be able to enjoy the everyday life of walking the dogs, travelling and having fun. After the initial change in food once you begin to feel so different it will be easier to continue and other things too – I found it an exciting experience. It takes slightly longer but it tastes fantastic. Try it and see for yourself. It's brilliant.*

To get an idea of exactly what we could be eating in processed foods, it is interesting to see what food additives are actually used in them. Some years ago the *Sunday Observer* ran a story about ice cream made naturally from eggs and cream in the home. It also listed all the ingredients in manufactured ice creams and explained their origins. The following list gives an idea of just what we may be eating in ice cream and other processed foods.

- Aldehyde C-17, for cherry flavouring, is a flammable liquid used in dyes, plastics and rubber. It is known to cause bladder cancer

- Amyl acetate, for banana flavouring, is a paint solvent

- Benzyl acetate, for strawberry flavours, is a nitrate solvent

- Butraldehyde, for nutty flavours, is an ingredient in rubber cement

- Diethyl glycol, used to emulsify eggs, is the same chemical which is used in anti-freeze and paint remover

- Ethyl acetate, used for pineapple flavouring, is used in the leather and textile industries. The vapours are believed to cause lung, heart and liver damage

- Piperonal, used to give a vanilla flavour, is a chemical which was used to kill lice. The body stores this substance in its cells as it cannot be excreted [68]

Looking at the above, our conclusion must be that it is always best to eat foods prepared from natural ingredients. Given the lack of available information, it is virtually impossible to surmise how damaging different combinations of food additives could be to the reproductive system.

Some short-term use of nutritional supplements may help correct imbalances in the digestive tract. Seek help from a qualified nutritionist.

If you suffer from stomach pains, diarrhoea, constipation, bloating, flatulence or anal irritation, you need to correct the digestive tract before health can be achieved. This is a key area to correct on the path to wellness. If you are malabsorbing nutrients, then no amount of good food or supplements can get you well. This area has to be healed first in order to allow nutrients to be absorbed so that they can help the reproductive system function. Herbal teas (mint, fennel or ginger) are helpful.

A selection of the following may be beneficial:

- Herbal colon cleanse
- Probiotics: acidophilus
- Slippery elm
- NAG
- Caprylic acid

- Prebiotics: FOS
- Digestive enzymes
- Milk thistle (silymarin)
- Butyric acid
- Multivitamin/mineral

## IRRITABLE BOWEL SYNDROME

Avoid all food intolerances, particularly wheat and dairy products, and citrus fruits. Some sensitive people may need to exclude all gluten grains. Obviously caffeine and sugars should be avoided and dietary fibre from fruits, vegetables and ground nuts should be increased gradually.

- Probiotics: acidophilus
- Slippery elm
- Multivitamin/mineral

- Digestive enzymes
- Mint, fennel or ginger teas

## BLOATING

Bloating is a problem in many women with endometriosis and may be due to an imbalance of gut flora. If too many antibiotics or hormones have been taken, it can increase the amount of bacteriodes bacteria in the gut (those which produce gases). By taking probiotics this balance may be restored and the bloating subside. As the state of the gut flora can affect hormone levels, these have to be corrected for women to get well. A recent international congress at the Royal College of Medicine in the UK on gut flora looked at all these problems. Gynaecologists may not know about this excellent research work. Pre- and probiotics and digestive enzymes may be tried; none have harmful side effects like those from many drugs.

Magnesium, zinc and vitamin B6 are natural diuretics as are proanthocyanidins (flavinoid family).

- NAG
- Digestive enzymes
- Zinc citrate
- Proanthocyanidins
- Multivitamin/mineral

- Acidophilus (dairy-free)
- Magnesium malate
- Vitamin B6 + B Complex (yeast-free)
- FOS
- TH207 (Biocare) or Kelp tablets

## SUMMARY

1  You are what your body can digest and absorb. It is important to eat nutrient-rich food and ignore calorie-laden junk.

2  Nutrition is essential to life. Your choice of food can make you ill or healthy. Analyse over four days exactly what you eat, then assess if you are giving your body the building blocks it needs to keep you healthy.

3  Your digestion is your first line of defence. Assess your digestion. If you suffer from heartburn, indigestion, stomach pains, gall bladder problems, flatulence and bloating, constipation or diarrhoea, something is wrong and it needs to be corrected before you can begin to get well. Introduce into your diet a digestive enzyme and acidophilus supplement to aid digestion and improve the gut flora. If you have been abroad where food and water are suspect, take some grapefruit seed extract which has an anti-bacterial and anti-parasitic effect.

4  The intestinal barrier's mucous membrane needs to be healthy. It is almost the size of a tennis court and protects us from

external elements. It also makes 80 per cent of the immunoglobulin-producing cells in the body. By acting to protect this membrane and rebalance your gut flora, you are strengthening your immune system. To help the gut membrane use slippery elm, NAG, glutamine, essential fatty acids, butyric acid and vitamin A and zinc.

5  Cleanse the liver regularly every three months or so by eating foods such as lemons, carrots, beetroot, cucumber, tomatoes, artichokes, chicory, celery, radishes, leeks, onions, cabbage, spring dandelion leaves, parsley, apricots, cold-pressed olive oil and grapefruit. The liver is the organ that degrades oestrogen and it needs to be efficient in women with endometriosis..

6  Drink three glasses of water each day and take three brisk 20-minute walks each week if possible to help stimulate the intestines.

7  To test for food intolerances cut out the suspect food from the diet for 30 days. Choose other foods as alternatives to ensure that your nutrient intake is maintained and take a multivitamin/mineral supplement to cover your change in diet. When you reintroduce the food, note any symptoms that you experience over the next 24 hours, e.g. faster pulse rate, flu-like symptoms, headaches, joint pains.

8  Insist upon tests for hypothyroid (tests for T3, T4, TSH and auto-antibodies to the thyroid), gut fermentation, gluten intolerance, and oestrogen and progesterone levels in the urine if you are suffering from fertility problems.

9  At least four vegetables, two fruits and some legumes plus a handful of nuts and seeds should be eaten each day along with some wholegrain cereal, as this will also speed up the transit time of food and provide the digestive tract with fibre which can bind to oestrogen and cholesterol and escort them from the body.

10  Spending money to service your car and repair your home seems natural. Your body is more important. You might consider giving your body a detoxification diet and spring clean. The body is designed to last us some 90 years or more and it is vital to maintain its health. Give it the tools it needs to give you a healthy old age. Endometriosis symptoms can be relieved, but it takes effort and patience.

# 9 Nutritional support for endometriosis and fertility

If the patient has been to more than four
physicians, nutrition is probably the answer
*Abraham Hoffer, MD, PhD*

Everything to do with nutrition is rather like the story of *Goldilocks and the Three Bears* in which Goldilocks settles for whatever is 'just right' for her. It implies that nothing should be eaten in excess, nothing should be eaten in deficient amounts, but that all food should be balanced: 'just right'. We hear so much about eating a 'balanced diet' that it all becomes a blur. After all, what is balanced for one person will not be correct for someone else, because of their differences in body build, health status and digestive and absorption capability. People rarely link what they eat with their state of health, although this is beginning to change. However, as we have seen in this book nutrients in food rule our state of health. But how does what you eat affect endometriosis and what should you eat to help reduce the symptoms of endometriosis?

What do we know so far? We know that endometriosis requires oestrogen in order to grow, and some women with endometriosis may have an oestrogen dominance, where oestrogen is out of balance with progesterone. We know that some pesticides may be a problem for us. Often the immune system does not function normally and remove the endometriotic implants as it should. We know too that the endometriotic implants are producing their own supplies of oestrogen and prostaglandins. There is inflammation around the implants which may cause extreme pain. There may be bowel and bladder involvement, some pain on intercourse, and women can suffer from a terrible leaden fatigue which prevents them from living the life they desire. Some women struggle terribly with a sense of loss if they are told they have infertility problems. Periods, ovulation time, even just vacating the bowels can be excruciating agony. All in all, endometriosis causes a lot of trauma.

Members of the medical profession often disbelieve the pains and other symptoms. Endometriosis is not as easy to treat as measles or a broken leg. It is a systemic disease, maybe an auto-immune disorder. When drugs and surgical treatment are used, they often just mask the symptoms and do not remove the cause. Women need to listen to the messages which their bodies give them. Illness is an imbalance and good nutrition can help to redress that imbalance. In previous chapters we have seen why and how nutrition can help to reduce the symptoms which we perceive as being triggered by endometriosis.

What you can do is try to help yourself. Living like a shadow of your former self is soul-destroying. You may wish to try the suggestions in this book. The nutrition path requires your co-operation. You have to make some changes to your life. You have to meet the needs of your body halfway. You have to feed it and you have to love it better, which takes time. You may have to work hard at this for up to six months. Inner strength may help you to reach this goal. Feeling well is a joy, particularly when you look back but now you can hardly remember what being well is like. Only you can make this decision. Become informed so that the choice can be made from the strength of knowledge. Read all the women's comments through this book again; they will help you and guide you. If they succeeded, then so could you. They were all ill, but they persevered because they believed that their bodies wanted to heal.

The main lessons to come from this book should be:

1  Eat as well as you can afford.

2  Buy the freshest food you can find.

3  Cook from fresh whenever possible or eat fresh food in salads daily once your digestion can tolerate raw vegetables.

4  Eat as wide a variety of foodstuffs as possible, remembering that 'variety is the spice of life'.


## THE MYTHICAL 'BALANCED' DIET

This chapter should help you to understand the difference between natural and unnatural foods and how their nutrient content differs wildly; and how different nutrients and supplements may be used to help the body through periods of illness. Maybe you can revise your food choice and give preventive medicine a chance. As you can see from the comments of women who have trodden the nutrition path, eating for health is not a fallacy. The link between diet and health is strong. Once the body begins to be replenished with the nutrient-based building blocks it needs to make the necessary hormones and immune cells, then it can begin to fight off the endometriotic implants.

Poor diet and/or poor absorption equals poor health. We cannot expect a sick body to begin to heal until it has the tools it needs from within. You can assess the nutrient content of your diet with the help of this chapter. Getting all the nutrients your body requires from your food can be helpful, but giving the body a boost from short-term supplementation may help to speed up this process. Caroline Walker, the dietitian, wrote in 1984 'that the importance of positively good food, above all when preparing for pregnancy, is a message vital to the health of the child as well as the mother'.[1] You can fight endometriosis and infertility by eating the best food available.

It is the *quality* of the foods eaten which can make all the difference in how our body cells function, including the cells in the reproductive system. By eating fresh, wholesome foods regularly you will give the body the fuel it needs to keep itself healthy. Fuel in this case includes the macro-nutrients (such as carbohydrates, proteins, fats and oils) and the micro-nutrients (the 52 known vitamins and minerals) plus the compounds known as phyto-chemicals. It is now recognized that dietary factors are closely linked with diseases. In fact the World Health Organization states that 'over 30 per cent of all cancers are diet related'.[2] The American National Academy of Sciences 'estimates that 60 per cent of women's cancers are related to nutritional factors'.[3]

The healthy choice should be the easy choice, but in our world of fast food and convenience meals, the healthy choice may be the hardest to make. It takes time and effort to eat well, and not resort to 'snatch and grab'-type meals. It takes conscious thought, 'Should I snack on fruit and nuts rather than cakes and cookies?' You should try to sit down and analyse all the foods you eat over the next four days. Write down absolutely everything you eat. It may be a surprise when you see the whole picture and analyse which vitamins and minerals are low in your diet. You will then be aware if you need to eat more of certain of the foods listed at the end of this chapter.

In 1991 research showed that 'older women were more likely to eat traditional foods like boiled potatoes, milk puddings, butter and preserves and bought more vegetables, while younger women ate out more and also ate convenience foods such as snacks and burgers more often'.[4] This calorie-laden food, as opposed to nutrient-rich food, leads to nutritional imbalances which have a domino effect on enzyme and hormone production. Despite the fact that so many of us eat junk food, most people today are aware of the importance of their diet: 'Seventy-one per cent of adults questioned believe that the most important thing that they do to protect their health involves eating.'[5] Choosing healthy food is the key we hold in our hands.

The word diet has connotations of limp lettuce leaves and starvation, but this is not what is meant. A healthy diet is a choice of fresh, natural, vibrant foods eaten in the appropriate quantities. And that is all you have to do – just choose to eat fresh foods every day. Giving the body the vital vitamins and minerals it needs is not difficult, and the next section looks at how to do just that.

That is all there is to it – just buying and eating the best quality and freshest foods available. In chapter 8 we looked at how the digestive system was so important in the breakdown of oestradiol, the oestrogen which causes cell proliferation and is involved with uterine and breast cancers. Why do women with endometriosis need to be so concerned with the balance of oestrogen and progesterone? What are their effects? Table 9.1 shows the effects of oestrogen and progesterone.

As with everything in the body, there is an action and an opposite reaction. Oestrogen and progesterone have to be in balance with one another, as body systems always try to create a balance. Your choice of food matters as it affects hormone production. You can help your body to heal itself.

Nutrients are those substances within the foods which we physically ingest and are used in order to maintain body cells, to provide materials for growth and repair, to promote energy and hormone production, or are used in order to regulate these processes. Some substances in food, such as caffeine and alcohol, are not looked upon as nutrients as they have no role in body maintainance and, indeed, may hinder the body's search for stability and health. They are stimulants that can cause internal stress, which is the last thing you need with endometriosis.

| Oestrogen effects | Progesterone effects |
|---|---|
| Causes the womb lining to thicken | Causes the endometrium to shed |
| Body fat deposits increase | Body fat is used for energy |
| Triggers depression and headaches | Acts as an antidepressant |
| Stimulates breast tissue | Protects breast tissue |
| Feeling less sexy | Normal feelings restored |
| Causes salt, sugar and fluid retention | Acts as a natural diuretic |
| Increases the risk of breast cancer | Helps prevent breast cancer |
| Counteracts thyroid hormone action | Aids thyroid hormone action |
| Causes copper levels to increase and zinc to decrease | Helps to balance copper and zinc levels |
| Reduces the supply of oxygen to all cells | Corrects the supply of oxygen to cells |
| Increases the risk of uterine cancer | Helps prevent uterine cancer |
| Increases the risk of blood clotting | Normalizes the risk of blood clots |
| Prolongs the menstrual bleed time | Normalizes the menstrual bleed time |
| Acts as an abortive | Maintains the pregnancy |
| High corticosterone | Precursor of corticosterone production |
| Reduces bone building by restraining osteoclast function | Stimulates bone building by stimulating osteoclasts |
| Stimulates the nervous system | Calms the nervous system |
| Reduces the tone of blood vessels | |
| Impairs blood sugar control | Normalizes blood sugar control |

Table 9.1
Effects of oestrogen and progesterone

# HEALTHY DIETS

As Hippocrates said in 460 BC, 'Let food be your medicine and medicine be your food.'

Your body is made from the foodstuffs you eat and the water you drink. We are almost 60 per cent water, 23 per cent protein, 14 per cent fats and 3 per cent minerals. The quality of what you put into

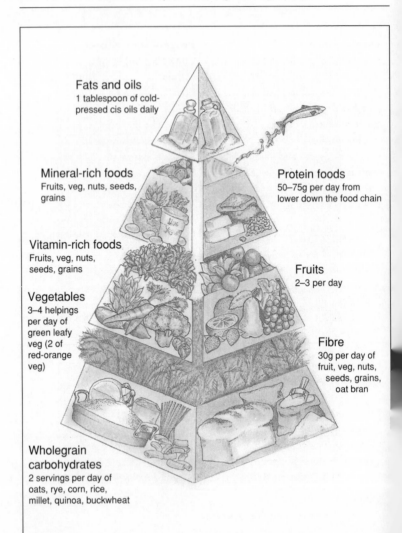

Figure 9.1

The Food Pyramid. A guide to the food groups from which you should pick your daily diet. By choosing the highest quality food you can ensure that the body can reach its optimum health potential. Remember that your body is entirely composed of the food you eat and the water you drink. Reproduced with kind permission of P Holford of ION from *Optimum Nutrition Magazine*, 9, p. 3, Autumn 1996 yourself is obviously a key to the health of the cells and tissues in your body.

What should we be eating to maintain good health? We hear constantly that if we eat a balanced diet we will be fine. But what exactly does that mean? For lots of us it would seem to involve confusion and effort: 'Many people regard healthy eating as difficult to achieve and that it requires great psychological effort to maintain a healthy change.'[6] People worry about time spent in food preparation, self-control, and the cost of fresh food, and the fact that 'the experts keep changing their minds' as another 'fad' comes into vogue. Sometimes mixed messages are given which can be totally confusing. In the end most people may feel bamboozled and give up. They continue eating the foods they have grown up with and those they enjoy without thinking.

In the UK the 'Balance of Good Health' logo used by dietitians and the Health Education Council shows a picture of a plate divided into five segments: fruit and vegetables; bread and other cereals and potatoes; milk and dairy foods; fatty and sugary foods; meat and fish; and alternatives. In the USA the fourth edition of *Dietary Guidelines for Americans* uses a Food Pyramid (figure 9.1) to emphasize the number of servings recommended from six food groups to meet the guidelines.[7] For our purposes we will use the Food Pyramid as it comes closer to the desired intake of nutrients. Chapter 10 will look at what foods should be eaten to maintain health, while chapter 9 concentrates upon nutrients and supplements. By looking at the diagram of the Food Pyramid it can be seen that we need to keep variety at the forefront of our choice of foods. The guidelines are as follows:

Drink one litre of fresh filtered water each day.

Eat 3–4 helpings of fresh green leafy vegetables per day, 2 servings of red–orange vegetables and 2 pieces of fresh fruit.

Eat 2–3 servings of wholegrain cereals such as rice, oats, rye, buckwheat, corn, millet, quinoa or wheat, unless you are grain-intolerant. Then you can use root vegetables, sago, tapioca or arrowroot, banana or chestnut flours.

Eat 30g of fibre foods each day. This comes from the fruit, vegetables and wholegrain cereals or nuts and seeds.

Eat some complex carbohydrate foods daily such as cereals, root vegetables, or pulse vegetables (legumes) as this supplies slow-releasing sugars into the body to sustain energy levels.

6  Eat 1 tablespoon of fresh cold-pressed cis oils each day from sesame, sunflower, safflower, olive or eat seeds and nuts, or use 1 tablespoon of ground linseeds with breakfast. Avoid trans fats.

7  Eat 50–75g of protein foods per day, choosing from a variety of sources so that you take in a wide range of amino acids, e.g. pulse vegetables (legumes), grains, nuts and seeds, eggs, dairy foods (cow, goat and ewes), and fresh fish or lean organic meats.

## Janet H of Berkshire

*I have found that a combination diet has helped over the last few years, i.e. not mixing starch and protein foods at the same meal.*

CASE STUDY

The foodstuffs we eat are divided into different groups by their chemical structure and the way in which they act when metabolized by the body. The main divisions are:

1  Macro-nutrients, composed of the proteins, carbohydrates and fats, and essential oils.

2  Micro-nutrients, consisting of tiny amounts of vitamins and minerals, essential oils and phytochemicals.

There are also the non-digestible fibres and water which we require to stay healthy. Eating a balanced diet means that we have to choose wisely from all these areas and maintain a variety.

## MACRO-NUTRIENTS

*Proteins*

Protein is Greek for 'I am first'. Proteins are the building blocks of life. Without them we cannot build new cells, tissues, enzymes, hormones, antibodies, macrophages and neurotransmitters. There are twenty-two known amino acids and in different combinations they build new cells. If you think of the 26 letters of the alphabet and the number of words in a dictionary, you can imagine the many uses of amino acids joined together in chains. The variety is almost endless. The quality of the protein you eat should be the best. Fifteen per cent of our daily food intake should be protein, around 75g (or 3 oz), depending on body build. This should come mainly from vegetable sources, with occasional meat, eggs, dairy foods and fish.

Animal protein foods are rich in saturated fats which need to be kept low. Include in the diet small amounts of organic pork, lamb and dairy produced from cows, sheep and goats to reduce your intake of saturated fats. Chicken, turkey, venison, game birds and eggs are good sources of protein and are lower in saturated fats. Fibrous foods bind to cholesterol and oestrogen to remove them from the body, so by balancing these fatty foods with oats and legumes you allow the body to maintain its homeostasis naturally.

Vegetable proteins are found in pulse vegetables (peas, beans and lentils), seed vegetables (broccoli, cauliflower), wholegrain cereals, and nuts and seeds. Nuts and seeds also contain the good quality cis oils which our cells so desperately need. If you are vegetarian or vegan, you need to take in sufficient vegetables and grains to meet your needs as well as ensuring you have adequate vitamin B12 supplements in your diet. Two helpings of vegetable protein each day would be adequate.

*Carbohydrates*

There are three forms of carbohydrate: simple sugars such as glucose, and fructose; double sugars such as sucrose (table sugar), maltose, lactose; and the long-chain carbohydrates such as cereal fibre and vegetables which are broken down slowly and release sugars steadily into the bloodstream. This is the way our bodies evolved to maintain a constant supply of energy production in cells.

Fast-releasing simple sugars dump too much glucose too quickly into the bloodstream for our pancreas and liver enzymes to deal with, and this can lead to illness. In 1907 people ate on average 7 pounds of sugar a year; by 1991 this had risen to 120 pounds per person, and our body cells and pancreas are not designed to deal with such vast amounts.

The eight pints of blood in the body require only two teaspoons of glucose to be circulating at any one moment. Insulin (which requires zinc) and glucose tolerance factor (which requires vitamin B3, chromium and manganese) help to maintain this fine balance.

But if you munch on bars of chocolates, cakes and cookies all day, you will use up all the zinc, B3, chromium and manganese, and end up with a stressed pancreas and liver. Eat these foods as occasional treats so that they stay special, rather than as everyday foods. When you are feeling hungry, the body is sending a message that it needs more nutrients. It does not want and cannot use sugars and fats in vast quantities. Eat nuts and seeds or fruits as snacks.

The body burns the carbohydrate glucose in every cell to provide energy, but we do not have to eat sweet foods to provide glucose. Our digestive system makes the enzyme amylase, which breaks down all the complex carbohydrate foods into simple sugars, but this is done at a steady rate so that the bloodstream carries a constant supply of glucose to the cells for energy production. Wholegrain cereals, root and pulse vegetables, and fresh fruits contain these slow-releasing carbohydrates, whereas sweets, cakes, cookies, pastries, honey and most refined foods are laced with sugars which release glucose into the blood too quickly. One Mars bar contains the equivalent of eight teaspoons of sugar, a small pot of yogurt may have seven, and a glass of alcohol has eight. Sugar excess can lead to problems like diabetes or low blood sugar (hypoglycaemia) where we suffer from high and low mood swings and dizziness. All refined sugars are unnecessary and should only be eaten occasionally as a treat, as our ancestors ate them when they found a honeycomb.

Complex carbohydrates come neatly packaged with vitamins and minerals combined in bananas, seeds and legumes, whereas refined sugars have been so processed that the essential vitamin and mineral content is depleted. Two-thirds of your daily carbohydrate diet should come from dark green leafy, legumes (peas, beans and lentils) and root vegetables (potatoes, parsnips, carrots, turnips, swedes), wholegrain cereals and fresh fruits.

*Fats and oils*

A well-balanced diet is composed of 30 per cent good quality fats and oils. The term 'good quality' means that they should be fresh and not rancid, and should be cold-pressed (the cis form). There are three main groups of fats: saturated fats from animals, mono-unsaturated and poly-unsaturated vegetable oils. Saturated hard fats from animal sources from meat, eggs and dairy foods should be eaten in small amounts. An excess can be bad for the heart and the arteries, and can lead to obesity. Too many fat cells equals too much oestrogen and with endometriosis this is undesirable. Your body weight should be within health guidelines for your height (*see* the section on body mass index in chapter 4).

The unsaturated oils come from nuts and seeds. Olive oil provides us with mono-unsaturated oil, and sunflower, safflower and sesame give us poly-unsaturated oils. The oil which you buy should never be hydrogenated, as this process turns them into undesirable trans fats which act just like saturated fats in the body, plus they lack valuable vitamin E. Only choose oils which say cold-pressed, unhydrogenated or unrefined on the label. As we have seen in chapter 3 the good quality cis oils are responsible for the production of prostaglandins, cell membranes, the all-important steroid hormones, brain cells, and skin cells. A good visual sign of deficiency is a dry skin.

Omega 3 oils, rich in alpha-linolenic acid, come from fish, pumpkin, flax seeds (*see* figure 3.4), while the omega 6 oils, rich in linoleic acid, come from sesame, safflower and sunflower oils (*see* figure 3.3). The body needs fresh supplies of both daily. As heat and light damage these oils, they are best eaten cold in salad dressings, or mixed into yogurt or soups. They should be stored in the fridge in a can or dark jar. The steroid hormones and prostaglandins are made from the oils you eat.

Two other substances which the body requires are not really 'nutrients' themselves but they do carry nutrients along with them.

*Fibre*

On average we should be eating around 30g of fibrous food daily, from fruits, vegetables, wholegrain cereals, nuts and seeds. Fibre is not digested by the body, but in transit through the intestines it absorbs water and binds with toxins as well as with oestrogens and cholesterol, to help remove them from the body. Oat bran fibre is the best. Wheat bran can be too harsh on the villi in the intestine. Fibre prevents constipation, diverticulitis and slow passage of food. Foods which are constipating are wheat, bananas, some cheeses and eggs. Speedy passage of waste prevents harmful toxins being absorbed into the body, where they can lead to a sluggish system and lack of energy. If we become constipated through lack of water and fibre, toxins build up and may lead to bowel cancers. Anyone who has suffered from constipation will know how toxic the body can feel and the feeling of freshness after relief is gained.

*Water*

Water is vital to life. After all, our bodies are two-thirds water. Fruits and vegetables have a high water content and, if we drink plenty of fluid, our body cells can detoxify more easily than if we are dehydrated. Try this test. Sit down and place your hand palm down on your thigh. Gradually you will see that the veins on the back of the hand puff up and stand out. As the veins become full of blood, slowly raise the hand and watch carefully what happens to the veins. If the veins go flat by chest level, the body needs another quart of fluid. If the veins take until chin level to go flat, you are one pint down. If the veins do not stand out when your hand rests on your thigh, you are dehydrating and need to drink water to replace your electrolytes.

Try to drink about 1 litre of fresh filtered water each day – 3–6 glasses full. Coffee, tea and alcohol are diuretics that cause water loss, removing minerals that are valuable for the reproductive system. Herb and fruit teas can be useful, especially mint, fennel, ginger, cinnamon (which aids digestion), limeblossom and chamomile (which are calmatives) and raspberry leaf tea (which relaxes the uterus muscle). One cup of green leaf tea daily is said to enhance the immune system. One cup per day of Pau d'Aco tea from South America, available in health food shops, has an anti-candidiasis effect. Always filter all water to remove chemicals. Never drink unfiltered tap water as it is high in chlorine and may contain fluorides, which are not helpful with endometriosis.

---

## Sarah G of Tyne and Wear

*I was diagnosed as having endo when I was 18, I am now 23. For as long as I can remember, I always had the most agonising period pains, but thought that this was normal. I would spend a good week each month practically overdosing on painkillers which never actually alleviated any of the pain.*

*Previous to my diagnosis, I started experiencing awful stinging pains in the bottom right of my abdomen. I was told I had a bladder infection and when I suggested endo I was promptly told I was 'far too young' and I specifically remember the comment 'oh, you'd know if you had it'. Know about it? I couldn't sleep because the pain was so bad. I eventually had a laparoscopy privately which revealed that, yes, I had*

C
A
S
E

S
T
U
D
Y

*endometriosis. I was unfamiliar with the disease, but was reassured by doctors that drugs could help. Luckily I already knew a nutritionist, who had been treating my brother with nutrition – he has ME. I have avoided taking any of the drugs given for endo. I was advised to change my diet considerably and to start taking a number of supplements. To be honest, at the time, I wasn't really convinced that changing my diet and taking a few supplements would help. It took a while, but finally I went on the diet programme free from yeasts, refined sugars, dairy foods and caffeine. Basically I ate fresh, natural food, nothing processed. I discovered after eliminating wheat from my diet, that I was particularly sensitive to it, to the extent that when I ate it I became tired, bloated and my stomach would hurt.*

*I also started taking a considerable number of supplements. There was one multivitamin/mineral, a vitamin C, a vitamin B complex, and acidophilus and four Efamol Marine capsules per day. This may sound like an awful lot to anyone who just takes one regular multi each day. I had also been put onto the contraceptive pill to stop the endo spreading and this leaves you deficient in a number of vitamins. [Author: It puts vitamin A and copper levels up and B vitamins and zinc down.]*

*Although this regime may seem pretty drastic, especially the diet, it's not, and it really helped me over the past five years. Not only has it helped with the pain, I've had the added bonus of losing a little weight, increased energy and fabulous skin, which everyone still comments on!! For me the most effective supplement was the evening primrose and fish oils, which is great for hair and skin, but most significantly, it acts as an anti-inflammatory, which has subsequently helped control the stomach pains. Since I was diagnosed I have had to have two laparoscopies and extensive laser surgery when my endo spread. However, the inflammation has calmed down, and my surgeon is most surprised.*

*Nutrition plays such an important part in controlling endo, it seems to me that very few doctors are aware of this fact, and that is why nutritionists can play such an important role in helping to control the symptoms of endo.*

*Endo is not something that has to rule your life, and from my experience you can at least control the awful pain which is so often associated with the disease. I still stick to the diet and take some supplements, but often I forget why I am taking them in the first place, since I have so few problems today.*

## MICRO-NUTRIENTS
*Vitamins and minerals*

Vitamins are used by the body in minute amounts. If you remember chemistry lessons, you often had to measure infinitesimal quantities of powders and mix them together. Then something amazing would happen and you ended up with a totally different substance – like making a cake!

Vitamins and minerals are catalysts of many reactions in the body, present in tiny amounts but precisely regulating what happens. The body suffers if it becomes vitamin depleted, as processes become unregulated and things can go haywire. They act as keys to our system. Lose the key and you can't open the door. The right key will trigger body processes, making the immune cells, neurotransmitters, enzymes and hormones work effectively. Endometriosis certainly feels like the body has gone haywire.

*Vitamins.* The vitamin B complex group and vitamin C are water-soluble, so the body cannot store them. Therefore they should be eaten every day. They are found in plant foods, and the fresher the plant the higher its nutrient content. Vitamins A, D, E and K are fat-soluble (in oily foods) and can be stored in the liver. Vitamins A, C and E are antioxidants which are protective against diseases and pollutants caused by free radical damage. Vitamin D (which is actually a hormone in its own right) ensures that our bones balance their calcium levels. Vitamin E protects our own oil-based cell membrane from going rancid, so it literally keeps us fresh. Vitamin A as retinol from animal foods and as beta-carotene from vegetable foods is vital for skin and tissue health.

Certain vitamins affect the reproductive and endocrine systems. The one everyone knows about is folic acid. Deficiency of folic acid is known to lead to spina bifida in the newborn. Folic acid is required by day 27 after conception and malformation of the fetus may occur if it is low. Many vitamin deficiencies are linked to malformations. Some vitamins work within the endocrine system and balance its workings. One study of 6,400 adults done in Basle, Switzerland, found that 22.8 per cent of women had low levels of thiamine (vitamin B1).

A deficiency of thiamine in animals begun 11–15 days before the mated caused 83 per cent of the embryos to be absorbed. If the deficiency had begun earlier, still most animals had no implantation and often ovulation was inhibited.[8] Clearly if this applied to mankind the function of the reproductive system would be damaged. A syndrome known as lutenizing unruptured follicle (LUF), where the egg remains trapped within the ovary follicle, has been reported in as many as 79 per cent of women with endometriosis.[9] It has been seen from research to correlate with anxiety. Our adrenal glands help us to cope with stress and anxiety. Vitamin B2 (riboflavin) is essential for adrenal gland function together with vitamin B5 and vitamin C.[10] Endometriosis 'thrives on stress-related immune system weakness, which can control a woman's body and her life'.[11] Riboflavin deficiency also causes hormonal imbalances and is essential for the homeostasis and liver clearance of oestradiol and progesterone. If these hormones accumulate in the liver they inhibit the release of LHRH from the hypothalamus and GnRH secretion from the pituitary which would result in infertility. In animals reproduction fails if enzyme levels of B2 and B5 are low.[12] Vitamin B6 encourages the production of progesterone. Some research indicates that the oestrogen and progesterone levels of women with endometriosis are slightly out of balance (there is not enough progesterone for the amount of oestrogen).[13]

Looking at many other pieces of research we can find thousands of pointers as to how vitamins are needed by the endocrine and reproductive systems. Thiamine is required for ovarian hormone production; a deficiency inhibits ovulation. Riboflavin helps the balance between oestrogen and progesterone. When supplies of B2 are low, production of GnRH in the hypothalamus is inhibited, which slows production of FSH and LH from the pituitary. If vitamin B3 is deficient, it causes a deficiency of folic acid and zinc. Vitamin B6 is essential in the hypothalamus to act as a coenzyme in the production of GnRH. It is also a precursor to progesterone and serotonin (a neurotransmitter in the brain). The macrophages of the immune system cannot do their work clearing endometrial implants if they are B6-deficient. You can see how important just the B vitamins are in keeping you healthy. The pill, HRT and antibiotics all have a harmful effect on the blood levels of B vitamins, so you could take a B vitamin supplement to help normalize levels while taking these preparations.

*Minerals*. Minerals are also needed in tiny quantities by cells: calcium for strong bones, teeth and the nervous system; magnesium for muscles and nerve cells; zinc for insulin and the brain and immune cells; chromium for blood sugar balance; iron to carry oxygen in the blood and for immune cells; and selenium for protection against free radical damage and disease.

Magnesium deficiency lowers thiamine levels in body cells and it works to produce energy. Research also shows it is very important in relaxing smooth muscle and may be of benefit in relieving menstrual cramps. It is used in the immune system for production of complement which helps to remove invading alien cells. Magnesium also promotes sleep, so insomniacs may find it useful. When thyroid function is low, you feel the cold, and magnesium works with iodine and selenium in the thyroid to help temperature regulation. The function of the ovary is also dependent on the body's supply of magnesium.

Zinc works alongside vitamin B6 in the hypothalamus to aid production of GnRH, which takes the message via the pituitary to tell the ovaries how and when to function. A high intake of wheat may reduce zinc levels, as wheat contains phytic acid which can bind to zinc and block its use by the body. White marks on the fingernails indicate zinc deficiency. Zinc is a component of insulin and may prevent ovarian cysts if balanced with copper, iron and manganese.

Chromium is essential for balancing the blood sugar levels and has been seen to help reduce cravings for sweet things. It is a part of glucose tolerance factor along with vitamin B3. Chromium deficiency causes excessive sweats, irritability, cravings and drowsiness during the day.

Hair mineral analysis is quite effective at showing if you have low levels of minerals which can then be rebalanced with short-term mineral supplementation. An audit of 150 women with diagnosed endometriosis has shown that they have a common pattern of deficiencies of vitamins C, B1 B3 and B6 and the minerals magnesium, zinc and chromium. Look at the charts at the end of this chapter (see p. 241) and ensure that your diet is rich in foods containing these nutrients. If it is, but you are still ill, look to healing your digestive tract which may have been compromised by stress, drugs or surgery. Malabsorption can be having a detrimental effect on your whole body's health. Read chapter 8 again and see what steps you can take to help improve your absorption of nutrients. Some women do not eat nutrient-rich food, but the vast majority try very hard to eat well. We know that endometriosis is systemic, it does not just affect the uterus and ovaries. To help yourself to heal you need to help your whole body. Plenty of fresh fruits, vegetables nuts and seeds should enhance your intake of vitamins and minerals. At the end of this chapter there is a section to explain the role of each vitamin and mineral in the reproductive system (*see* p. 241).

## POOR NUTRIENT INTAKE

Diets are easily unbalanced. Many people cook the same tried-and-tested dishes day after day, year after year and do not eat a varied diet. This reduces the amount of nutrients and phytochemicals eaten. And this, in turn, reduces the strength of the immune army, the production of hormones, enzymes and gastric juices, neurotransmitter function etc. This amounts to a 'domino effect': being low on some nutrients in the diet has a profound effect on the body's production of these vital messengers. Liken it to a large hall in Japan, where for fun they often set out long, swirling lines of dominoes. Someone flicks a switch and the dominoes begin to fall one by one creating amazing patterns, twists and turns. Our body's metabolism flows rather like this. Creation of one enzyme triggers production of a hormone, which causes a gland to produce another hormone – but only if the nutrient is present to help the enzyme key that hormones need. It is as complicated as a road map. But poor nutrient uptake is like removing some of the dominoes in the patterns. For instance, if you remove some of the zinc you could not make the enzymes, therefore the hormone could not be produced, and so the cells cannot work at their optimum level, and they become ill. This is called subclinical deficiency – we function below par. What we need is to reach 'enzyme saturation' level, where every cell has all the vitamins and minerals it needs in order to work efficiently.

Zinc, for instance, is required by over 200 enzymes. Imagine 200 enzyme-dominoes in a row. If you absorb sufficient zinc, all 200 of the dominoes will pass on their energy to a hormone or enzyme. If you absorb insufficient zinc, some of the dominoes may not fall, so the production of a zinc-dependent hormone will fail. Effective production of proteins for hormones, enzymes within body cells will also begin to fail and the body fall ill. Magnesium works over 300 enzymes. If we are deficient in zinc or magnesium, some of the body systems may begin to fail or at least work erratically. This would mean that hormones and immune cells will not be produced at the optimum level to make all the body systems function normally. Vital messages could not be sent or may be garbled, which changes normal cellular functioning.

Vitamins and minerals are synergistic with one another (they balance one another's reactions), or they may be antagonistic, so that if one is too high the other may be forced too low, or if one is deficient, it may trigger deficiency in anothe or each may amplify the effect of another. For instance, if vitamin E is deficient 'this depletes the body of zinc, which in turn raises copper levels [...] high copper levels have been related to high oestrogen levels, and this in turn has been connected with ovarian cysts and depression'.[14] Research shows that 'deficiency in vitamin B6 automatically lowers vitamin B2 levels, that impairs the metabolism of folic acid, B5 and zinc. In turn vitamin C and A uptake are affected. Low vitamin C will prevent efficient absorption of iron, again allowing excess copper into the system which harms zinc even more.'[15] Folic acid is not absorbed well without zinc, but excess folic acid reduces all the other B vitamins. It is like a vicious circle, and it has profound effects on the production of hormones for the reproductive system. As we have seen, vitamin B6 and zinc are vital to the production of GnRH in the hypothalamus and their levels affect pituitary production of FSH and LH which trigger the ovarian function.

## ANTI-NUTRIENTS

Caffeine, alcohol, cigarettes and heavy metals have detrimental effects on our intake of nutrients, as they can act as diuretics and remove nutrients from the body, or they may block nutrient uptake.

### Caffeine

Studies have shown that 'women who were heavy coffee drinkers before pregnancy (seven or more cups per day) had, either before or after adjustment, almost a doubled chance of difficulty in becoming pregnant compared with the women who drank little or no coffee (less than one cup)'.[16] Caffeine is also found in colas, tea and chocolate and some painkillers. Other chemicals associated with caffeine are theophylline and theobromine, both of which are known to be nervous system stimulants. Caffeine robs the body of thiamin (vitamin B1), inositol, biotin, zinc, calcium and iron. It appears to have an effect on ovarian function.

Things which matter most must never be at the mercy
of things which matter least.

*Goethe*

*Alcohol*

Research revealed that 'the risk of endometriosis was roughly 50 per
cent higher in women with any alcohol intake than in control
subjects in research. In the body we know that alcohol is converted
into fat for storage and that all fat cells in the body in turn produce
oestrogens. Moderate alcohol use may contribute to the risk of
specific types of infertility'.[17] Alcohol robs the body of the vitamins
A, D, E, K, and all the B complex group and magnesium. The latest
research suggests that women should give up all alcohol if they want
to become pregnant. Women who drank less than five units a week
were twice as likely to get pregnant as those who consume ten. Dr
Tina Kold Jensen, of the National University Hospital in Denmark,
reported the research in the *British Medical Journal*. Women had the
best chance of conceiving when they did not drink at all. It was felt
that alcohol disrupted the ability of the fertilized egg to implant in
the womb. So although women conceived, the body would abort a
pregnancy.[18] Those women with endometriosis who are attempting
to become pregnant should note this information.

*Smoking*

It is common knowledge that smoking causes cancer but less well
known that it also affects reproductive health: 'Current and past
smokers have reduced gonadotrophin-stimulated ovarian function.
Tobacco exposure is associated with decreased oestrogen, and
decreased numbers of oocytes. Smoking has an adverse effect on
ovarian function.'[19] Research also suggests that 'women with
prenatal exposure to their own mother's cigarette smoking had
reduced fecundity; that is they found it less easy to become pregnant
themselves'.[20] If you smoke, you may damage your future daughter's
ovaries and her chances of achieving a pregnancy. Nicotine robs
cells of vitamin C, B1, calcium and the whole B complex family. For
each cigarette smoked the body uses 25mg of vitamin C! Recent
research reported by the American Chemical Society found 'a by-
product of cancer-causing chemicals (known as NNK) in the urine

of babies born to mothers who smoked. These compounds passed through all of the babies' cells and were present in 22 out of 31 urine samples taken from newborn babies whose mothers smoked, while none were found in the urine of babies whose mothers did not smoke'. As endometriosis cells behave similarly to cancer cells, women with endometriosis may wish to refrain from smoking before and during pregnancy and lactation.[21]

*Heavy metals*

A diet which is rich in calcium, magnesium, selenium, iron and zinc protects us from the bad effects of 'heavy' metals such as lead, mercury and cadmium. These latter metallic elements are damaging to body cells. Lead is known to be mutagenic, causing abnormalities in the fetus. Contact with these metals should be avoided where possible. Lead is found in paints and petrol and cadmium comes from cigarettes. Dr Bryan Hellewell, advisor on toxic metals to the Environmental Health Agency in the UK warns that, 'In the face of mounting evidence of danger and an absence of evidence of safety, it is my duty to advise that the use of mercury dental amalgam tooth fillings in the mouths of women who are pregnant should be discontinued.' Research shows that 'mercury is seen to cause birth defects and nervous system disorders and it is best to avoid dental fillings while pregnant'[22] and 'copper in excess can also cause problems in the liver and digestive tract'.[23] Eating an excess of chocolate can be a problem for some: 'The total dietary copper intake by males and females was positively associated with the consumption of chocolate foods.'[24] High copper correlates with high oestrogen and women with endometriosis and those attempting pregnancy need to keep oestrogen in balance. High copper is also related to ovarian cyst formation.

## ASSESSING YOUR NEEDS

Using the Food Pyramid on p. 212, the vitamin and mineral listings at the end of this chapter, and the chart provided, you can analyse the foods you eat over the next two days. With endometriosis, infertility and pain, we are trying to target the nutrients to begin a healing process. It is therefore very important that you assess your diet in order to work out if you do take in the B vitamins, magnesium, zinc and essential oils etc., which the reproductive system requires. It may take a little time, but as you work through this you will begin to see just which foods you need to add to your diet and which you need to reduce or exclude. Wanting to feel well again can act as the spur. Photocopy the chart on pages 228 and 229 two times and write down absolutely everything you eat over the next four days. *Be honest with yourself* in order to get the best picture. Use the vitamin and mineral charts at the end of this chapter to help you. Try to judge whether or not you are eating a good range of vitamins and minerals. Two examples are given to guide you, one of a good diet and the other of a sub-optimal diet.

**DAY ONE**

**Breakfast:** ....................................................................................
....................................................................................

**Lunch:** ........................................................................................
....................................................................................

**Dinner:** ......................................................................................
....................................................................................

**Snacks:** ......................................................................................
....................................................................................

**DAY TWO**

**Breakfast:** ....................................................................................
....................................................................................

**Lunch:** ........................................................................................
....................................................................................

**Dinner:** ......................................................................................
....................................................................................

**Snacks:** ......................................................................................
....................................................................................

## Self-analysis chart
(transfer the nutrient details to analyse intake and highlight wheat in yellow, dairy in blue)

| Food group | Breakfast | Lunch | Dinner | Snacks |
|---|---|---|---|---|
| Protein | | | | |
| Carbohydrate | | | | |
| Fats/oils | | | | |
| Water | | | | |
| Fibre | | | | |
| Vitamins | | | | |
| Minerals | | | | |

**Sub-optimal diet**. From a woman who was referred by her gynaecologist and was on her third IVF attempt.

**Breakfast**: Sugar-coated cereal, milk, toast and chocolate spread. Two cups of black coffee with sugar.

**Lunch**: Chips and beefburger with ketchup and fried onions. Two cans of fizzy drink and a bar of chocolate.

**Dinner**: Crisps and chocolate cake, black coffee and two cans of lager.

| Food group | Breakfast | Lunch | Dinner |
|---|---|---|---|
| **Protein** | milk | beef | |
| **Carbohydrate** | sugar/cereal chocolate spread sugar in coffee | bread roll chips ketchup onion | crisps/chocolate cake |
| **Fats/ oils** | chocolate spread cream in milk | beef fat chip fat onion cooked in oil bar of chocolate | crisps fat chocolate cake |
| **Water** | in coffee | in canned drink | coffee/lager |
| **Fibre** | cereal | potato/onion | crisps |
| **Vitamins** | A&D in milk cereal fortified with B vitamins | vitamin C in potato and onion folic acid B6 | |
| **Minerals** | calcium in milk | potassium calcium | copper in chocolate |

You can see that the above diet is too high in refined starches, sugars and hydrogenated trans oils. There is no fresh fruit and the only vegetable is the onion. The coffee and alcohol are diuretics and take the few minerals being eaten out of the body. This diet is lacking in vitamin C, B complex and magnesium and zinc. There is no nutrient intake from fresh fruits, vegetables and nuts. The chosen protein source is high in saturated fats. No good quality cis oils are present, only the poor quality trans oils. The high refined starch and sugar content could lead to low blood sugar and would not sustain energy levels and stamina. This woman was experiencing peaks and troughs in energy levels throughout the day. It took some time to improve her health due to the long-term poor nutrient intake. However, she persevered and improved her eating pattern, and had a successful pregnancy.

**Ideal diet**. From a woman with severe endometriosis who had tried many drug treatments and also had extreme irritable bowel syndrome. In other words her digestive tract was probably inflamed and malabsorbing nutrients, despite her seemingly good diet.

**Breakfast**: Muesli with nuts, seeds, banana and natural yogurt, lemon and ginger tea.

**Lunch**: Mackerel salad with rye crackers, fresh fruit salad. Still water with lemon.

**Dinner**: Stir-fry vegetables with tofu and brown rice, apple. Limeblossom tea.

| Food group | Breakfast | Lunch | Dinner |
|---|---|---|---|
| **Protein** | nuts, seeds, yogurt | mackerel | tofu<br>brown rice |
| **Carbohydrate** | wheat, oats, rye, millet flakes | Ryvita | brown rice |
| **Fats/oils** | in nuts and seeds | mackerel | stir-fry olive oil |
| **Water** | herb tea | still water | herb tea |
| **Fibre** | muesli<br>banana | salad veg<br>rye<br>fruit | brown rice<br>vegetables<br>apple |
| **Vitamins** | A,D, C, B6, E | A, B complex, E, C | B complex, A, C, E |
| **Minerals** | calcium<br>magnesium<br>zinc | selenium<br>zinc<br>calcium<br>potassium | calcium<br>magnesium<br>zinc<br>potassium |

This person was receiving more vitamins and minerals each day. She was eating more good quality cis oils from the olive oil, the fish and the nuts and seeds, as well as vegetable protein sources and a good range of fibre foods. All the carbohydrate foods were complex, thus releasing sugars gradually into the bloodstream, keeping energy levels even throughout the day. She also ate a wide range of fresh fruits and vegetables. She was sensitive to wheat and, once that was removed and the digestive tract inflammation had been corrected with supplements, this woman's symptoms eased.

## NUTRITIONAL SUPPLEMENTS

Why should we need supplements at all if our diet is balanced? After all, if we eat a balanced diet we should stay healthy. The trouble is that most of us have diets that are unbalanced. If your diet is well balanced and you are healthy, then taking supplements may not be necessary. However, if you are ill and your diet is not the best it can be, then taking supplements for the short term to give the body cells a boost can be beneficial to the healing process. Also digestive problems do affect absorption. Being ill shows that the body is not coping, so short-term supplementation for 3–4 months to correct imbalances can be tried, while the diet or digestion are being corrected.

## *Jo R of Slough*

*I am 25 years old and have had painful periods for as far back as I can remember. By the age of 18 the period and pre-period pains worsened and I found myself suffering for 2 weeks of my cycle, leading up to my period. My pre-period symptoms were stomach cramps, tiredness, water retention and extremely volatile moods, which would last up until my bleeding began. Once my period came, for the first 2-3 days, the pain in my lower abdominal area would be so excruciating, that at the time I found it difficult to stand up straight. My bleeding would be so heavy that I found it difficult to function at all. Once the first few days had passed, I would have a fairly normal period, which lasted, for approx. three more days and then two fairly pain-free weeks until the cycle began again.*

   *This became increasingly more difficult as it not only affected my*

•

C
A
S
E

S
T
U
D
Y

•

*work, as I was incapable of working for 3 days a month, but my social relationships were also affected, as I was so lethargic and irritable.*

*My doctor's response to my repeated pleas for help were, 'Do you think you're the only woman who has ever had period pains.' Typical.*

*Out of desperation I changed my doctor and set about the many elimination tests, scans and examinations until finally, following a laparoscopy, I was diagnosed as having a classic case of endo in my pelvis and lower abdominal area.*

*I was advised that my only form of treatment would be a hysterectomy or hormone treatment. As you can imagine I opted for the latter of the two and began taking Provera 3 times daily.*

*After about 3 weeks of this treatment my body shook so ferociously that I found it difficult to hold a cup of tea without spilling it. Huge boils appeared on my back and shoulders, and hair began to sprout from my neck, face and lower body. I returned to my consultant who immediately took me off Provera treatment. We discussed the other possibilities but I still kindly refused a hysterectomy! I then tried taking the pill continuously with a break every 3 months. My mood swings remained and the rest of my body eventually gave up, and I had problem after problem with headaches, haemorrhoids, to greasy hair and acne.*

*It was at this time that a friend read an article written by Dian. I drove down for a nutrition consultation and found that I gained more answers and satisfaction in the hour I had with her, than the entire time I had been under the various consultants and GPs.*

*I started a nutrition programme which incorporated diet, exercise and vitamin supplements. I cut out wheat, alcohol and caffeine and supplemented my diet with a multivitamin/mineral, evening primrose oil, vitamin B6, fish oils, acidophilus, vitamin C and magnesium. Within 2 months I felt and looked like a new person. My energy returned, my mood swings ceased, my periods regulated themselves and my skin cleared up. Not only did I feel 110 per cent better, but people commented on my appearance!*

*I will not pretend that this initial step was easy; in fact I found it extremely difficult. But once I came to terms with this fact and changed my way of thinking, it became much easier.*

*I followed the diet for over a year and now I have reduced my vitamins to evening primrose oil and a multivitamin and magnesium. I now take the pill 2 monthly and my periods remain pain-free.*

## SUPPLEMENT CHOICE

When you first walk into a health food shop or pharmacy, the vast array of nutritional supplements lined up on the shelves can be daunting. You feel overwhelmed in choosing the right one for your needs. The body is a chemical factory and has a need for each nutrient and, although they should be in our food, we have to absorb them efficiently. We have also seen that poor farming with depleted soils have reduced the mineral content of foods (*see* pp. 156–7).

Rest assured that no supplement company is going to produce any tablets containing an unsafe dose. If you stick to the exact recommendations on the label, you can't go wrong. Some people feel that if one tablet is good for you, two must be even better – this is a very dangerous idea. Doses are always very carefully gauged, so you must stick to them. A table of safe doses is given on page 237. For instance, if you are taking a multivitamin/mineral tablet and an antioxidant tablet make sure that you do not overdo the selenium (no more than 150µg per day).

Always check with a nutritionist or nutrition-trained health professional if you need extra guidance. They are trained to find out, through various tests, exactly what your specific nutrient requirements will be. In nutrition consultations, which usually last for an hour, every person is treated as a unique individual and no two people leave with the same 'prescription' of supplements. Very few people absorb the level of nutrients their bodies need to function, and taking the correct ones at the correct dose for your needs can help to get your body biochemistry up and running again at its optimum range.

Keep in mind that the recommended dietary allowances (RDAs) are for healthy people and that they do not allow for those whose needs are affected by illness: 'In the USA alone 100 million people suffer from allergies, arthritis, diabetes, heart disease, etc.'[25] For many people the RDAs are too low.

When endometriosis strikes, it is often a fact that the body's digestive tract is malfunctioning, and that the immune, nervous, endocrine and reproductive systems are undernourished. Short-term supplementation may help your body cells to begin functioning again at an optimum level. Dr Anthony J Verlangieti, Director of the Artherosclerosis Research Laboratories and Professor of Pharmacology and Toxicology at the University of Mississippi

School of Pharmacy states that 'it is a myth that we get all the vitamins we need in our daily diets'. He suggests that everyone should take supplementary vitamins. Several economists have estimated that by increasing our intake of vitamins and minerals, we would reduce health-care costs for cardiovascular disease by 25 per cent.

Subclinical deficiencies would 'not normally be discovered in routine physical examinations but subclinical deficiencies affect the body's well-being and do show up with hair mineral analysis and blood tests done at specialist clinics.'[26] The health service presently makes no attempt to check the vitamin and mineral levels of sick and dying people in order to treat them and correct their body balance/homeostasis. Instead, drugs are given which mask the symptoms. With good nutrition you begin to heal the tissues the natural way.

Begin to feed your body with the nutrients it needs both from foods and supplements and, in the first three to four months, you may well feel your health begin to improve slowly but surely.

As we have seen from the numerous case histories, supplements alone are not sufficient – you must combine them with a healthy diet. Supplements are only used to kick-start the body, to help cells to reach enzyme saturation levels, where all cells have the nutrients they require to make enzymes work effectively. But the need for good quality food is paramount. Natural, fresh foods contain nutrients if they have been grown in nutrient-rich soil. Processed foods and those grown on overfarmed soils are depleted. It is your choice of nutrient-rich food that counts the most. Try to broaden your horizons and be bold, try different foods to add a wider variety of nutrients to your repertoire. As James I of England (1566–1625) said: 'He was a bold man who first swallowed an oyster'.

To continue to eat low-nutrient high-calorie foods and take supplements alone will not lead to good health. We hope that this book will be a working guide for you to achieve a feeling of total well-being again.

Good supplements will tell you the exact form of the minerals (citrates, picolinates, amino acid chelates are best; oxides and carbonates are a waste of time), and they should be wheat-, dairy-, yeast- and sugar-free. *If they are not, do not buy them.* Avoid yeast-based B vitamins, chronium and selenium. If you are intolerant of yeasts, they will make your symptoms worse. Your body is like your car. Would you put cheap inferior oil or petrol into your car and risk it being damaged? Treat your body in the same way; after all, it has to stay healthy for at least 80 or 90 years. 'Picking the right supplements is an art in itself', says Patrick Holford, founder of the Institute for Optimum Nutrition. Choose from the most reputable companies, or ask your local consumer council which companies have the best labelling policies. If in doubt, write directly to the manufacturer. Read up about nutrients from other books. A good health food shop should help to guide you in your choice. Some mail order companies produce good quality supplements, and their addresses are at the end of this book (*see* p. 335).

Carl Pfeiffer, MD, PhD, of the Brain Biocentre, NJ, says: 'Vitamins and minerals play a crucial role in preserving and maintaining health and restoring it in diseased patients.' Supplements of vitamins, minerals and essential fatty acids taken for three to six months will help to replenish body cells. When the body is ill, it requires the building blocks of life to restore its vitality and renew failing cells. By taking supplements you can support the digestive, immune and reproductive systems and improve the body's healing potential. Remember that the body is striving to be well all the time. The only way the body has to heal itself is through the nutrients we eat. If the diet is depleted in nutrients or the digestive tract is damaged, the body cells will sustain damage. The following is a basic programme for everyone to try. For an individually tailored programme, consult a qualified nutritionist and get a full assessment of your personal needs.

Take each of the following daily, for 2–3 months:

- Multivitamin/mineral (yeast-, sugar-, gluten-, dairy-free)
- Vitamin C with bioflavinoids
- Evening primrose and fish oils (combined)
- Acidophilus (dairy-free)
- B complex 50mg (yeast-free) (optional)
- Selenium and vitamins A, C and E (yeast-free) (antioxidants) (optional)
- Magnesium taurate or malate
- Zinc methionine or citrate
- Digestive enzymes with each meal

Table 9.2 provides a guide to safe levels of supplements. Always err on the side of caution and take the lower doses in the optimum range to begin with. Higher doses may not be necessary unless you are properly assessed and instructed by a nutritionist to take certain nutrients in higher quantities. The maximum figures come from

| Vitamins | Optimum range | Maximum safety level |
|---|---|---|
| A | 7,500–20,000iu** | 33,333iu* |
| D | 400–1,000iu | 2,000iu |
| E | 100–1,000iu | 1,500iu |
| C | 1,000–4,000mg | 6,000mg |
| B1 | 25–100mg | 140mg |
| B2 | 25–100mg | 160mg |
| B3 | 50–150mg | 180mg |
| B5 | 50–300mg | 400mg |
| B6 | 50–100mg | 300mg |
| B12 | 5–100μ | 300μ |
| Folic acid | 50–400μ | 2,000μ |
| Biotin | 50–200μ | 10,000μ |

\* For women of child-bearing age the maximum safety level for long-term use is 10,000iu per day.
\*\* When attempting pregnancy or while pregnant take no more than 2,000iu of vitamin A per day in total.

**Minerals**

| Calcium | 400–800mg | 3,000mg |
|---|---|---|
| Magnesium | 300–500mg | 1,000mg |
| Iron | 10–25mg | 50mg |
| Zinc | 15–30mg | 50mg |
| Copper | 1–3mg | 5mg |
| Manganese | 5–25mg | 100mg |
| Selenium | 50–250μ | 500μ |
| Chromium | 50–250μ | 500μ |

Table 9.2
Vitamins and minerals – how much is safe? Reproduced with kind permission of P Holford of ION, from *Optimum Nutrition*, ION Press, p. 141, 1994.

research on the level at which supplements cause adverse side effects in some individuals. (*See* p.296 for rules when taking supplements.)

## TAKING ACTION

Think positive. Take control. Consider what you may gain – better health, and improved quality of life. If you have to give up wheat or dairy foods for a time, so what? Providing you use all the alternative foods suggested to maintain the supply of nutrients from other sources, there should be no problem. The benefits far outweigh the disadvantages, as can be seen from the various case studies throughout this book. Once you develop a new set of menus to follow and know which stores to buy from, life all becomes easy again. In fact, easier. Once you start feeling healthier and happier, coping skills improve.

Knowledge is power. If you know that some foods are making you ill and that using supplements occasionally with the right diet makes you well, then you and those around you will benefit if you put this into practice. Try this for one month and see if there is a difference in how you feel. Then we can put your success on our World Wide Web bulletin board (http://www.endometriosis.co.uk) and let other people know how to regain their health. Remember at football games watching 'the Mexican wave' go round the arena? Well, we can send this wave round the world via this book and cyberspace. Your story is just as important as those already in this book.

## PRACTICALITIES

• Give yourself one month from now as a goal to try the programme.
• Assess your diet, exclude whatever food you think is upsetting you for one month, eating the alternatives suggested.
• Eat the healthiest, freshest foods you can afford.
• Take some basic supplements each day while you are ill.
• Report how you fare onto our World Wide Web page (http://www.endometriosis.co.uk).
• Join in and let us combat this disease.
• Encourage more research into how nutrients affect endometriosis and infertility and pain.

As Mary Lou Ballweg, President of the International Endometriosis Association, headquartered in America, states, 'Together we make a difference'. The more of you who try this path and achieve good results, the more we can help each other regain health in this way.

The eminent Professor of Nutrition John Yudkin says, 'The health of the majority of humans depends more on their nutrition than it does on any other single factor. However important and dramatic the advances in hygiene, medicine and surgery have been, proper nutrition has a more important effect on human morbidity and mortality. For this reason, I believe that the ultimate objective of nutritionists must be the nutrition education of the public.'[27] We owe it to the next generation to encourage research in this vital area. We must save the next generation of women from this disease.

Some supplement regimes seem to help to deal with the many symptoms which we perceive as being triggered by endometriosis. The following regimes may be useful for those with endometriosis and also for those who also experience premenstrual tension.

## ENDOMETRIOSIS

Correction of imbalances of steroid hormones, too much oestrogen in proportion to progesterone, and correction of prostaglandin levels appear to be key factors in improving health, and nutrition is key to controlling hormone levels. The liver requires a constant supply of B vitamins to deal with hormones, as do the immune cells, together with vitamin C, magnesium, zinc and the antioxidants. The recommendations are:

- Evening primrose and fish oils (2000mg per day)
- B complex vitamins (yeast-free and optional)
- Vitamin C with bioflavinoids (1000-2000mg per day)
- Multivitamin/mineral (yeast-, wheat-, sugar-, dairy-free
  – 1 per day)
- Magnesium malate for fatigue/muscles or magnesium taurate for oestrogen breakdown (300mg per day)
- Zinc methionine (15mg per day)
- Selenium ACE antioxidants (yeast-free and optional)
- Probiotics (dairy-free acidophilus, 4-8 billion viable cells daily)
- Digestive enzymes (glandular-free; one with each meal)

## PREMENSTRUAL SYNDROME

Four distinct types of premenstrual syndrome are recognized. (Often with extreme endometriosis we seem to have them all!)

1   PMS type A – anxiety, nervous tension, mood swings and irritability. Sufferers need vitamin B6 and magnesium-rich diets.

2   PMS type B – hydration, weight gain, swollen legs, breast tenderness, abdominal bloating. Sufferers need diets rich in vitamin E, B6 and magnesium.

3   PMS type C – cravings, headaches, increased appetite, heart pounding, fatigue. Sufferers need diets rich in B6, magnesium and chromium.

4   PMS type D – depression, forgetfulness, crying, confusion, insomnia. Sufferers need diets rich in vitamin B6, magnesium and vitamin C.

The recommendations are:
- Vitamin C with bioflavinoids
- Vitamin B6 as pyridoxine 5 phosphate
- Magnesium EAP2
- Chromium polynicotinate
- Evening primrose and fish oils
- Vitamin B complex (yeast-free)
- Multivitamin/mineral
- Zinc methionine
- Vitamin E

## SUMMARY

Eating well can enhance your body's ability to heal and may well aid its recovery from endometriosis, infertility and pain.

1   Eat as well as you can afford.

2   Buy the freshest food you can find and eat while it is still fresh.

3   Cook from fresh wherever possible, and eat some raw vegetables and fruit every day.

4   Eat a wide variety of foods every day, not just usual old favourites. Make it fun to try new dishes and expand your horizons.

5   Use 1 tablespoon of cold-pressed cis vegetable oils daily and try to avoid trans fats.

6  Follow the Food Pyramid as your guide to daily choices of foods. Ensure that you eat good quality protein foods every day.

7  Avoid caffeine, refined sugars and alcohol while you are trying to recover from illness.

8  Drink 1.5 litres of fluid daily. Avoid fizzy canned drinks and use diluted fruit juices or fresh water.

9  Include 30g of fibre from fruits, vegetables, nuts, seeds, legumes and cereals in your daily diet in order to keep your intestines healthy.

10  Use only good quality supplements while you are ill. Use them wisely. Stick to the dose on the carton or bottle. They will only help you if your eating pattern is healthy and once you have corrected your digestive problem.

'It is only with the heart that one can see rightly; what is essential is invisible to the eye.'

*The Little Prince*

## VITAMINS AND MINERALS

Our first line of defence against endometriosis may come from our food.

*Dian Shepperson Mills*

### DEFINITIONS

*Good sources*. Foods with the highest nutrient levels per calorie are listed in descending order. So the first foods are the best. All foods listed are excellent sources of these vitamins.

*Deficiency*. When the body lacks optimal levels of vitamins it cannot work efficiently. Early warning signs, such as joint pains, headaches, rashes, bloating, etc., suggest your nutrient intake from diet and supplements may need increasing.

*RDA*. These Recommended Dietary Allowances are based on the European Union figures, and in cases where they don't exist on

McCance and Widdowson. These are the levels designed to prevent serious vitamin deficiency. They are not necessarily optimal intakes.

*Optimum intake.* These are optimal nutrient allowances derived from research testing the level of vitamins needed for optimal health taken from the book, *What is Optimum?* by Dr Cheraskin.
N.B. You should only ever take a B-complex supplement, never just one B vitamin on its own, as they tend to compete with each other. If you need more of one, say B6, you should take a B complex plus an extra amount of B6.

*Helpful.* Vitamins and minerals need each other in order to work. Eat a healthy, wholefood diet as priority and, if you are ill, supplement a good multivitamin and mineral, before adding extra nutrients.

*Harmful.* Our diet and environment expose us to 'anti-nutrients'. The more of these you are exposed to, the higher your need for supplements.

## VITAMIN C – ASCORBIC ACID

*RDA.*                 Adults: 60mg
*Optimum intake.*      Adults: 500mg

*Effects.* Antioxidant, antiviral, antibacterial, antihistamine. Used for immune system. Fights infection. Needed for collagen for skin, muscles, joints. Detoxifies pollutants. Protects against cancer. Necessary for energy and stress resistance. Supports adrenal function. For white blood cell function. Used in cells for energy production. Used for sperm production. Thins blood. Potentiates Clomid. Increases absorption of nutrients in the gut. Softens stools. Removes heavy metals from the body. Enhances phagocytosis. Needed for antibody production. Reduces pain. Analgesic.

*Deficiency.* Frequent colds and infections, lack of energy, bleeding gums, easy bruising, nosebleeds, slow wound healing. Causes poor uptake of iron.

*Helpful.* Bioflavinoids. Works with B vitamins, Co Q10 and iron to produce energy within cells. Vitamin E. Take with food. Iron is more effectively absorbed when vitamin C is present.

*Harmful.* Smoking (every cigarette burns up 25mg of vitamin C), alcohol, pollution, stress, fried food.

*Good sources.* Blackcurrants, berries, peppers, lemons, watercress, strawberries, oranges, grapefruit, new and sweet potatoes, cauliflower, broccoli, melon, spinach, tomatoes, savoy cabbage, green leafy vegetables, jacket potatoes, kale, cantaloupe and honeydew melons, turnip, peas, apples.

## VITAMIN B1 – THIAMINE

*RDA.*                    Adults: 1.4mg
*Optimum intake.*         Adults: 7.1mg

*Effects.* Energy production in cells. Brain function. Used in digestion by protein. Strengthens heart muscle alongside magnesium. Reproductive system, enriches womb lining, needed for ovarian hormones. Works liver enzymes which degrade oestrogen. Suppresses pain. Analgesic.

*Deficiency.* Tender and weak muscles, eye pains, irritability, poor concentration, 'prickly' legs, poor memory, stomach pains, constipation, tingling hands, rapid heartbeat. Reduces fertility. Depression, insomnia. Reduces endorphin production. Inhibits ovulation. Increases pain.

*Helpful.* B5, B complex vitamins, magnesium, manganese.

*Harmful.* Antibiotics, tea, coffee, stress, birth control pills, alcohol, alkaline agents, e.g. baking powder, sulphur dioxide (preservative), destroyed by cooking/food processing.

*Good sources.* Peas, red kidney beans, milk, lamb, brown rice, oatmeal, peanuts, pork, lamb, chicken, legumes (peas, beans, lentils), potatoes, watercress, mushrooms, most vegetables, lettuce, cauliflower, tomatoes, Brussels sprouts, spring cabbage.

## VITAMIN B2 – RIBOFLAVIN

*RDA.*              Adults:1.6mg
*Optimum intake.*   Adults: 2.0mg

*Effects.* Turns fat, sugar, protein into energy. Repairs skin. Regulates body acidity. Hair, nails and eyes. Works liver enzymes which degrade oestrogen. Needed for ovarian hormones.

*Deficiency.* Hormonal imbalances of oestrogen and progesterone, inhibits GnRH production for FSH and LH, burning/gritty eyes, sensitivity to bright lights, sore tongue, cataracts, dull/oily hair, eczema or dermatitis, split nails, cracked lips.

*Helpful.* B5, B vitamins and selenium. Take as B complex with food.

*Harmful.* Alcohol, contraceptive pill, tea, coffee, alkaline agents (baking powder, sulphur dioxide [preservative]), food processing.

*Good sources.* Mackerel, mushrooms, potatoes, broccoli, muesli, natural yogurt, skimmed milk, whole milk, green leafy vegetables, watercress, wholemeal bread, spring cabbage, blackcurrants, beans, eggs, fish, tomatoes.

## VITAMIN B3 – NIACIN

*RDA.*              Adults: 18mg
*Optimum intake.*   Adults: 25mg

*Effects.* Energy production. Brain function. Skin. Balances blood sugar. Adjusts cholesterol levels.

*Deficiency.* Lack of energy, diarrhoea, insomnia, headaches or migraines, poor memory, anxiety, depression, irritability, bleeding gums, acne, eczema/dermatitis. Causes deficiency of folic acid and zinc.

*Helpful.* Works with B complex vitamins and chromium. Best taken with food.

*Harmful.* Antibiotics, tea, coffee, contraceptive pill and alcohol, refined sugars.

*Good sources*. Canned tuna, smoked mackerel, roast turkey, roast chicken, steamed salmon, lamb chops, wholemeal bread, cornmeal, potatoes, broccoli, mushrooms, tomatoes, carrots, fish, eggs, peanuts, avocado, prunes, cauliflower, cod, new boiled potatoes, cabbage.

## VITAMIN B5 – PANTOTHENIC ACID

*RDA.*                    Adults: 6mg
*Optimum intake.*        Adults: 25mg

*Effects*. Energy production. Fat metabolism. Improves function of brain and nerves and anti-stress hormones. Skin and hair. Anti-allergy vitamin. Supports adrenal function. Needed for ovarian hormones.

*Deficiency*. Muscle tremors/cramps, apathy, poor concentration, burning feet/tender heels, nausea, lack of energy, exhaustion after light exercise, anxiety, teeth grinding, nervousness.

*Helpful*. Other B complex vitamins. Biotin and folic acid. Best taken with food. Magnesium.

*Harmful*. Stress, alcohol, tea, coffee. Destroyed by heat, food processing.

*Good sources*. Boiled eggs, mushrooms, grilled pork chops, lean meat, green leafy vegetables, nuts, chicken, sea fish, wholemeal bread, celery, strawberries, tomatoes, boiled potatoes, baked cod, cabbage, beans, peas, watercress.

## VITAMIN B6 – PYRIDOXINE

*RDA.*                    Adults: 2mg
*Optimum intake.*        Adults: 10mg

*Effects*. Protein digestion. Brain function. Sex hormone production GnRH in hypothalamus. Reduces symptoms of PMS, menopause. Antidepressant and diuretic. Precursor to progesterone and seretonin. Needed for macrophage function. Works enzymes in liver which degrade oestrogen. Natural diuretic. Needed for ovarian hormones. Improves immune function. Healthy blood and blood vessels. With zinc works in metabolism of EFAs. Analgesic.

*Deficiency.* Infrequent dream recall, water retention, tingling hands, depression due to low serotonin levels, irritability, muscle cramps, lack of energy. Causes deficiency of B3 and B2. Anaemia. Poor immune system response. Causes cracks around the mouth and dermatitis on the face. Macrophages cannot remove cell debris in the abdomen.

*Helpful.* Works with B complex vitamins, plus zinc and magnesium. Take with food and zinc.

*Harmful.* Alcohol, smoking, birth control pill, high protein intake, processed foods, penicillin, stress.

*Good sources.* Bananas, turkey, oat bran, egg yolk, leeks, cod, trout, salmon, sardines, herrings, mackerel, tuna, kale, red kidney beans, broccoli, Brussels sprouts, lamb chops, watercress, cauliflower, spring cabbage, carrots, beans, chicken, peas, potatoes, spinach, cantaloupe melons, onions, almonds.

## VITAMIN B12 – CYANOCOBALAMIN

*RDA.*  Adults: 1μ
*Optimum intake.*  Adults: 2μ

*Effects.* Use of protein. Helps blood carry oxygen. Essential for energy/nerves. Synthesis of DNA. Detoxifies tobacco smoke. Improves sperm count and motility. Analegsic action on pain.

*Deficiency.* Poor hair condition, eczema or dermatitis, mouth oversensitive, sterility.

*Helpful.* Works with folic acid. Best taken within B complex, with food. PABA.

*Harmful.* Alcohol, smoking, lack of stomach acid.

*Good sources.* Lamb's liver, sardines, tuna, plaice, Edam cheese, shrimp, eggs, lamb chops, whole milk, cheese, pork, miso paste, herrings, mackerel, cod, chicken legs. Vegetarians may need to take a supplement.

## VITAMIN B COMPLEX – FOLIC ACID

*RDA.*            Adults: 200μ
*Optimum intake.*  Adults: 800μ

*Effects*. Early development of brain and nerves, by 27th day of fetal development. Energy production. Reduces inflammation. Oestrogenic action. Improves immune function. Promotes cells to divide.

*Deficiency*. Eczema, cracked lips, prematurely greying hair, anxiety or tension, poor memory, lack of energy, poor appetite, stomach pains, depression.

*Helpful*. Works with other B complex vitamins, especially B12. Best supplemented as part of B complex with food. Zinc and folic acid levels must be balanced.

*Harmful*. High temperature, light, food processing, contraceptive pill.

*Good sources*. Peanuts, spinach, green leafy vegetables, carrots, egg yolk, apricots, melons, beans, pumpkin, hazelnuts, broccoli, walnuts, cauliflower, wholemeal bread, tuna, avocado, dark rye flour, corn tortilla.

## VITAMIN B COMPLEX – BIOTIN

*RDA.*            Adults: 150μ
*Optimum intake.*  Adults: 200μ

*Effects*. Important in childhood. Essential fats use, healthy skin, hair and nerves. Made by bifido bacteria to support immunoglobulins.

*Deficiency*. Dry skin, poor hair condition, premature greying hair, sore muscles, poor appetite/nausea, eczema.

*Helpful*. Works with other B vitamins, magnesium and manganese. Best supplemented as part of a B complex with food.

*Harmful*. Raw egg white, fried food.

*Good sources.* Almonds, oatmeal, eggs, herring, smoked mackerel, whole milk, lamb, chicken, cheese, rice, tomatoes, boiled cauliflower, grapefruit, lettuce, peas, cherries, apples, white cabbage.


## VITAMIN A – RETINOL AND BETACAROTENE

| *RDA.* | Adults: Retinol 800μ | betacarotene 2,000μ |
|---|---|---|
| *Optimum intake.* | Adults: Retinol 800μ | betacarotene 5,000μ |

*Effects.* Healthy skin and cell membranes. Protects against infections. Antioxidant. Immune system. Protects against cancers. Essential for night vision. Reduces menstrual cramps.

*Deficiency.* Mouth ulcers, poor night vision, acne, frequent colds/infections, dry flaky skin, dandruff, thrush or cystitis, diarrhoea, menstrual cramps. Used inefficiently if thyroxine is low. Abnormality of sperm.

*Helpful.* Works with zinc. Vitamin C and E help protect it. Best taken within a multivitamin with food.

*Harmful.* Heat, light, alcohol, coffee and smoking. Low fat diet.

*Good sources. Retinol*: butter, single cream, hard cheeses, boiled eggs, whole milk, fish liver oils. *Betacarotene*: carrots, watercress, green and yellow vegetables, cantaloupe melons, tomatoes, broccoli, dried apricots, white cabbage, tangerines.


## VITAMIN D – ERGOCALCIFEROL

| *RDA.* | Adults: 5mg |
|---|---|
| *Optimum intake.* | Adults: 10mg |

*Effects.* Strong and healthy bones by retaining calcium. Precursor to cholesterol (which is the precursor to progesterone).

*Deficiency.* Joint pain or stiffness, backache, tooth decay, muscle cramps, hair loss.

*Helpful*. Exposure to sunlight (vitamin D is made in the skin). Under these conditions dietary vitamin D may not be necessary. Vitamins A, C and E protect D.

*Harmful*. Lack of sunlight, fried foods. Low fat diet.

*Good sources*. Herrings, salmon, smoked mackerel, boiled eggs, salmon, tuna, butter, hard cheeses.

## VITAMIN E – D-ALPHATOCOPHEROL

*RDA*.                 Adults: 10mg
*Optimum intake*.      Adults:100mg

*Effects*. Antioxidant, protecting cells from damage, including cancer. Helps to oxygenate red blood cells, preventing blood clots. Improves wound healing and fertility. Promotes healthy skin. Reduces hot flushes. Improves breast tenderness. Aids sperm. Thins blood. Anti-inflammatory action. Needed for antibody production. Aids egg implantation.

*Deficiency*. Lack of sex drive, exhaustion after light exercise, easy bruising, slow wound healing, varicose veins, loss of muscle tone, infertility. Low testosterone.

*Helpful*. Vitamin C and selenium.

*Harmful*. High temperature cooking, especially frying. Air pollution, contraceptive pill, excessive intake of refined or processed fats and oils. Low fat diet.

*Good sources*. Sunflower seeds, soya beans, cold-pressed olive oil, safflower and sunflower oils, broccoli, sprouts, green leafy vegetables, spinach, wholegrain cereals, rye, hazelnuts, almonds, peanuts, avocados, salmon, eggs, asparagus, tuna, bananas, brown rice, oatmeal, carrots, peas, pilchards, runner beans.

## VITAMIN K – PHYLLOQUINONE

*RDA.*               Adults: 1μ/kg/day. Sufficient amounts made by beneficial bacteria in the gut.
*Optimum intake.*    Adults:10μ

*Effects.* Controls blood clotting. Anti-inflammatory effect. Strong bones.

*Deficiency.* Haemorrhage (easy bleeding), osteoporosis.

*Helpful.* Healthy intestinal bifido bacteria, then no need for dietary source.

*Harmful.* Antibiotics, hormone treatments. For infants, lack of breastfeeding. Low fat diet.

*Good sources.* Cauliflower, Brussels sprouts, lettuce, beans, peas, broccoli, cabbage, potatoes, watercress, corn oil, tomatoes, milk.


# MINERALS

## CALCIUM

*RDA.*            Adults: 800mg
*Optimum intake.*  Adults: 1,000mg

*Effects.* Health of the heart, nerves, muscles, skin, bones and teeth. Relieves aching muscles, bones, menstrual cramps. Classic complement pathway. Needed for ovarian hormones. Speeds up macrophages' ability to fight infections when the body runs a fever.

*Deficiency.* Muscle cramps, insomnia or nervousness, joint pain, arthritis, tooth decay, high blood pressure. Menstrual cramps.

*Helpful.* Works with magnesium and vitamin D, boron. Phosphorus must be in ratio to calcium.

*Harmful.* Caffeine depletes the body of calcium. Stress causes excretion. Hormone imbalances, alcohol. Phytic acid in wheat. Phosphates in fizzy drinks.

*Good sources.* Kelp, Gouda cheese, hard cheese, sardines, almonds, whole milk, sunflower seeds, green beans, wholegrain bread and cereals, boiled cabbage, natural yogurt, carob flour, rhubarb, corn, prunes.

## MAGNESIUM

*RDA.*                           Adults: 300mg
*Optimum intake.*               Adults: 300mg

*Effects.* Strong bones and teeth. Regulates and relaxes smooth muscles, uterine muscle, heart muscle. Central nervous system calmative. Energy production. Carbohydrate metabolism. Alternative complement pathway. Strengthens cell membranes. Used by 300 enzymes (30 enzymes for cell growth). Promotes sleep. Regulator of temperature in thyroid function. For red blood cells. Natural diuretic. For ovary function. For myelin sheath. Softens stools. Needed for antibody production. The anti-allergy nutrient.

*Deficiency.* Muscle spasms, insomnia, nervousness, high blood pressure, irregular heartbeat, constipation, fits/convulsions, hyperactivity, depression, miscarriage, mutagenic changes in sperm, infertility, mitral valve prolapse.

*Helpful.* Vitamins B1, B5 and B6, and zinc.

*Harmful.* Large amounts of calcium, vitamin D, proteins and fats decrease magnesium absorption. Fizzy drinks. Alcohol. Phytic acid.

*Good sources.* Kelp, sunflower seeds, wheat germ, buckwheat, millet, green beans, barley, crab, bananas, yams, blackberries, broccoli, cauliflower, carrots, sweetcorn, dried figs, aubergines, chicken, onions, apples, celery, lettuce, fresh peas, almonds, Brazil nuts, peanuts, oatmeal, wholemeal bread, soya beans, brown rice, garlic, raisins, peas, baked potatoes in skin, crab, tuna.

## IRON

*RDA:*             Adults: 14mg
*Optimum intake.*  Adults: 15mg

*Effects.* Iron helps transport oxygen to all cells for energy production. Red blood cells. Precursor for interleukin 1 production. Needed by macrophages to work. Needed for ovarian hormones. Needed for antibody production.

*Deficiency.* Pale skin, sore tongue, fatigue or listlessness, loss of appetite or nausea, heavy periods or blood loss, infections, impairs cell-mediated immunity, natural killer cells stop recognizing tumour formation.

*Helpful.* Vitamin C increases iron absorption, and vitamin E, also calcium if balanced but not in excess. (Iron EAP2 is well absorbed and does not cause constipation.)

*Harmful.* Oxalic acid in spinach, tea, antacids, soya protein, wheat bran, high zinc intake, phosphates in soft fizzy drinks, food additives.

*Good sources.* Sunflower seeds, almonds, dried prunes and apricots, raisins, Brazil nuts, walnuts, oat bran, pumpkin seeds, millet, parsley, almonds, cashews, dried dates, pecans, eggs, lentils, tofu, peas, brown rice, pork, lamb chops, red kidney beans, sesame seeds, wholemeal bread, cottage cheese, apples.

## ZINC

*RDA.*             Adults: 15mg
*Optimum intake.*  Adults: 25mg

*Effects.* Works over 200 enzymes in the body (20 in the brain). Protein synthesis. Carbohydrate metabolism. DNA synthesis. Healing – skin health. Strong antibodies. Insulin production. Healthy sperm and ova. Alcohol metabolism. Sex hormone production (GnRH in hypo-thalamus, testosterone in testes). For ovarian function. Stomach acid production. Helps with dyslexia and anorexia. For cell-mediated immunity. Helps convert EFAs to prostaglandins. Natural diuretic. Anti-inflammatory. Healthy sperm. Allows egg to implant in the womb.

*Deficiency*. Poor sense of taste or smell, white marks on fingernails, frequent infections, stretch marks, acne/greasy skin, low fertility, pale skin, tendency for depression, loss of appetite. Infertility.

*Helpful*. Vitamin B6 and magnesium, vitamins A and C.

*Harmful*. Phytic acid in wheat prevents uptake, high calcium intake, low protein intake, alcohol, white sugar prevents uptake, stress. Lead, cadmium, aluminium, iron, manganese. High copper. High oestrogen. Fizzy drinks. High meat and dairy food intake.

*Good sources*. Fresh oysters, ginger root, lamb chops, pecan nuts, haddock, green peas, shrimps, turnip, parsley, potatoes, Brazil nuts, boiled eggs, wholemeal bread, rye crispbread, oatmeal, peanuts, almonds, walnuts, sardines, chicken, buckwheat, hazelnuts, tuna, garlic, carrots, corn, grape juice, olive oil, cauliflower, spinach, cabbage, lentils, butter, lettuce, cucumber, spices, chicken legs.

## CHROMIUM

*RDA.*               Adults: 25μ
*Optimum intake.*    Adults: 100μ

*Effects*. Strengthens heart. Balances blood sugar. Improves life span. Balances cholesterol. Turns glucose into energy. Makes insulin work effectively. Aids building of new proteins. Improves weight loss when on a diet.

*Deficiency*. Excessive/cold sweats, irritability after six hours without food, need for frequent meals, cold hands, drowsiness during the day, excessive thirst, 'addicted' to sweet foods, problems with cell renewal.

*Helpful*. Vitamin B3, improved diet and exercise.

*Harmful*. Refined sugars and flours, additives and pesticides, petroleum products, processed foods.

*Good sources*. Wholemeal bread, rye bread, oysters, potatoes, wheat germ, green peppers, eggs, chicken, apples, butter, parsnips, cornmeal, lamb chops, Swiss cheese, bananas, spinach, pork, carrots, shrimps, lettuce, oranges, green beans, cabbage, mushrooms, strawberries.

## SELENIUM

*RDA.*               Adults: 60μ
*Optimum intake.*    Adults: 100μ

*Effects.* Protects against cancer. Disarms FoRs, Boosts the immune system. Needed by thyroid gland. Potentiates iodine. Anti-inflammatory effects. Antioxidant. Needed for prostaglandin production. Sperm production. Ovarian function. Antibody production. Protects the liver. Detoxifies pollutants.

*Deficiency.* Family history of cancer, signs of premature ageing, cataracts, high blood pressure, frequent infections, infertility, low sperm count, low thyroid function (hypothyroid).

*Helpful.* Vitamins A, C and E, iodine.

*Harmful.* Mercury, cadmium, lead.

*Good sources.* Butter, herrings, wheat germ, Brazil nuts, cider vinegar, scallops, barley, wholemeal bread, lobster, shrimps, kippers, tuna, shrimps, oats, crab, whole milk, oysters, broccoli, cod, brown rice, lamb, turnips, garlic, orange juice, egg yolks, chicken, Swiss cheeses, cottage cheese, radishes, pecans, almonds, hazelnuts, green beans, onions, carrots, cabbage.

## IODINE

*RDA.*               Adults: 150μ
*Optimum intake.*    Adults: 500μ

*Effects.* Essential for thyroid glands (controls the body's metabolism), vitality, stable weight, sex organ development, ovarian function, strong teeth, good circulation, temperature regulation, ovarian function.

*Deficiency.* Breast cancer, lack of energy, hypothyroidism, weight gain, bulging eyes, brittle nails, low resistance to infection, fuzzy brain, obesity, persistent cough and sore throat, constipation, hair loss. Relieves fibrocystic breast with selenium and vitamin E.

*Helpful.* Selenium, magnesium, copper, manganese.

*Harmful.* Low fish diet, low vegetable intake, imbalance of calcium and phosphorus, low selenium intake.

*Good sources.* Shrimps, scampi, haddock, halibut, oysters, cod, salmon, sardines, pineapples, strawberries, tuna, boiled eggs, peanuts, natural yogurt, hard cheeses, pork chops, lettuce, spinach, green peppers, butter, cream, cottage cheese, lamb, raisins, fried onions.

## MANGANESE

| | |
|---|---|
| *RDA.* | Adults: 2.5mg |
| *Optimum intake.* | Adults: 15mg |

*Effects.* Used in energy production, bone formation, protein metabolism, metabolism of fats and cholesterol production. SOD (superoxide dismutase) needs manganese to fight FoR damage and protects the cell membrane. Formation of thyroxine. Protects mitochondria. Required by liver. Helps fertility.

*Deficiency.* Reduced fertility due to defective ovulation, rheumatoid arthritis, cancer, leads to calcium deposition in arteries and soft tissue, abnormal bone and cartilage, backaches, sore knees, glucose intolerance, birth defects, growth retardation, inner ear balance, convulsions, epilepsy, irregular heartbeat, weight loss, dermatitis, loss of hair colour, reduced levels of dopamine, high copper levels, testicular degeneration, inhibits synthesis of cholesterol.

*Helpful.* Lecithin, choline, increase liver uptake.

*Harmful.* Excess calcium, phosphorus, iron, cobalt, zinc and copper, pesticides and insecticides, milling process for grains, soya protein.

*Good sources.* Pecans, Brazil nuts, almonds, barley, rye, buckwheat, split peas, wholewheat, walnuts, fresh spinach, peanuts, oats, raisins, Swiss cheese, corn, cabbage, peaches, butter, tangerines, peas, eggs, beets, coconut, apples, oranges, pears.

## BORON

*RDA.*                  Adults: none given
*Optimum intake.*       Adults: 3mg

*Effects.* Boron works very much like oestrogen to prevent the loss of minerals from bone. It is useful combined with vitamin D, calcium and magnesium to help improve bones in menopause to prevent osteoporosis.

*Deficiency.* None have been identified.

*Helpful.* Vitamin D, calcium, magnesium, zinc.

*Harmful.* Caffeine, alcohol.

*Good sources.* Fresh fruits and vegetables.

# 10 Food – the best choice for health

Nothing becomes real until it is experienced.
*John Keats*

## WHAT TO EAT?

This is easy. You just have to eat the freshest food available. If you are vegetarian, buy fresh fruits, vegetables, beans, peas, lentils, nuts and seeds and organic dairy foods. If you are carnivorous, choose organic meat which is hormone- and antibiotic-free and find the most unpolluted source of fish (deep-sea fish is probably the best). Then you cook from fresh as often as possible. Try to avoid foods with additives and flavour enhancers and preservatives unless they are natural ones like vinegar or vitamin C. The healthier your food, the healthier you will become.

In *Gulliver's Travels,* Jonathan Swift writes, 'He had been eight years upon a project for extracting sunbeams out of cucumbers.' Indeed this is what our food really is – trapped rays of light and energy from the sun. Plants grow by using the energy of the sun directly to convert nutrients from the soil and elements from the air into plant tissues. The secret to this miracle is the chlorophyll molecule found in plants. Chlorophyll is magnesium-based and it captures the energy of the sun and uses it to synthesize new carbohydrates, proteins and fats in the plants. The plants are eaten by herbivores and we consume plants and/or herbivores. So we are all dependent upon the sun as our major source of energy. Vital energy allows our cells to work at their best.

The Soil Association (*see* p. 352) can provide a list of suppliers in your area who deliver organic vegetables weekly. If you buy foods which have been sprayed with pesticides, herbicides and fungicides, peel them; scrubbing will not be effective. You need to reduce the load of oestrogenic (xeno-oestrogens) chemicals which you take in.

We should not be anxious about food, but by being aware we can make more informed choices about what we choose to buy and eat.

Health is such a precious commodity. We do not realize until we lose it, how much it should be treasured and valued. However, food is not a commodity, although great profits are made by food manufacturers and retailers. Your food should be seen as something which can bestow good health.

Think of our ancestors. What did they eat? When times were hard and it was survival of the fittest, you grew what you ate or bartered food, which had to be eaten fresh as storage was a problem. Crops were rotated and fields were allowed to lie fallow to renew the soil. You ate what was in season. Obviously we cannot go back to this, but we should eat from fresh whenever possible. We all have manic days when we arrive home shattered from work and need to take short cuts, but we should try to eat fresh food as often as possible. Meals do not have to take a long time to prepare. Some recipes are given later on in this chapter to help you.

## Avril G of Sussex

*When I have managed to stick to a natural diet of fresh fruits and vegetables I do definitely feel less sluggish and ill. As soon as I eat something 'unnatural', such as chocolate or sweets, I almost immediately feel ill again. I feel like the substance is poisoning me, which being totally unnatural to the human body, it probably is. I am now expecting a baby in June! Thanks for all your help.*

## SHOPPING STRATEGIES

Many people shop once a week at the local supermarket. They push trolleys laden with food. But stop and think. Those vegetables and that fruit – how many days ago were they picked? We take them home and they sit at the bottom of the fridge for how many more days? This is not good. Most of the vitamins oxidize as they sit around. We need to eat fresh foods. Our grandparents grew their own or bought fresh local produce so it was still vibrant and full of nutrients. They did not have fridges so could not store food as we do. We should shop for fruits and vegetables every two days to ensure they are still full of vitamins.

Boring diets can also lead to poor intake of nutrients; we need to be more adventurous when cooking. Dishes which are quick to prepare do not have to be the convenience foods we throw in the microwave after an exhausting day. Salads and soups take very little time to prepare. Once you have sorted out your digestive system and begun to absorb nutrients efficiently, you need to keep your body supplied with a wide variety of nutrients, which means a wide variety of foods. Use the weekends to experiment with new recipes – there are some in this book for you to try. Some are wheat- and dairy-free for those who wish to try sensible exclusion diets. The word 'diet' is misleading; this is not a diet, it is eating for health.

Stock your store cupboard up with useful items. You will need some balanced mineral salt, black pepper, spices and herbs for lots of lovely flavours. When you try a wheat-free diet, you need to stock all the alternatives for when you are hungry. Alternatives to wheat include rye crispbreads, 100% rye bread, rye pasta, oatcakes, porridge oats, corn tortilla and tacos, corn pasta, rice pasta, lentil pasta, buckwheat pancakes, ricecakes, brown rice, millet, millet flakes, pastry (made from brown rice flour, ground almonds and margarine in equal proportions), potato-based pizza, and poppadoms.

Unflavoured crisps would also be fine, in moderation. Tins of tuna, salmon, beans, vegetable soups and tomatoes for occasional use are handy. Frozen vegetables and fruits are also useful, as are sugar-free jams. A tour around your local health food store will yield a lot of foodstuffs – a yeast-free vegetable stock powder, organic rice and corncrisps.

If you are trying a dairy-free regime, stock up with various soya 'milks', rice dream or oat milks, soft soya cheeses, vegetable pâtés (carrot, mushroom, chestnut) or use nut butters or black olive paste. Alternatives to dairy foods from cows are tofu, nut milks, soya yogurt, ewe's or goat's milks and yogurts, hummus, avocado and egg pâté, tuna, mackerel or crab pâté.

Choose some organic fruit and nut bars, dried apricots and carob bars to snack on, if you crave anything sweet. Keep some nuts and seeds or sesame sticks in your desk drawer at work. Look at other grains, such as quinoa and millet, and look for wheat-free muesli. Try goat's and ewe's milk yogurts and ice creams, like yummy Tofutti. There are so many alternatives to try, you need never feel hungry. Just look around the shelves of your local health food store for other alternatives. You won't starve.

## RULES FOR A HEALTHY DIET

1 **Eat two fresh fruits and four fresh vegetables daily.**
Whenever possible, eat fruit and vegetables raw, as they are rich
in vitamins and minerals needed by the body. Cooking destroys
many of the vitamins, and breaks down the fibre in the food
making it less effective in the intestines. Green leafy vegetables
are rich in the B vitamins and magnesium which are needed by
the reproductive system daily. Red-orange vegetables and fruits
are rich in vitamin A. Dried apricots are a good source of iron.

2 **Eat wholegrain cereals and unrefined foods**. Include a
variety of cereals in your diet, not just wheat. Use oats, rye, spelt,
barley, millet, rice, corn, quinoa or buckwheat. If you have a
problem with gluten use the last five cereals only. Nuts and seeds
are rich in vitamins and minerals, as well as important cis
vegetable oils. As far as possible use only fresh unprocessed foods
as a basis for your meals, e.g. lean meat, poultry, fish and game.
Oily fish, such as herrings, tuna, mackerel, sardines, salmon,
pilchards and trout contain essential oils which your body needs
to build healthy tissues, so eat them twice a week.

3 **Drink at least a litre of fresh water daily.** Try diluting
unsweetened fruit juices, or various herb teas. Chamomile helps
sleep, lime blossom aids relaxation, mint, ginger and fennel aid
digestion. Dandelion tea is a diuretic. Carrot juice also helps
digestion. V8 vegetable juice helps to cleanse the liver.

4 **Use only cold-pressed vegetable oils.** Our bodies require
essential cis oils to strengthen cell walls and to build the anti-
inflammatory prostaglandins of series 1 from vegetable oils and
series 3 from fish oils. It is very important to use unprocessed
vegetable oils which have not been chemically or heat treated.
The jar should say unrefined, unhydrogenated, or cold-pressed
for sunflower, safflower, corn and olive oils. Evening primrose oil
is a good source but is expensive. Edible food grade linseed oil
from a health food shop is also useful. Try grinding one
tablespoon of linseeds each day and mix into muesli or salad
dressings. Butter can be used in moderation (organic butter can
be found) or choose unhydrogenated margarine from your health
food store.

5 **Half your diet should consist of alkaline-forming foods**, such as vegetables, fruits, sprouted seeds, live yogurt, almonds, Brazil nuts and buckwheat. The other half should be acid-forming foods, such as grains, pulses, nuts, seeds, eggs, cheese, fish and poultry. This helps to balance your digestive enzymes.

6 **Reduce your intake of sugary foods.** Try to avoid needless refined sugar consumption as it can cause fluid retention and may prevent other vital nutrients from being absorbed. Sugar also thickens the blood and stops immune cells from working efficiently for four hours after intake. Avoid chocolate, sweets, biscuits, cakes, puddings, ice cream, sugary fizzy drinks, sweet tea or coffee, jams and honey. Find other treats to give yourself instead. Chocolate can be saved as a special treat for birthdays, anniversaries, Christmas and Easter. Try Green & Black's organic chocolate. Carob bars or fruit and nut bars are far more nutritious snacks.

7 **Avoid excess salt intake.** Too much salt causes fluid retention and some PMS symptoms. Reduce the amount of salt added to cooked foods and avoid eating salty crisps, nuts, bacon and kippers. Use herbs, spices, lemon juice or root ginger to impart flavour instead. You require only 3g salt per day (0.1oz) and most diets allow up to 10g (0.3oz). If you suffer from low blood pressure, then a little salt is fine; it is a danger with high blood pressure.

8 **Cut down your intake of tea, coffee, alcohol and tobacco.** Caffeine and excess alcohol are thought to impair ovarian and testes function and so affect fertility. Tobacco and alcohol can aggravate some PMS symptoms. Try herb teas or coffee substitutes. Caffeine and alcohol are diuretics and literally throw out of the body some of the precious minerals needed by our reproductive system.

9 **Avoid excess fatty foods,** e.g. beef, lamb and pork. Red meat supplies the pro-inflammatory series 2 prostaglandins, so should be eaten in moderation. Game is often less fatty meat. Use white meat and fish. Avoid fried foods, and grill or bake instead. If you must fry, use very little cold-pressed olive oil and butter and gently cook on a low heat. Steam vegetables whenever possible. Eat a sensible amount of dairy foods. If eaten to excess, the calcium in them can prevent absorption of magnesium, which helps muscles to relax. Balance dairy foods with lots of fresh, green leafy vegetables. If you are a vegetarian use more legumes.

10 **Exercise regularly.** Gentle exercise and exposure to fresh air
and sunshine are vital in maintaining health. Take walks, go
swimming or cycling if you are able. Gentle exercise helps the
body produce endorphins (natural painkillers) and stimulates
the digestive tract.

11 **Eat a high-fibre diet.** We need to include more fibre in our
diet to ensure the stools are well-formed and that waste can pass
through us at an even rate, avoiding the build-up of harmful
toxins in the intestines. Fibre of the type provided by fructo-
olligosaccharides (FOS) also helps to maintain the good bifido
gut flora which produce the B vitamins needed by the liver
enzymes. The fibre in the diet also stimulates peristalsis, and
binds to cholesterol and oestrogens to escort them from the body.
Fibre can be from wholegrain cereals (especially oats), nuts, seeds
or from fruits and vegetables. Only 30g (1oz) of fibre is needed
each day, and a diet rich in plant fibre easily supplies this.

12 *Candida Albicans.* If you think you have an overgrowth, or
allergy or sensitivity to the yeast *Candida albicans* in your digestive
tract and suffer abdominal bloating after meals, then remove
the foods which are 'feeding' the yeast for 2 or 3 months: refined
sugars, yeasts, wheat, fermented foods, dried fruits and dairy
foods. The following foods have anti-yeast properties and should
be used frequently – garlic, onions, cabbage, broccoli, Brussels
sprouts, kale, watercress, mustard cress, cauliflower, turnips,
cinnamon, olive oil, aloe vera juice and Pau d'Arco tea.

SUGGESTIONS FOR WEEKLY MENU PLANS
(Recipes are given for those in bold type)

The following suggested weekly menus can act as a starter for a new
nutrition plan. They can also act as a guide for food exclusion diets.

## Wheat-free diet – week 1

| | BREAKFAST | LUNCH | TEA/DINNER |
|---|---|---|---|
| **1** | Prune juice<br>Ricecakes & hummus<br>Mint tea | **Potato & leek soup**<br>Oatcakes & apple<br>Figs | Turkey breast<br>Rice, broccoli, carrots |
| **2** | Sheep's yogurt with<br>ground almonds, oat bran<br>banana<br>Prune juice<br>Fennel tea | Mackerel<br>Mixed salads<br>Baked potato<br>Dates | Chestnut pâté<br>Pumpernickel rye bread<br>Tomato & celery<br>Apple |
| **3** | **Breton<br>pancakes**<br>Blueberries<br>Mint tea | **Chicken with<br>lemon & olives**<br>Boiled rice<br>Broccoli, carrots<br>Figs | **Carrot & almond<br>soup**<br>Corn tacos<br>Apple |
| **4** | **Rye bread** &<br>poached egg<br>Carrot juice & herb tea | Grilled chicken<br>Green beans, swede<br>Jacket potato<br>Dates | Vegetable &<br>lentil soup<br>Rye crackers<br>Pineapple |
| **5** | Potato cakes<br>Sugar-free baked beans<br>Mint tea | Stuffed aubergine<br>(eggplant)<br>Grilled tomato, green<br>salad<br>Pear | Turkey breast<br>Boiled potato<br>Brussels sprouts,<br>beetroot |
| **6** | Greek sheep's yogurt<br>with banana, oatbran<br>and almonds<br>Herb tea | **Bean & rice casserole**<br>Green salad<br>Soya yogurt with mint,<br>cucumber | Salmon pâté &<br>ricecakes<br>Tomato, celery<br>Apple |
| **7** | Oatcakes & hummus<br>Prune juice<br>Fennel tea | **Vegetable cobbler**<br>Cabbage, carrots<br>Potato | Green leafy salad<br>**Tuna pâté** &<br>cornbread<br>Pear & figs |

## Suggestions for week 2 – menu plans

| | BREAKFAST | LUNCH | TEA/DINNER |
|---|---|---|---|
| **1** | Scrambled egg<br>Ricecakes<br>Herb tea | **Cream of water-<br>cress soup**<br>Apple<br>Beverage | **Chickpea & spinach curry**<br>Rice<br>Oat crumble |
| **2** | Soya yogurt with<br>dates, ground almonds,<br>banana<br>Tea | Chicken<br>Spinach salad<br>Jacket potato<br>Figs | **Avocado pâté** & ricecakes<br>Salad |
| **3** | Rye bread and<br>spreads<br>Herb tea | **Nut loaf**<br>Boiled new potatoes<br>Broccoli, carrots<br>Banana | Courgette (zucchini) &<br>spinach soup<br>Oatcakes<br>Apple |
| **4** | Rye crackers &<br>poached egg<br>Herb tea | Poached salmon<br>Green beans, sweetcorn<br>Jacket potato<br>Melon | **Lentil & apricot<br>soup**<br>Rye crackers<br>Dates |
| **5** | Potato cakes<br>Scrambled egg<br>Tea | **Potato-based pizza**<br>Watercress salad<br>Grilled tomato, peas<br>Pear | Grilled pork chops<br>Boiled potato<br>Green beans<br>red cabbage<br>Kiwi |
| **6** | Soya yogurt<br>with banana<br>Herb tea | **Aubergine loaf<br>(eggplant)**<br>Green salad &<br>jacket potato<br>Soya yogurt<br>with mint, cucumber | Tuna pâté & rye crackers<br>Tomato, celery<br>Apple |
| **7** | Oat crackers &<br>nut butter<br>herb tea | **Tuna &<br>sweetcorn flan**<br>Broccoli, carrots<br>Melon | **North African salad<br>Tomato salad**<br>Pear |

*Snacks between meals:*

Nuts
Sunflower seeds
Date & fig bars
Raisins & sultanas
Savoury popcorn
Hazelnut butter on crispbreads
Replace cow's milk with soya milk in recipes

These are merely suggestions to give you an idea of how several days' meals can be wheat- and dairy-free, should you want to try an exclusion-style diet. There are so many alternatives and you need not feel hungry. In fact the meals are very tasty. Experiment with some of the following recipes at weekends and get a feel for what you like. Wander round the local health food shop and see what they have to offer as alternatives to crisps and bars of chocolate. Try some of their corn pastas and rice couscous. The following recipes should give everyone something to try, many are quick and easy to prepare, and we hope that you enjoy eating them. (All recipes are for 4 people.)

> Happiness: a good bank account, a good cook, and
> a good digestion
>
> *Jean-Jacques Rousseau, Philosopher*

## SOUPS

### Lentil and apricot soup

| | |
|---|---|
| 50g/2oz red lentils, washed | ½ lemon juice |
| 50g/2oz dried apricots, washed | 1tsp ground cummin |
| 1 large potato | 3tbsp chopped parsley |
| 1.2l/2pt vegetable stock | seasoning |

*Method:*
1  Put lentils and apricots in large saucepan.
2  Chop potato and add to pan with remaining ingredients.
3  Bring to the boil, cover and simmer for 30 minutes.
4  Leave to cool.
5  Place in a blender and liquidize until smooth.
6  Reheat, adding seasoning to taste.

## Carrot and almond soup

| | |
|---|---|
| 400g/1lb carrots | 1 tbsp chopped parsley |
| 1 potato | 1tsp vegetable stockpowder |
| 1 large onion | $\frac{1}{2}$ lemon juice |
| celery leaves | 1tsp mixed herbs |
| 1 large cooking apple | 50g/2oz ground almonds |
| 2tsp wholegrain mustard | |

*Method:*
1  Dice all the vegetables.
2  Cook in 1.2l/2pt of water, simmering gently. Add the apple last of all.
3  After 25–30 mins remove from the heat. Cool for 5 mins.
4  Add the mustard, vegetable stock powder, lemon juice and herbs.
5  Blend or liquidize until smooth.
6  Add the ground almonds and reheat.
7  Garnish with flaked almonds and parsley to serve.

## Potato and leek soup

| | |
|---|---|
| 1kg/2lb potatoes | $\frac{1}{2}$oz butter |
| 400g/1lb leeks | Seasoning |
| 0.7l/1 pt milk (soya) | Parsley to garnish |

*Method:*
1  Peel and boil the potatoes until soft.
2  Clean the leeks, finely chop and fry gently until soft.
3  Mash the potatoes with some of the milk and butter.
4  Mix in the leeks and rest of milk. This may be liquidized.
5  Bring to the boil and serve garnished with parsley.

## Cream of watercress soup

| | |
|---|---|
| 1 medium onion | 0.35l/$\frac{1}{2}$pt milk (soya) |
| 1 small potato | 0.35l/$\frac{1}{2}$pt vegetable stock |
| 25g/1oz butter | salt and pepper |
| 1 bunch watercress | 4 tbsp single cream (optional) |

*Method:*
1  Chop the onion and potato.
2  Melt the butter in a saucepan and sauté the onion until transparent.

3   Add potato, watercress, milk and stock. Bring to boil, cover and simmer for 20min.
4   Allow to cool slightly, then blend until smooth.
5   Return to pan, season to taste, stir in cream and reheat to serving temperature.

## Avocado soup/dip

| | |
|---|---|
| 1 ripe avocado | 2 tbsp cream |
| 6 spring onions (scallions) | salt and pepper (optional) |
| 175g/7oz sheep's milk | |
| or soya yogurt | |

*Method:*
1   Peel and stone the avocado.
2   Slice into a tall jug.
3   Add the chopped onions, milk or yogurt, cream and seasoning.
4   Liquidize or blend to make a dip.
5   Add 0.35l/½pt water to make a cold soup.

## MAIN MEALS

## Chicken with lemon and olives

| | |
|---|---|
| 2tbsp olive oil | 1¼tsp turmeric |
| 3kg/6.5lb chicken | ½tsp salt |
| cut into 8 pieces | black pepper |
| 100g/4oz chopped onions | 2 fresh lemons, quartered |
| 1½tsp paprika | 0.3l/⅜pt water |
| 1tsp ground ginger | 24 small green olives |

*Method:*
1   Warm the olive oil and brown the chicken pieces. Place in a dish with the stock they make.
2   Pour off the remaining oil from the pan and fry the onions gently until soft and brown.
3   Stir in the paprika, ginger, turmeric, salt and pepper.
4   Add the fresh lemon, chicken pieces and the stock.
5   Add the water and bring to the boil, then reduce the heat and cover and simmer for 30min until the chicken is tender.
6   Add the olives and cover and simmer for 5min. Taste for seasoning.
7   Serve with rice and green salad or steamed vegetables.

## Potato-based pizza

| | |
|---|---|
| 225g/8oz boiled potatoes | salt and freshly ground black |
| 50g/2oz butter | pepper |
| 100g/4oz rye flour/ | |
| buckwheat/cornmeal | |

*Topping:*

| | |
|---|---|
| 2 tbsp olive oil | ½ level tbsp oregano |
| 225g/8oz onions (thinly sliced) | 2 tsp lemon juice |
| 1 red pepper (thinly sliced) | salt and freshly ground black pepper |
| 1 clove garlic (crushed) | 2 tbsp tomato purée |
| 50g/2oz frozen sweetcorn | 175g/6oz feta or buffalo milk |
| | mozzerella cheese |

*Method:*

1  Boil the potatoes until they are soft and then mash them to a pulp with the butter.
2  Sift in the flour and a little salt and pepper. Now mix to a dough.
3  Transfer to a floured surface and knead lightly until the mixture becomes soft and elastic.
4  Roll out to a 10in round. Place on oiled baking sheet.
5  Heat the olive oil in a large frying pan and fry the onions, red pepper and garlic for 5min.
6  Stir in the sweetcorn, oregano and lemon juice and a seasoning of salt and pepper.
7  Spread the tomato purée on the pizza base and then top with the onion mixture.
8  Place the cheese on top and bake on a high shelf at Reg. 6 or 400F or 200C for 40min.


## Bean and rice casserole

225g/8oz black beans, soaked overnight and drained (or cheat and use tinned kidney beans)
2 tbsp cold-pressed sunflower oil
1 medium onion, peeled and chopped
1 clove garlic, peeled and crushed
1 green pepper, cored, seeded and sliced
1 red pepper, cored, seeded and sliced
1 red chilli, finely chopped (optional)
4 large tomatoes, skinned and sliced

1 tsp coriander                     300ml/½pt. chicken stock
225g/8oz long grain brown rice  Salt and pepper

*Garnish:*
Fresh coriander leaves, avocado slices, lemon juice

*Method:*
1  Cook the beans in fast boiling, unsalted water for 15min. Reduce
   heat and simmer for 45min until tender. Drain.
2  Heat oil, fry onion over moderate heat for 3min. Add garlic,
   peppers, chilli. Stir well. Cook for 2min.
3  Add tomatoes, salt, pepper, coriander and cook for 1min. Add
   rice, stock, beans. Bring to boil.
4  Cover pan. Simmer for 45min until rice is cooked and stock is
   absorbed.
5  Garnish.


## Tuna and sweetcorn flan

100g/4oz ground almonds       100g/4oz tub margarine
50g/2oz brown rice flour          (Vitaseig or Vitaquell)
50g/2oz oatbran               salt and pepper

*Filling:*
2 eggs                        1 175g/7oz tin tuna
150ml/¼pt soya milk or small  1 175g/7oz tin sweetcorn
  carton sheep's or goat's yogurt 1 tbsp fresh parsley (chopped)

*Method:*
1  Mix the ground almonds, brown rice flour and oatbran with a
   little salt and pepper.
2  Mash together with margarine to form a soft dough.
3  Grease a pie/flan dish. Press the mixture to form a solid base and
   walls.
4  Beat the eggs and yogurt together.
6  Place the tuna, then the sweetcorn evenly in the dish. Season.
6  Sprinkle over the chopped parsley. Pour over the egg mixture.
7  Bake until pale gold. Oven Reg. 5 or 375F or 190C for 30min.

Shortcrust pastry may be used for the base (150g 6oz flour/75g 3oz
margarine rubbing in method).

## Aubergine loaf (eggplant)

1 large or 2 medium aubergines
100g/4oz cooked millet or rice
2 tbsp parsley
1 clove garlic
a few drops Worcestershire
  sauce
salt and pepper

3 eggs
75g/3oz grated cheese
  (feta/mozzarrella)
150ml/¼pt olive oil
2 tbsp tomato purée
75g/3oz flaked almonds or
pine nuts

*Method:*

1  Wash aubergines. Cut in half lengthways. Sprinkle with salt, leave for ½ hour to sweat.
2  Place all the other ingredients, except the nuts, into blender and liquidize until smooth.
3  Rinse the aubergine and chop roughly.
4  Place the aubergine and nuts into the mixture and stir.
5  Grease a 1kg/2lb loaf tin with oil. Pour in the mixture.
6  Cook for 20min at Reg. 6 or 400F or 200C. Reduce heat to Reg. 4 or 350F or 180C and cook for a further 20min.
7  Test with a skewer. Leave for 10min to cool, loosen gently and turn out.
8  Serve with rice or jacket potato and a crisp salad. Garnish with apple slices. Lovely cold too!

## Nut loaf

1 onion
75g/3oz butter
4 tbsp medium oatmeal
350ml/½pt milk (soya)
2 beaten eggs (or 1 egg + 2 yolks)

100g/4oz sweetcorn
8oz/225g nuts
  (peanuts/cashew) or dried,
  soaked chestnuts/almond
1 tbsp oat bran or sesame seeds

*Method:*

1  Peel and chop onion finely.
2  Melt the butter in a pan. Add the onions. Fry 5min.
3  Add the oatmeal, stir well.
4  Add the milk, stir until thickened. Allow to cool.
5  Stir in the beaten eggs and the sweetcorn.
6  Add the ground nuts and mix well. Season.
7  Oil tin. Line with oat bran or sesame seeds.
8  Place mixture in tin, bake for 1 hour in oven Reg. 4 or 350F or 180C.

## Chickpea and spinach curry

2 onions
1 tsp chopped root ginger
1 clove garlic chopped
1 tsp mild curry powder or
  spices: salt and pepper;
  cummin; coriander;
  cinnamon; ginger;
  ¼ tsp of each
0.25l/10 fl oz natural yogurt

2 tbsp tomato purée
1 15oz can tomatoes
1 tsp creamed coconut
450g/1lb chickpeas (soak
  overnight. boil 10min, simmer
  2h) (or tin)
450g/1lb fresh spinach
  (250g/8oz frozen)

*Method:*
1  Chop the onions finely and fry until soft in 2 tbsp olive oil with ginger and garlic.
2  Add curry powder and fry 2–3 min. Lower heat.
3  Add most of the yogurt a little at a time. Cook gently until the oil separates out.
4  Add the tomatoes and paste. Cook gently 30min until a rich curry sauce is produced.
5  Add the chickpeas and spinach. Simmer gently for 20min (add a little water if the sauce becomes too dry).

Any meat, fish or vegetables or beans may be used in the curry sauce, or it may be used to stuff aubergines and peppers (capsicum).

Serve with mango chutney, banana slices, brown rice or millet, yogurt and mint, lime pickle and tomato slices.

## To cook millet:

1 cup millet to 4 cups water. Simmer 15min. Can also be used with stir-fry vegetables. This is the most nutrient-rich grain of all and the only one which is alkaline.

## Vegetable cobbler

*Base:*
3 medium carrots
½ small cauliflower
50g/2oz butter
3 leeks

50g/2oz sweetcorn
1 tbsp cornflour
150ml/¼pt chicken stock
2 tbsp fresh parsley

*Topping:*

| | |
|---|---|
| 40g/1.5oz margarine | 50g/2oz feta cheese |
| 175g/6oz rye flour | 1 egg |
| ½ tsp baking powder | 2 tbsp natural soya yogurt |
| 75g/3oz oat bran | |

*Method:*

1  Cook carrots and cauliflower in boiling water for 5min.
2  Drain. Place into a casserole dish.
3  Melt 25g/1oz butter. Fry leeks and sweetcorn 4min. Stir.
4  Melt 25g/1oz butter. Stir in cornflour to form a roux paste.
5  Remove from heat. Slowly blend in the stock. Season.
6  Boil. Simmer 3min. Add chopped parsley. Stir continuously.
7  Place all vegetables in the casserole dish. Pour sauce over top. Put in oven for 40min at Reg. 4 or 350F or 180C.
8  Scones: Rubbing-in method. Rub the margarine into the sieved flour and baking powder. Add the bran and ¾ grated cheese.
9  Add the beaten egg and yogurt to form a firm dough.
10  Roll out. Cut 15 scones. Arrange over the vegetables.
11  Sprinkle with rest of cheese. Bake for 15min at Reg. 6 or 400F or 200C, till golden.


SNACKS

## Tuna pâté

| | |
|---|---|
| 1 tbsp live soya yogurt (level) | ¼ tbsp tomato purée. |
| ½ tbsp mayonnaise (level) | 1 small tin tuna |

*Method:*

1  Mix the yogurt, mayonnaise and tomato purée together.
2  Add the tuna and mix in.


## Avocado pâté

| | |
|---|---|
| 1 hard-boiled egg | ½ lemon |
| 1 avocado | salt, pepper, paprika |

*Method:*

1  Chop the hard-boiled egg finely into a bowl. Add salt and pepper.
2  Cut the avocado flesh into the bowl.
3  Chop together. Add the lemon juice.
4  Place in a small dish. Garnish with paprika.

## Tomato salad

| | |
|---|---|
| 4 tomatoes (peeled and thinly sliced) | Salt and freshly ground black pepper |
| 2 tbsp olive oil | 1 tbsp chopped fresh chives |
| 2 tsp lemon juice | |

*Method:*
1  Place the tomatoes in a shallow salad dish.
2  Mix together the oil, lemon juice and salt and pepper to taste.
3  Pour over the tomatoes. Sprinkle with the chives. Chill for at least 1 hour before serving.

## North African salad

| | |
|---|---|
| 175g/6oz long grain rice | 4 tbsp olive oil |
| 1 small cucumber (sliced) | 4 tsp lemon juice |
| 2 medium bananas (peeled and sliced) | large pinch ground coriander |
| 1 avocado (peeled and diced) | large pinch ground cummin |
| 1 tbsp pine nuts or almonds | salt and pepper |

*Method:*
1  Cook the rice in boiling salted water for 15min or until it is tender. Drain and allow to cool.
2  Put the rice, cucumber, bananas, avocado and pine nuts in a salad bowl and stir well.
3  Mix together the oil, lemon juice, coriander, cummin, salt and pepper in a bowl and beat well.
4  Pour dressing over the rice mixture and mix well. Serve with tuna pâté.
2 tbsp raisins can be used in place of the avocado)

## Celery, apple and walnut salad

| | |
|---|---|
| /2 medium head of celery (finely chopped) | juice of ½ lemon |
| red eating apples (cored and diced) | 1 tbsp mayonnaise |
| tbsp live yogurt | 25g/1oz shelled walnuts or pecan (chopped) |

*Method:*
1  Mix together the celery, apples, yogurt, lemon juice and mayonnaise in a salad bowl.
2  Chill for 30 minutes.
3  Just before serving, stir in the walnuts or pecans.

## Salad niçoise

½ small lettuce
  (separated into leaves)
2 tbsp olive oil
juice of ½ lemon
150g/6oz French beans
  (cooked)
3 medium potatoes
  (cooked and diced)

3 tomatoes
  (peeled and quartered)
1 75g/3.5oz can tuna
  (drained and flaked)
black olives (stoned)

*Method:*
1  Arrange lettuce leaves on a shallow serving dish.
2  Mix the oil and lemon juice together to form a dressing.
3  Cut the beans into 1in lengths and mix together with the potatoes, tomatoes, dressing and tuna.
4  Toss gently to combine. Spoon the mixture over the lettuce leaves and garnish with the black olives.

## Green tossed salad

Lettuce
Celery
Watercress

Chopped spring onions
  (scallions)
Baby spinach leaves

*Method:*
Choose a selection of the above and toss together with a mixture of olive oil and lemon juice. For flavourings add honey mustard or tahini or black olive pâté.

# BREADS

## Shaker corn bread

1 cup cornmeal (polenta)
$^1/_3$ cup soya flour
$^1/_4$ cup oatmeal
3 tsp baking powder

$^1/_2$ tsp salt
1 egg
1–1$^1/_4$ cups soya milk

*Method:*
1  Heat the oven to 190C.
2  Grease a 20cm x 10cm loaf tin.
3  Mix the dry ingredients in a bowl.
4  Beat the egg and milk together.
5  Whisk the egg milk mixture into the dry ingredients and pour into the tin.
6  Bake until golden (30min approx).
7  Eat hot or cold or toasted.
8  For a lighter texture add 2 whisked egg whites after the milk and egg, or 4tbsp grated cheese.

## Flat rye bread

2 cups rye flour
2 tsp baking powder
$^1/_2$ tsp salt

2 tbsp melted butter
1 tbsp honey
1 cup milk

*Method:*
1  Heat the oven to Reg.6 or 400F or 200C.
2  Mix the dry ingredients together.
3  Melt the butter and honey and add to the milk.
4  Beat the liquid ingredients into the flours until a smooth dough forms.
5  Oil a round pizza baking sheet and spread the dough.
6  Prick with a fork.
7  Bake until golden (approx 20 min).

## Breton pancakes

cup buckwheat flour
beaten egg

1 cup cornmeal
1$^3/_4$ cups soya milk

*Method:*
1  Mix the dry ingredients.
2  Beat the egg and milk together.
3  Add the egg and milk mixture and beat well.
4  Heat a knob of butter on a hot griddle.
5  Pour in ⅓ cup mixture and fry one side until brown and then the other.
6  Keep warm under a low grill (makes 6–8 crisp-edged pancakes).
7  Serve with maple syrup and stewed blueberries for breakfast or dessert.

Serve with tuna or salmon in parsley sauce or with chicken in mushroom sauce for a savoury meal.


## BE AWARE

Read product labels carefully when buying foods.

1  Any of the following could indicate the presence of wheat or a derivative: modified starch, dextrins, wheat flour, thickening, bran, wheat germ, cereal filler, couscous, semolina, rusk.

2  If you are gluten-sensitive, avoid: wheat, barley, oats, rye, spelt, bran, malt.

3  Any of the following could indicate the presence of milk:
   lactose, casein, whey, caseinates, ghee, hydrolized casein, milk solids, non-milk fat solids, skimmed milk powder, whey protein/sugar, yogurt.

4  If you are sugar-sensitive, watch out for:
   corn syrup, dextrose, fructose, fruit sugar, glucose, glucose syrup, golden syrup, honey, invert sugar, malt syrup, maple syrup, molasses, sucrose, treacle.

5  If eggs affect you, watch out for:
   albumen, conalbumen, egg white, egg yolk, ovalbumen, ovomucoid, ocoglobulin, vitellin, vitellenin.

6  If you are yeast-sensitive, avoid: breads, wines, dried fruits, Marmite, B vitamins and selenium obtained from yeasts, vinegars, pickled and fermented foods.

There are many good wheat-free, dairy-free and Candida recipe books around. Make or buy soda breads or sour-dough breads. Explore your diet and, if the changes you make help you, then stick with them for three months and then gradually introduce a 'new' food every fourth day. It can take up to four days to react to a food so leave at least that time between different foodstuffs. You may wish to try a rotation diet of rye on the first day, potato on the second day, oats on the third day, rice on the fourth day and corn on the fifth day.

This is a quest which you can try to see if a particular food is upsetting your digestion or immune system. Allergy Care and Lifestyle (*see* Useful addresses) have mail order catalogues which may help you to find the alternative foods if you live far from a good health food shop.

## SUMMARY

1  Eat organic fruits and vegetables if you can.

2  Eat more foods from lower down the food chain, such as fruits, vegetables, nuts, seeds and cereals. Avoid an excess of animal foods, so less pesticides will be absorbed from animal fat.

3  Stock up your cupboard with interesting foods, especially when undergoing an exclusion diet. Ensure that you have corn tacos, oatcakes, rye crispbreads, ricecakes on hand. Add exciting dishes to your repertoire and try some of the recipes included here.

4  Look around health food shops for all the alternative foods and healthy cis cold-pressed oils and organic grains, nuts and seeds. Find out about organic food delivery services from the Soil Association.

5  Try to cook most of your meals from fresh food, so you have control over their content.

6  Make the changes and give your new 'diet' three months to help your body renew itself and to stimulate the cells to work efficiently at producing hormones, enzymes and prostaglandins.

If you suspect one or two foods are upsetting you, exclude them one at a time for one month. If it makes a difference to the way you feel you are halfway there, and the second half of the journey gets much easier. Once you begin to taste that feeling of wellness, there is no going back.

Variety is the spice of life!

# 11 Furthering research: let's find the cure

> There is no medicine like hope, no incentive so great, and no tonic so powerful as expectation of something better tomorrow.
>
> *Orison Swett Marden*

Endometriosis has the dubious distinction of being one of the major enigmas of modern gynaecology. It rightly deserves this honour of being classified as an enigma for the simple reason that science has yet definitively to determine the cause of the disease and, more importantly, has yet to develop a permanent cure. It is especially enigmatic since it is not a newly discovered disease. Sampson gave an elegant description of endometriosis in the early 1920s and we have not made much progress in medically understanding this disease for the 50 years following his landmark observations. However, since the 1980s, things are beginning to happen at a rapid pace. Over the past 10 years, more and more scientists have taken on the challenge of uncovering the nature of these rogue implants and hopefully in our lifetime we may see the development of a cure for endometriosis.

The reason for the absence of a cure for one of the most prevalent gynaecologic disorders of our society can be summed up in one statement: 'nobody dies from endometriosis'. Although women may at times feel like they could die from the pain, there have been rare reports of serious complications. Endometriosis is a benign disease. Because of this, most governments are not willing to give much financial backing for scientific investigations of endometriosis. Just 15 years ago you could count on your fingers the number of scientists around the world who were actively engaged in research on endometriosis. But the good news is that this attitude has abruptly changed over the past 10 years, primarily through the 'grassroots' efforts of afflicted women. Working through organizations like the International Endometriosis Association, headquartered in the USA, who aid associations in countries all over the world, and the separate National British Endometriosis Society and the Endometriosis Association of Australia and New Zealand Endometriosis Foundation (and fertility self-help groups like the American Resolve and British Issue groups), more money has recently become available to scientists through the lobbying of governments to release more money for this specialized research. Often women are too ill to raise money on their own behalf to give to drug companies for research. This new research has begun to shed light on the cause and development of endometriosis, and will hopefully lead to an understanding of the disease that will eventually evolve into a medical cure. It would be so wondrous to have at our disposal a one-application cure that would rid womankind of the pain and infertility of endometriosis, though healthy eating relieves symptoms.

The authors would like to share with you some of the promising areas of scientific investigation that may lead to the cure that women so desperately crave. Current scientific research seems to be centred on investigations of the cause of endometriosis, the biochemistry of the endometriotic implant and therapies, and the design of new drugs to suppress the disease or new surgical techniques to cut out damaged organs. More thought needs to be applied to finding the cause in order to elicit the cure. Only by actually knowing what is triggering this disease can we hope to develop a real cure, instead of just suppressing symptoms. Nutrition is a key player in this discovery.

## THE CAUSES OF ENDOMETRIOSIS

In chapter 2 we discussed the current theories of what causes endometriosis. The theory with the most support is that proposed by Sampson in the early 1920s. He noted that endometriosis may be a result of endometrial tissue falling into the abdominal cavity, instead of flowing out of the uterus at the time of the menstrual period. This endometrium attaches to the walls of the abdomen and grows under the influence of the ovarian steroids. However, there is a problem with this theory. It seems that nearly all women have free-floating endometrium in their abdomen at the time of the menstrual period, yet many women do not develop endometriosis. The obvious question thus arises – 'Why do some women appear to be "immune" to endometriosis while other women readily develop the disease?' To answer this question scientists have been actively examining what mechanisms are involved in the attachment of endometrial tissue to the abdominal wall.

## ATTACHMENT OF CELLS

The most exciting research has been on molecules that allow two cells to attach or become integrated into each other. The three major types of substances involved in the attachment and growth of endometriotic implants are growth factors, remodelling enzymes and integrins.

The growth factors are hormone-like substances that stimulate cellular growth. They are required for normal cells to divide to form new cells and therefore they allow for tissue growth.

The remodelling enzymes are compounds that enzymatically digest away the connections between cells. These are the enzymes that some cells secrete to digest away the cement that allows cells to be attached to each other. They must be secreted in order for cells, like endometrial cells, to invade or wiggle their way in between the cells of the abdominal cavity.

The physical attachment of cells to each other involves the third type of molecules, the integrins. Integrins are molecules on the surface of cells that allow cells to attach to each other. They are like the glue that allows the endometriotic implant to become permanently attached within the abdominal cavity.

### Growth factors

Many cells of the body produce a class of stimulatory molecules that have been called growth factors and cytokines. These factors are very diverse and have been given names which would seem unusual to most people. Since these names can be confusing we will use their initials as we describe them. In women with endometriosis, growth factors and cytokines are secreted primarily by the endometrium itself and also by immune cells (*see* chapter 7). These factors are dumped into the fluids of the abdominal cavity and stimulate the cells of the endometriotic implant to grow.

The five major growth factors and cytokines found in the fluids of the abdominal cavity are IGF (insulin-like growth factor), EGF (epithelial growth factor), VEGF (vascular epithelial growth factor), IL-1 (interleukin-1) and TNF (tumor necrosis factor).[1] Laboratory experiments have shown that abdominal fluid and some of these compounds stimulate the growth of the endometrium. Furthermore, the abdominal fluid of women with endometriosis contains more VEGF, IL-1 and TNF than that of women who do not have the disease. We have not yet investigated all of the growth factors/ cytokines, but by understanding these substances better we may come up with a means of preventing growth of endometriotic implants.

## Remodelling enzymes

As the endometrial tissue attaches to the abdominal wall, the cells of the abdominal wall must be separated to allow the endometrial cells to wedge themselves in between the cells of the abdominal wall. This remodelling of the cells of the abdominal wall is controlled by two groups of proteins, the MMPs (metalloproteinases) and TIMPs (tissue inhibitors of MMPs). MMPs (which are based upon minerals) digest the connections between cells, and TIMPs inhibit this action. As the endometrium attaches to the wall of the abdomen MMPs are secreted, and the endometrium worms its way into the abdominal wall. TIMP molecules are secreted at the same time to prevent the digestion of the abdominal tissue next to the endometrium. For endometrial tissue, the production of the remodelling enzymes is controlled by the ovarian steroid hormone progesterone.[2] This may be why the endometriosis re-attaches and gets worse with each menstrual cycle. The oestrogen and progesterone produced in each menstrual period is conducive to endometrial implantation into the abdominal wall. Another exciting bit of laboratory research has been the discovery that suppression of MMPs prevents the attachment of endometrium to abdominal cells.[3] This has not been tested in humans, but if a form of treatment could be developed that did not have bad side effects, the potential therapeutic benefits would be great. Remember that magnesium, vitamins A, E and C and cis fatty acids give cell membranes their integrity so harmful drugs are unnecessary.

## Integrins

Each cell has to be able to 'stick' to another and the surrounding tissue to form our body structure. This adhesion material is collectively known as 'integrins'. In addition to maintaining the structure of our body, integrins are important in the healing of wounds and for the development of the embryo. Once again the 'stickiness' has to be just right. The mesh formed by integrins is made of gel-like chains of sugars and proteins, as well as collagen. It is rather like the cell having velcro made of proteins on the outside. This velcro surface sticks to the protein scaffold on the next cell wall, which makes up the connective tissue known as collagen (using vitamins A, C and zinc).

Over 20 different types of integrins have been found so far and the number of integrins discovered in the human endometrium and in endometriosis continues to grow.[4] Additionally, the integrins of the endometriotic implant are different from those of the endometrium of the uterus.[5] The role of these differences is still under investigation.

The integrins can have a very powerful effect on cells. If these contacts are lost, dividing cells stop proliferating and die. The messages passed via integrins from outside and inside all cells depends upon the quality of integrins. If we could selectively inhibit the integrins of the endometriotic implant, it would cause the death of the endometriosis. There is some evidence that the function of integrins is modulated by lipids, so again the type of cis oils in the diet may play a role.

By studying the molecules involved in the growth and development of the endometriotic implants, scientists may be able to better understand why some women get endometriosis and others do not. It is hoped that we can mimic the effects seen in the abdomens of the women without endometriosis as a cure for women who develop endometriosis.

## THE IMMUNE SYSTEM

One of the more promising areas of research has been the role of the immune system in the development and maintenance of endometriosis. As we discussed in chapter 7, the immune system of the endometriosis patient appears to be altered, and this alteration may be one of the main reasons why some women develop endometriosis while others do not. The first indication that the immune system may have gone awry was the observation in the early 1980s that the macrophages of the abdominal cavity were different in patients with endometriosis to those in disease-free patients.[6, 7] We now know that these macrophages make some of the growth factors/cytokines mentioned above and that they stimulate endometrial growth and therefore the endometriotic implant.[8] More recently, laboratory experiments were presented at the international endometriosis meetings in Yokohama, Japan, that suggest that implant growth will not progress in the absence of macrophages.[9] The administration of a compound that inhibits the activation of macrophages (pentoxyphyline) prevented the invasion and development of endometriotic implants. These studies have not been tested in long-term human studies but the initial results are encouraging, though a loss of macrophages, and weakening the immune system could lead to major health problems and death.

## THE ENDOMETRIOTIC IMPLANT

One of the reasons why very little progress has been made in endometriosis research is related to the fact that most research over the past 30 years has dealt exclusively with treatment. Very little work was directed towards the study of the pathology and physiology of the disease. Money can only be made by drug companies in developing drugs so the crucial basic cellular science work is neglected. However, there has been a recent interest in studying how the endometriotic implant functions. In particular, the implants have been examined for their capacity to secrete substances that may be of physiological importance. We have already seen from the above discussion that many scientists have examined the implants' ability to produce a variety of substances (e.g., growth hormones, cytokines and integrins). There has also been an interest in examining the proteins produced by implants. Drs Sharpe and Vernon have shown that endometriotic implants are prolific in manufacturing proteins and that they produce hundreds of different proteins.[10] However, when they compared the implant with the endometrium, they noted that two unique proteins were produced by the implant and not by the endometrium of the uterus. These two proteins were called endo 1 and endo 2 (endometriotic implant proteins 1 and 2). Dr Sharpe has purified, isolated and determined that these proteins are TIMP (see pp. 69, 280) and a large protein called haptoglobin. These are exciting discoveries since these proteins may serve as markers of the disease. It may be possible some day to collect a blood or abdominal fluid sample to determine if a person has endometriosis and maybe even be able to tell how severe the disease is. This would be much better than performing a laparoscopic examination under general anaesthesia.

## PRION PROTEINS

Strange prion proteins, responsible for 'mad cow disease', have been cast as 'social deviants' because their only known function was to wreak havoc. But new research is beginning to show that prion proteins may have an important role to play in health. A geneticist at the National Institute of Health in Washington DC has discovered prions in yeasts. Some researchers believe that prion proteins may help the fertilized egg to become a multicellular organism. At some point in this transformation the embryo cells decide whether to become liver, muscle or other tissue. Once they have made that decision, all their progeny have to stick with it. Yet all cells carry the same genetic code, so it is unclear just how these cells pass on this vital information. Prions could be responsible. Cells in different tissues manufacture different types of protein, some of which keep the correct genes for that tissue turned on. If these regulatory proteins had the ability to spread their influence as prions do, then dividing cells within a tissue would automatically know which genes to turn on. Some of these phenomena could be to do with prions.[11]

When a group of cells in the developing animal begin to change into a different type of tissue, large amounts of regulatory proteins appear in a cascade which later subsides. Researchers have identified these prion proteins which allow yeasts to change between the two types, though it is too early in the research to see specifics. This new area of research may show why normal endometrium tissue within the uterus turns into endometriotic implants outside the uterus, producing its own oestrogens and proteins.

## NUTRITION RESEARCH

There has been a lack of well-controlled experiments involving sufficient numbers of women with the specific condition o endometriosis. However, there have been other trials which have looked at the role of nutrients in relation to symptoms of pain fatigue, heavy periods and fertilization. There have been numerou studies on nutrition and its effects on reproduction and the uterus, bu to our knowledge there has only been one endometriosis study tha has looked at women's health and symptomatology with regard to th use of supplements and diet. Research into the nutritional status c the endometriosis patient looked at 20 women diagnosed wit endometriosis and 10 women with no history of female complain (acting as controls), for a three-month period. The women were matched in pairs according to deficiency symptoms; each pair was then randomly split into two groups – A and B. A placebo or nutrition supplement containing thiamine (100mg), riboflavin (100mg), pyridoxine (100mg), magnesium amino acid chelate (300mg) and zinc orotate (20mg) was taken for three months. During the three months the women with endometriosis in the placebo group showed no statistically significant change in their symptoms, whereas the women with endometriosis on the supplement showed a statistically significant (98 per cent) improvement of their symptoms. The study suggests that nutritional supplementation and/or an improvement in the diet may offer significant alleviation of some of the symptoms which we perceive to be linked to endometriosis.[12] Much of this information is included in this book and it is hoped that this information will stimulate an increase in awareness of the importance of doing nutritional research on endometriosis.

Further detailed research assessing the vitamin and mineral status of women with endometriosis may well show up certain anomalies in body biochemistry that we may be able to use to our advantage in treating the symptoms of endometriosis. Whether these anomalies are due to a poor diet, malabsorption or a genetic enzyme failure may hold a clue to the elusive cure for endometriosis. By assessing B vitamin levels, red cell, magnesium, white cell, zinc, liver enzyme status, hair mineral analysis, thyroid profile, thyroid auto antibodies, allergy screen, gluten sensitivity evaluation, gut fermentation study, liver profile, chlamydia species specific antibody screen, and hormone profiles, we may find a commonality to help research follow the right path. Research has shown ways in which nutrients and changes in diet may be used to alleviate pain, inflammation, fatigue and PMS symptoms. We can harness that information to help improve our health. Orthodox treatments currently fall short of curing the disease; correcting the basic body biochemistry of each individual may be a start. We are at a crossroads when a combination of research in different fields may combine to provide the cure.

## THE ELUSIVE CURE

The bottom line for endometriosis research is to develop a cure. It should be evident from the above discussion that there is much hope for a cure. What we should learn from the study of endometriosis is that the body is not a set of disparate organs. We can no longer compartmentalize the organs into the separate digestive, immune and endocrine systems as they all work together. Gynaecologists need to become immunologists and gastroenterologists, and vice versa, or work very closely together. Nutrition helps the body as a whole; it is true holistic and preventive medicine for the future. Orthodox medicine has not yet reached this point of knowledge but it must if we are to find a cure. Nutritional assessment should be a major part of the cure.

The main driving force behind the development of a cure is the procurement of the funds required by nutritionists to continue their research. Through the efforts of many 'grassroots' groups, funding has increased for endometriosis research, but we must guard against slowing down our efforts when we are so near having a potential cure. We must unite to encourage increases in the government funding of endometriosis research. Our daughters must not have the threat of this illness hanging over them like the sword of Damocles; it is currently estimated that 'one in 20 sufferers will be teenagers'.[13] How could we ever want any of our children to suffer what we are going through? Present statistics demand action: 'With the present world population of 6 billion, not less than 200 million women should therefore have endometriosis. By the year 2025 the world population could reach 10 billion with the potential of half a billion women suffering from this disease.'[14] Women need to push forward the research effort on endometriosis.

Let us all hope that a second edition of this book will not be needed because of the development of a cure. What a pleasant thought!

> There is nothing so far removed from us to be beyond our reach, or so hidden as to be that we cannot discover it
>
> *René Descartes, French Philosopher*

## SUMMARY

1   Encourage government funding of basic research to find a cure.

2   A cure will only come when we know why endometriosis occurs. Suppression by drugs is not a cure. When the drugs are stopped the endometriosis comes back, often within 18 months.

3   Encourage research which shows how cells function.

4   Support your local endometriosis charity, even if you do not attend the meetings. Stay in contact with the group leader to encourage and support research. Local companies may be willing to give to the charities. Persuade family members to leave a legacy in their wills. (Look up www.endometriosis.co.uk.)

5   Watch little girls at play. Do you really want them to grow up and experience what women with endometriosis have to go through? The answer is always NO. No one should have to endure this pain. Make yourself heard either through your local group or at a national level.

6   The interest in medical research has increased greatly over the past 10 years. However, relative to other areas of science, very few governmental resources have been applied to endometriosis research.

7   Some promising areas of research include those which look at growth factors, the immune system, integrins and specific proteins which are excreted, as well as looking at basic body biochemistry.

8   Although nutrition can have an amazing impact on endometriosis there has been a lack of well-controlled research. By looking at a large group of women and comparing their basic body chemistry, we may be able to find exactly what imbalances exist in body cells which could be common to us all. This could point to a cure and treatment for the source of the problem. Healthy eating often alleviates the symptoms.

9   Nutrition affects all body systems, the reproductive, immune, digestive and nervous systems, which are all interlinked. We have to move away from the idea that just the womb and ovaries are involved in endometriosis. As we have seen in this book, this disease is systemic. It affects the whole body.

10   Become informed of research and the choices open to you. You can only make a true choice for your own treatment if you have been given an informed choice. If access to some orthodox and holistic treatments are being hidden or even denied you, then be suspicious. Ask questions until you are happy with the answers. Ulterior motives abound, usually to do with profit, not your health.

# 12 Conclusion

There's no elevator to success
You have to take the stairs
*Live and Learn and Pass it On,*
*quote from the Central Baptist Hospital*
*1997 calendar*

Endometriosis is a serious, debilitating disease which can manifest itself in so many ways. This is the crux of the problem. Every woman's endometriosis pain is different. The whole condition remains a mystery to the medical profession and lay people alike. Women need a cure. This is the cry of distressed women the world over. Drugs and surgery can allay some symptoms, but often bring others. Getting to the root of the problem and working with the body are all-important. After all, we are what we eat. To help the body heal requires good food rich in nutrients. The body is trying to heal itself all the time. Look at the speed with which it can work, given the right building blocks:

- Blood circulates through the body every 20 seconds. In one minute it has travelled through the liver 3 times!
- You produce 100 billion red blood cells every day.
- Over 2,000 immune cells per second are produced by the body.
- Touch something and you send a message to your brain at 124 mph.
- You make one litre of saliva each day.
- Every four days the whole lining of the GI tract is renewed.
- When you smile, you exercise 30 different muscles.

Seek happiness in the present, and you'll find it in
the future

*Kazuo Suzuki, Karate Master*

We need to work with the body, not against it. The environment contains harmful substances, as do some foodstuffs. We have to try to avoid these to give our immune and reproductive systems a fighting chance. Health can be regained, as you have read in this book.

We are all unique and we can only do our best. Eating well gives your body the ability to heal itself. Remember, the main nutritional premises of this book are:

1  Eat as well as you can afford.
2  Buy the freshest food you can find.
3  Cook from fresh whenever possible, or eat fresh, raw food in salads daily.
4  Eat as wide a variety of foodstuffs as possible, remembering that 'variety is the spice of life'.

Nutrition is not an easy option, as some of the women have stated in the case studies. It requires some determination and perseverance. You can but try. Women can all help one another through this healing process. The support network is on the Internet. Log into: http://www.endometriosis.co.uk and http://www.makingbabies.com. The web page offers a holistic approach including both orthodox and complementary ideas, information on medical ethics, and contacts around the world in order to answer the questions you seek help for and to give you an informed choice.

Being positive in the face of an illness for which no cure is offered requires a lot of faith and hope and the will to be well. Helping yourself along the path to recovery is a start. Let this book be a guide; we want to take you on a journey back to wellness.

This book should help to lead you into discovering the power of good nutrition. Use it well and pass the message on. When women meet at endometriosis symposia all over the globe, we try to metaphorically hold hands around the world, because we are all a part of a whole. Never feel alone with endometriosis – women are all guides for one another. There are many roads back to wellness, and when you have the strength you will find the right combination for you. Have faith in the body's ability to heal.

> We only grow when we push ourselves beyond what we
>     already know
> Every great achievement was once considered impossible
>
> *Live and Learn and Pass it On, quote from the Central Baptist*
> *Hospital 1997 calendar*

## TWENTY ESSENTIAL THINGS TO DO WHEN YOU HAVE BEEN DIAGNOSED AS HAVING ENDOMETRIOSIS

Patient empowerment helps those suffering from ill health to regain their sense of well-being; therefore empower yourself. Research ways you can help yourself. Self-help techniques can bridge the gap between suffering from the debilitating effects of illness and regaining your health. When you have been diagnosed as having endometriosis, find out about complementary therapies which can be combined with or used separately from drugs or surgery that you can use on your road to recovery. Never assume anything. Always ask questions. Ask your consultant, ask your doctor, ask other women with endometriosis about the condition – and keep on asking. The answers you are after will be out there somewhere. Collect together the pieces of the jigsaw and find your own key to good health. Here follows a list of 20 things that will help you.

1   While endometriosis is not a fatal illness, the pain is real and we have to learn to control it. Learn about pain and methods of pain relief to ease it with the treatments that are right for you.

2   Take charge of your treatment. Ask yourself what you want and devise a strategy to get it. Choose your healing team and work with them towards your goals, be those the goals of pain reduction or regaining your fertility.

3   Ask your doctor questions such as the following:
   • Where is my endometriosis growing?
   • Have you performed biopsies?
   • What stage is my endometriosis at, according to the ASRM? (*see* appendix.)
   • What additional tests are needed?
   • What are my options for treatment?
   • Would laser surgery be the best option?

   Be active and ask all the questions that you need answers to.

4   If necessary, get a second opinion. If you feel unhappy about what is being recommended to you, seek help elsewhere. It is not a crime to want the best for your body. Women in your local support group/chapter or at a charity office may be able to

recommend consultants who carry out specialist research, if that is what you need. Talk to them. Be sure of their competence.

5 Read, talk about and review your treatment options. Only then can you know which treatment is right for you and give informed consent. Find out as much as you can from other women. Many women use a combination of orthodox and complementary therapies to help them heal. You must choose what feels right for you as an individual.

6 Be sure of your doctor. If you are wracked with pain or feeling depressed because you have not been able to conceive, you need the best doctor you can find to help you. Find a doctor with good interpersonal skills – someone you can talk to, who listens and works with you. Your doctor should be your friend and guide, never an enemy.

7 Think hard about your treatment decision. Check that you have been given consistent information. You must be satisfied that you have gathered all the information available. Listen to the women who have become well – then decide.

8 Give informed consent. You need to know in detail the risks from taking courses of drugs, from having surgery, from the effects of anaesthetics, and so on. *Never* sign a consent form unless you are completely clear about the procedures involved in your treatment. Make sure that the procedure is described to you before you consent. Cross out statements that you do not wish to consent to. Write in your own statements if necessary, such as 'I do not wish to have any organs removed without having being consulted after exploratory surgery'.

9 Have faith. If you believe in and are happy with your choice of treatment, this will make a difference. Optimism is infectious – if the treatment feels right, go for it wholeheartedly. If not, review your options.

10 Make the most of your appointments with your doctor. If you wish, take a friend or partner with you. Appreciate that the information you and your doctor share forms an important part of your recovery. Trust and honesty play key roles. Be open and assertive about your needs and expectations. Show your appreciation when your doctor responds in kind. Your doctor should be your healing partner.

11   Your lifestyle is your personal choice, but remember that some of the keys to healing include following a healthy diet, enjoying gentle exercise, relaxation and stress reduction. Do what you can to make these factors play an important role in your healing.

12   Aim for total well-being. Enjoying life and feeling content are important. You have to take care of yourself. Decide to be well, make this your goal. Aim straight and true.

13   Eat well. It is important to give your body the best quality food available. Choose the freshest options and give up manufactured foods. Go for gold – the best nutrient intake possible!

14   Avoid stressors. Substances which stress your body the most include coffee, tea, chocolate, fizzy drinks, alcohol and cigarettes. Decide what your priorities are when you are trying to get well.

15   Drink fresh water and replace your body fluids frequently. The optimum amount of water every day is eight cups. Use a water filter or drink bottled water.

16   Use nutritional supplements to boost yourself up. Be cautious, read and study to find out what you need. Consult a nutritionist who specializes in women's problems. Combined with a healthy diet for three to four months, supplements may speed your body's ability to heal.

17   Rest, sleep and exercise. All are important. Give yourself permission to be ill and allow your body the time it needs to heal. Go for gentle walks; visit your local pool and allow the water to take your weight. Sleep when your body tells you it is tired.

18   Read books for pleasurable relaxation and learn about how your body can heal itself. Endometriosis is a challenge but adequate rest and relaxation can give you more energy to help yourself heal.

19   Use visualization techniques. As the saying goes, 'imagination sets you free to be just what you want to be'. Create mental pictures of yourself bouncing with health. Visualize your uterus and ovaries as pink and glowing with health. Imagine your cysts and endometriotic implants shrinking away. Be positive. Women

have healed and there is no reason why you will not be one of them.

20  Learn to laugh and play again. Whenever we are ill, in pain, or trying desperately to become pregnant we lose a part of ourselves in the trauma. Find your smile again. Watch funny films, do things which bring pleasure into your life. Choose to spend time with people who fill you with joy.

Strive to be well again; it is your future.

## ADJUSTING YOUR EATING PATTERN

To help to guide you down the right path to health, we have some suggestions for supplements which you may wish to use while you adjust your eating pattern. No woman requires exactly the same supplements as another, owing to our unique biochemical individuality. Just as our endometriosis manifests itself in a different way in each of us, the pattern of nutrients needed by each of us will be subtly different. As a nutritionist assesses your specific needs they will be different from the next person's. Tests will show the vitamin and mineral status of your tissues, gut fermentation and food intolerances, and from these any deficiencies can be seen and adjusted. This is why no two women who come for nutrition consultations ever leave with the same dietary advice or 'prescription' for supplements.

It is important to understand that the nutritional regimes in this book are not like orthodox or complementary medicine. Both of these approaches require you to take a medicine, be it a pharmaceutical drug, a herb or a homeopathic tablet, until you are well. Nutrition works when you assess your present lifestyle and nutrient intake. The changes you make hopefully will improve the integrity of the digestive tract and thus the absorption of the vital nutrients which the body requires in order to heal. You may need to take supplements for a short time to speed up this healing process. Many of the changes you make will stay with you for a long time, once you are eating foods which supply the nutrients your reproductive system needs. Knowing how good it can feel when you are well again often keeps one focused on the goal of maintaining that sense of wellness, and continuing a healthy eating habit.

Often the author has been asked to formulate a little tablet for everyone to take. This is impossible. Endometriosis is too multifactorial and the sufferers have symptoms which are so varied. And not all symptoms may be caused by endometriosis, some may be vitamin and mineral deficiencies, enzyme failures or genetic weak links. Everyone has to be treated according to their individual needs. The treatment is individually tailored and that uniqueness is followed up each visit. Over a period of two to six months your diet can be adjusted and supplements taken to improve nutrient absorption until the body biochemistry has been corrected. The healthy eating pattern should then be maintained and supplements may be used only as necessary. The body should be able to correct itself and maintain this balance while good quality food is eaten, with supplements only taken if ill health strikes again. Some people like to take a maintenance dose of supplements at weekends only.

The role of nutrition should be to correct imbalances. Once health has been obtained the body should, given a good quality, nutrient-rich, balanced diet and an efficient digestive system, maintain that health without the constant need for supplements. Supplements alone will not suffice; what you eat is all-important. The two need to be combined at first in order for the body to recover its equilibrium, its balance. Just taking supplements alone and continuing to eat an over-processed, high-sugar, high-fat, low-fibre diet will not improve health.

One should always take a low dose multivitamin/mineral supplement as a base upon which to build. Remember that if a single specific B vitamin is required, then a B complex should be taken either alone or as part of a multivitamin and mineral supplement. Then the single B vitamin can be added on top. All the supplements you buy should be hypo-allergenic, yeast-, wheat-, gluten-, sugar- and dairy-free. Many can be obtained by mail order if a good supplier is not available locally. The quality is very important. Cheaper supplements may have less absorbable forms of minerals or yeast-based vitamins. Never begin a treatment until you have consulted a qualified nutritionist.

All substances are poisonous if taken in excess, even water. Manufacturers always put safe doses in their products. The danger comes when people think they know better and that if one is good, two must be even better. It is NOT! Follow the instructions and check with the table in chapter 9 (*see* p. 237) as to safe levels. Never exceed these. Always err on the side of caution.

Earlier chapters have listed supplements which may be helpful in the treatment of pain, infertility and endometriosis. Here follows a list of those supplements, a selection of which may assist in the reduction of additional symptoms which are associated with endometriosis.

## FATIGUE

Low energy reserves are common with endometriosis, when you are constantly fighting pain and anxiety from wondering what is going to happen next. The emotional toll from the stress of it all wears out the nerves.

- Coenzyme Q 10 (ubiquinone)
- B vitamin complex
- Iron EAP2 or citrate
  (for one month)
- Chromium polynicotinate
- Evening primrose and fish oils
- Magnesium malate
- Pantothenic acid (B5)
- Vitamin C with
  bioflavinoids
- Zinc citrate

## DEPRESSION

Deficiencies of various vitamins and minerals are associated with depression, e.g calcium, magnesium, potassium, iron, vitamin C, biotin, folic acid, pyridoxine, thiamin and B12, plus an excess of copper or magnesium. Balance is all-important with all nutrition. Certain food allergies can be problematic, especially sugar and wheat with susceptible people. Some foods become addictive, and often it is the food which you are craving which is doing you the most harm.

- B complex vitamins
- Folic acid
- Magnesium EAP2
- Vitamin C
- Chromium polynicotinate
- Multivitamin/mineral
- Biotin
- Calcium citrate
- Iron EAP2
- Evening primrose and fish oils
- DL phenylalanine or L
  tyrosine

## MITRAL VALVE PROLAPSE

This has been found to be fairly common in women with endometriosis. The heart requires vitamin B1 (thiamin) and magnesium to help the muscle relax. Avoid phosphorous fizzy drinks and all foods containing caffeine. Potassium levels should be checked, and eat plenty of fresh fruits and vegetables.

- Magnesium EAP2
- Coenzyme Q 10

- Vitamin B1 (thiamin)
- Multivitamin/mineral

## OSTEOPOROSIS

As oestrogen levels decline we may be liable to osteoporosis. Also some hormone treatments may provoke this condition if they simulate menopause. Maintaining a healthy diet containing all the nutrients required by bone can be a start. Bone is living tissue with nutrients constantly flowing in and out. It needs magnesium, phosphorus, boron, manganese, silicon, strontium, zinc, copper, sodium, vitamins K, D and B6, folic acid and protein, as well as calcium. The balance is all-important. Three brisk 20-minute walks each week helps to put calcium into bone. Avoid caffeine.

- Boron (3mg day)
- Magnesium malate
- Vitamin D

- Calcium gluconate
- Multivitamin/mineral tablet

## HOT FLUSHES

Research has shown vitamin E to be very effective in reducing the frequency of hot flushes and painful breasts. If you have wheat intolerance, look for a vitamin E which is not from wheatgerm oil.

- Vitamin E
- Vitamin C with bioflavinoids

- Multivitamin/mineral
- Evening primrose oil

## INSOMNIA

Foods high in the amino acid L tryptophan may be helpful as this amino acid is the precursor to serotonin, a neurotransmitter which is important in inducing sleep. Evening meals containing turkey, milk, soya, cottage cheese, peanuts, lentils, etc. can be helpful. Never take B vitamins at night as they keep you awake!

- Magnesium malate
- Chamomile or lime blossom tea

- Vitamin B3 (niacinamide)
- Multivitamin-mineral

**There are a few rules to remember when taking supplements:**

1  Always consult a doctor before you try to get pregnant or if you

are planning to lose weight. Choosing supplements on these occasions requires expert advice from a nutritionist, not a doctor with no nutrition training.

2  Ask for various tests (thyroid and coeliac checks) to be done. Never undertake a course of supplements if you are already taking orthodox medications unless interactions have been ruled out.

3  Vitamin E should only be taken at 100iu dose if you have high blood pressure. It should not be taken with magnesium, as they are antagonistic and cancel one another out. Similarly never take zinc and iron together.

4  Always take folic acid with zinc. Take a B vitamin complex with a single B vitamin, otherwise the single B vitamin stays high, while the others are knocked down low. Vitamin C taken with iron helps its absorption; calcium uptake is improved when evening primrose oil is taken; likewise boron improves calcium uptake.

5  Evening primrose oil should not be taken by anyone prone to epilepsy.

6  Most supplements are designed to be taken with food.

7  Prebiotics, probiotics and digestive enzymes should be taken with a cold drink. You must heal the digestive tract first.

8  All the supplements you buy should be hypo-allergenic, yeast-, wheat-, gluten-, sugar-, and dairy-free.

We wish you well in your quest for health. Be sensible and eat as well as you are able, taking supplements only when necessary. Two to three months should be adequate if you have milder symptoms, but some women may need to follow a sensible eating pattern for longer (six months to one year). It all depends how ill you are to begin with.

Listen to what your body tells you about foods and supplements. There is life after endometriosis, and you can regain good health by making your body as strong as possible. Take heed of the comments of women throughout this book. They have trodden this path before you. Let them lead the way. We must thank all of them for their trust and perseverance. Good luck with your quest. May good health be yours; it is the most precious thing you own.

> Eat well, sleep well – deeply. For tomorrow comes and
> it's all yours.
>
> *Ancient proverb*

## SUMMARY

1  Your body is trying to heal itself. Have faith in your body's ability to heal.

2  You can give your body the building blocks it needs. Changing your eating pattern will help. Taking supplements will enhance the healing process, but just taking supplements without improving digestion and nutrient intake will have no effect.

3   Heal your digestive tract first.

4  You are unique and, as such, you need individual treatment. What works for one person will not work in the same way for another.

5  You need to muster some determination and perseverance in your quest for good health. It takes some time to heal a body which has been ill for some time. Use this book's nutritional suggestions as a guideline.

6  Never feel alone with endometriosis. Know that all over the world women are sharing your pain and working to overcome it.

7  Assess your present lifestyle and nutrient intake carefully and honestly.

8  Eat healthy food and avoid greasy, fatty, sugary, starchy processed junk – it will make you ill. Cook from fresh often.

9  Be sensible about nutritional supplements. They are a support while you improve your eating pattern and/or correct your digestion.

10  Let the women who have trodden this path before you lead the way. Health is a pleasure we should grasp in both hands.

'Never doubt that a small group of thoughtful, committed people can change the world. Indeed, it is the only thing that ever has.'

*Margaret Mead, Anthropologist*

Join us on our web pages:
www.endometriosis.co.uk
www.makingbabies.com

# Appendix A

American Society for Reproductive Medicine Revised Classification of Endometriosis

| Patient's Name | | | | Date | |
|---|---|---|---|---|---|

| Stage I | (Minimal) | - | 1-5 | Laparoscopy _____ Laparotomy _____ Photography _____ |
|---|---|---|---|---|
| Stage II | (Mild) | - | 6-15 | Recommended Treatment _____ |
| Stage III | (Moderate) | - | 16-40 | |
| Stage IV | (Severe) | - | >40 | Prognosis _____ |
| Total | _____ | | | |

| | ENDOMETRIOSIS | | <1cm | 1-3cm | >3cm |
|---|---|---|---|---|---|
| **PERITONEUM** | Superficial | | 1 | 2 | 4 |
| | Deep | | 2 | 4 | 6 |
| **OVARY** | R | Superficial | 1 | 2 | 4 |
| | | Deep | 4 | 16 | 20 |
| | L | Superficial | 1 | 2 | 4 |
| | | Deep | 4 | 16 | 20 |

| POSTERIOR CULDESAC OBLITERATION | Partial | Complete |
|---|---|---|
| | 4 | 40 |

| | ADHESIONS | | <1/3 Enclosure | 1/3 - 2/3 Enclosure | > 2/3 Enclosure |
|---|---|---|---|---|---|
| **OVARY** | R | Filmy | 1 | 2 | 4 |
| | | Dense | 4 | 8 | 16 |
| | L | Filmy | 1 | 2 | 4 |
| | | Dense | 4 | 8 | 16 |
| **TUBE** | R | Filmy | 1 | 2 | 4 |
| | | Dense | 4* | 8* | 16 |
| | L | Filmy | 1 | 2 | 4 |
| | | Dense | 4* | 8* | 16 |

*If the fimbriated end of the fallopian tube is completely enclosed, change the point assignment to 16.

Denote appearance of superficial implant types as red [(R), red, red-pink, flamelike, vesicular blobs, clear vesicles], white[(W), opacifications, peritoneal defects, yellow-brown], or black[(B) black, hemosiderin deposits, blue]. Denote percent of total describe as R____%, W____% and B____%. Total should equal 100%.

| Additional Endometriosis: | Associated Pathology: |
|---|---|

To Be Used with Normal Tubes and Ovaries

L          R

To Be Used with Abnormal Tubes and/or Ovaries

L          R

**EXAMPLES & GUIDELINES**

**STAGE 1 (MINIMAL)**

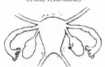

PERITONEUM
| Superficial Endo | - | >3cm | 2 |
| R OVARY |
| Superficial Endo | - | <1cm | 1 |
| Filmy Adhesions | - | <1/3 | 1 |
| | | TOTAL POINTS | 4 |

**STAGE II (MILD)**

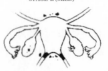

PERITONEUM
| Deep Endo | - | >3cm | 6 |
| R OVARY |
| Superficial Endo | - | <1cm | 1 |
| Filmy Adhesions | - | <1/3 | 1 |
| L OVARY |
| Superficial Endo | - | <1cm | 1 |
| | | TOTAL POINTS | 9 |

**STAGE III (MODERATE)**

PERITONEUM
| Deep Endo | - | >3cm | 6 |
| CULDESAC |
| Partial Obliteration | | | 4 |
| L OVARY |
| Superficial Endo | - | 1-3cm | 16 |
| | | TOTAL POINTS | 26 |

**STAGE III (MODERATE)**

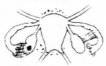

PERITONEUM
| Superficial Endo | - | >3cm | 4 |
| R TUBE |
| Filmy Adhesions | - | <1/3 | 1 |
| R OVARY |
| Filmy Adhesions | - | <1/3 | 1 |
| L TUBE |
| Dense Adhesions | - | <1/3 | 16* |
| L OVARY |
| Deep Endo | - | <1cm | 4 |
| Dense Adhesions | - | <1/3 | 4 |
| | | TOTAL POINTS | 30 |

**STAGE IV (SEVERE)**

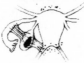

PERITONEUM
| Superficial Endo | - | >3cm | 4 |
| L OVARY |
| Deep Endo | - | 1-3cm | 32** |
| Dense Adhesions | - | <1/3 | 8** |
| L TUBE |
| Dense Adhesions | - | <1cm | 8** |
| | | TOTAL POINTS | 52 |

\* Point assignment changed to 16
\*\* Point assignment doubled

**STAGE IV (SEVERE)**

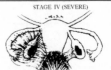

PERITONEUM
| Deep Endo | - | >3cm | 6 |
| CULDESAC |
| Complete Obliteration | | | 40 |
| R OVARY |
| Deep Endo | - | 1-3cm | 16 |
| Dense Adhesions | - | <1/3 | 4 |
| L TUBE |
| Dense Adhesions | - | >2/3 | 16 |
| L OVARY |
| Deep Endo | - | 1-3cm | 16 |
| Dense Adhesions | - | >2/3 | 16 |
| | | TOTAL POINTS | 114 |

Determination of the stage or degree of endometrial involvement is based on a weighted point system. Distribution of points has been arbitarily determined and may require further revision or refinement as knowledge of the disease increases.

To ensure complete evaluation, inspection of the pelvis in a clockwise or counterclockwise fashion is encouraged. Number, size and location of endometrial implants, plaques, endometriomas and/or adhesions are noted. For example, five separate 0.5cm superficial implants on the peritoneum (2.5 cm total) would be assigned 2 points. (The surface of the uterus should be considered peritoneum.) The severity of the endometriosis or adhesions should be assigned the highest score only for peritoneum, ovary, tube or culdesac. For example, a 4cm superficial and a 2cm deep implant of the peritoneum should be given a score of 6 (not 8). A 4cm deep endometrioma of the ovary associated with more than 3cm of superficial disease should be scored 20 (not 24).

In those patients with only one adnexa, points applied to disease of the remaining tube and ovary should be multiplied by two.
\*\*Points assigned may be circled and totaled. Aggregation of points indicates stage of disease (minimal, mild, moderate, or severe).

The presence of endometriosis of the bowel, urinary tract, fallopian tube, vagina, cervix, skin etc., should be documented under "associated pathology." All pathology should be depicted as specifically as possible on the sketch of pelvic organs, and means of observation (laparoscopy or laparotomy) should be noted.

Property of the American Society for Reproductive Medicine 1996

For additional supply write to: American Society for Reproductive Medicine,
1209 Montgomery Highway, Birmingham, Alabama 35216

American Society for Reproductive Medicine          *Revised ASRM classification: 1996*          *Fertility and Sterility* ®

# Notes

(References to medical journals use standard abbreviations of journal titles.)

## CHAPTER 2

1 Hedge G H, Colby H D and Goodman R L, Chapter 9 'Female Reproduction' in *Clinical Endocrine Physiology*, W B Saunders, Philadelphia, London, 1987

2 'Human Reproduction' 10: 101, 1995, quoted in: Leiberman S and Bruning N, *The Real Vitamin & Mineral Book*, Avery Press, New York, p. 265, 1997 (2nd Ed)

3 Ziegler E E and Filer L J, *Present Knowledge in Nutrition*, ILSI Press Washington, DC p. 174, 1996 (7th Ed)

4 Fredericks C, *Guide to Women's Nutrition: Dietary Advice for Women of all ages*, Perigree Books, New York, 1989

5 Ambrus J L, 'Estrogens and clotting factors' in *Consensus on Menopause Research*, eds P A Van Keep, R B Greenblatt and M Albeaux-Fernet, MTP Press, Lancaster, 1976

6 Katchadourian H, *The Biology of Adolescence*, W H Freeman, San Francisco, 1997, p. 18

7 Vernon M W, IVF Center, Central Baptist Hospital, Lexington, Kentucky (Personal Communication) 1996

8 Oliker A J and Harris A E, 'Endometriosis of the bladder in a male patient' in *Journal of Urology*, 106: 858, 1971

9 O'Connor D T, *Endometriosis: Current Review in Obstetrics and Gynaecology 12*, Churchill Livingstone, p. 20, 1987

10 Sampson J A, 'Peritoneal endometriosis due to menstrual dissemination of endometrial tissue into the peritoneal cavity' in *Am J Obstet Gynae*, 14: 422, 1927

11 Halme J M G, Hammond J F, Hulka S J, Raj S J and Talbert L M, 'Retrograde menstruation in healthy women and in patients with endometriosis' in *Obstet & Gynaecol*, 64 (4): 151–4, 1984

12 Vernon M W, 'Animal Models in Endometriosis Research' in *Infertility and Reproductive Medicine Clinics of North America*, W B Saunders, Philadelphia, London, p. 565, 1987

13 Meyer R, 'Uber Endometrium in der tube, sowie uber die hierausentstehenden wirklichen sacomatosa' in *Zentralbl Gynakol*, 51, p. 1482, 1927

14  Hurst B S and Rock J A, 'Anatomic and functional considerations in the development of a classification for endometriosis and pelvic pain and infertility' in *Proc. of the Vth World Congress on Endometriosis*, eds X Minaguchi and O Sugimoto, Parthenon Press Publishing Group, New York, London, 1997

15  Kolberg R, 'NEWS: Endometriosis Enigma: Do the cells themselves hold the crucial clues?' in *J NIH Research*, Vol 9:23–5, February 1997

16  Ibid.

17  Vernon M W, Beard J S, Graves K and Wilson E A, 'Classification of endometriotic implants by morphological appearance and capacity to synthesize prostaglandin F' in *Fert. Steril.*, 46:801, 1986

18  Passwater R A and Cranton E M, *Trace Elements, Hair Analysis and Nutrition*, Keats Publishing, New Canaan p. 66, 1983

## CHAPTER 3

1  Bradley D, *Hyperventilation Syndrome*, Celestial Arts Publishing, Berkeley CA, 1992

2  Kronhausen E, Kronhausen P and Demopoulos H B, *Formula for Life*, William Morrow, New York, p. 95, 1989

3  Kohlmeier L, Rehm J and Hoffmeister H, 'Lifestyles and trends in worldwide breast cancer rates' in *Annals of the New York Academy of Science*, 609: 259–68, 1990.

4  Hawkes N, 'Margarine linked to breast cancer' in *The Times*, 5 September 1997

5  Kassis V, 'The prostaglandin system in human skin' in *Danish Medical Bulletin*, Univ. Copenhagen, Dept Dermato-Vererolgy, pp. 320–42, 1983

6  Ibid

7  Lieberman S and Bruning N, *The Real Vitamin and Mineral Book*, Avery Publishing, p. 315, 1997 (2nd Ed)

8  Covens A, Christopher P and Cusper R F, 'The effect of dietary supplementation with fish oil fatty acids on surgically induced endometriosis in the rabbit' in *Fertility & Sterility*, 49: 698–703,1988

9  Taraye J P and Lauressergue H, 'Advantages of a combination of proteolytic enzymes, flavinoids and ascorbic acid in comparison with non-steroid inflammatory drugs' in *Ameim Forsch*.27(1): pp. 1144–9, 1977

10  Hanck A and Weiser H, 'Analgesic and anti-inflammatory properties in vitamins' in *Int J Vit & Nutri Res*, 27:189–206, 1985

11  Cathcart R F et al, 'Leg cramps and vitamin E' in *J Am Med Assoc*, 219 216–17, 1972

12  Kammura M, 'Anti-inflammatory effects of vitamin E' in *J Vitaminol*, 18 204–9, 1972

13  Greenwood J, 'Optimum vitamin C intake as a factor in the preservation o disc integrity' in *Med Ann DC*, 33: 274, 1964

14  Misra A L et al, 'Differential effects of opiates on the incorporation of (14C) thiamine in the central nervous system of the rat' in *Experimentia*, 33: 372–4, 1977

15  Hieber H, 'Die Behandung vertebragener Schmerzen und Sensibilitatsstorungen mit Hochdosiertem Hydroxoxcobalamin' in *Med onatsschr*, 28: 545–8, 1974

16  Muller P, *First International Symposium on Magnesium Deficit in Human Physiology*, 1971

17  Marone G et al, 'Physiological concentrations of zinc inhibit the release of histamine from human basophils and lung mast cells' in *Agents Action*, 18: 103–106, 1986

## CHAPTER 4

1  Hasson H M, 'Incidence of endometriosis in diagnostic laparoscopy' in *J Reprod Med*, 16: 135, 1976

2  Ballweg M L, *Overcoming Endometriosis*, Congdon and Weed, New York, Chicago, p. 76, 1987

3  Ward, N, 'Preconceptual care and pregnancy outcome' in *J Nutrition and Environmental Medicine*, 5: 205–8, 1995

4  Vernon M W, 'Biochemical activity: differential responsiveness of endometriotic implants' in *Proc 3rd Congress on Endometriosis*, eds I Brosens and J Donnez, Parthenon Publishing, Carnforth, 1993

5  Ibid.

6  Sharpe K L and Vernon M W, 'Polypeptides synthesized and released by rat endometriotic tissue differ from those of uterine endometrium in culture' in *Biology of Reproduction*, 48: 1334, 1993

7  Tummon I S, Maclin V M, Radwanska E, Binor Z and Dmwoski W P, 'Occult ovulatory dysfunction in women with minimal endometriosis or unexplained infertility' in *Fertility & Sterility*, 50: 716, 1987

8  Donnez J and Thomas K, 'Incidence of the luteinizing unruptured follicle syndrome in fertile women and in women with endometriosis' in *Eur J Ob Gynae Reproductive Biology*, 14: 187, 1982

9  Wardle P G, McLaughlin E A, McDurmott A, Mitchell J D, Ray B D and Hull M G R, 'Endometriosis and ovulatory disorder: Reduced fertilization in vitro compared with tubal and unexplained infertility' in *Lancet*, 2: 236, 1985

10  Naples J D, Batt R E and Sadigh J, 'Spontaneous abortion rate in patients with endometriosis' in *Obs Gynae*, 57: 509, 1986

11  Pittaway D E, Vernon C, and Fayex J A, 'Spontaneous abortion in women with endometriosis' in *Fertility & Sterility*, 50: 711, 1988

12  Barlow D H, Kennedy S H, Fernandez-Shaw S and Starkey P M, 'Changes in humoral immunity in endometriosis' in *The Current Status of Endometriosis: Research and Management*, eds I Brosens and J Donnez, The Proceedings of the 3rd World Congress on Endometriosis, Brussels, June 1992, : 235–48, 1992

13 Swann K, Lai T and Parrington J, 'Life starts with a new conception' in *The Sunday Times*, 12 May 1996

14 Price W A, *Nutrition and Physical Degeneration*, Price-Pottinger Foundation, La Mesa, p. 397, 1945

15 Esther 2:8, *Good News Bible*, Collins, London, 1978

16 Genesis 30:14, *Good News Bible*, Collins, London, 1978

17 Judges 13:3–4,*Good News Bible*, Collins, London, 1978

18 Whorton M D and Milby T H, 'Recovery of testicular function among DBCP workers' in *J Occup Med*, 22: 177–9, 1980

19 'Help yourself to a healthy pregnancy', *She Magazine*, Tommy's Campaign Tesco leaflet, October 1996

20 Higgins I M, 'Nutrition and maternal health' in *Proceedings of the First Conference on Human Nutrition*, Ohio State Department of Health, Columbus, Ohio, 1971

21 Price Weston A, *Nutrition and Physical Degeneration*, Price-Pottenger Foundation, La Mesa, p. 397, 1945

22 Pottenger F M Jr, *Pottenger's Cats*, Price-Pottenger Foundation, La Mesa, 1983

23 McCarrison R, *Nutrition and Health*, McCarrison Society, London,1984

24 Williams R J, *Biochemical Individuality: The Basis for the Genetrophic Concept*, Wiley, New York, 1956

25 Wynn A H A and Wynn M, *The Case For Preconceptual Care in Men and Women*, AB Academic Publishers, Bicester, p. 84, 1991

26 Ward N, 'Preconceptual care and pregnancy outcome' in *J Nutrition and Environmental Medicine*, 5: 205–8, 1995

27 Wynn A H A and Wynn M, *The Case For Preconceptual Care in Men and Women*, AB Academic Publishers, Bicester, pp. 68–70, 1991

28 Watteville H, Jurgens R and Pfalz H, 'Einfluss von Vitaminagel auf Fruschbarkeit, Schwangerschaft und Nachkommen' in *Schweiz Med Wochenschr*, 84: 875–82, 1954

29 Russell L B and Russell W L, 'The sensitivity of different stages in oogenesis to the radiation induction of dominant lethals and other changes in the mouse' in *Progress in Radiobiology*, eds J S Mitchell, B E Holmes and C C Smith, Oliver & Boyd, Edinburgh, pp. 187–92, 1956

30 Wynn A H A and Wynn M, *The Case For Preconceptual Care in Men and Women*, AB Academic Publishers, Bicester, pp. 32–3, 1991

31 Ibid

32 Gregory J, Foster K, Tyler H and Wiseman M, *The Dietary and Nutritional Survey of British Adults*, London, HMSO, p. 29, 1990

33 Abraham S, Mira M and Llewellyn-Jones D, 'Should ovulation be induced in women recovering from an eating disorder or who are compulsive exercisers?' in *Fertility & Sterility*, 53: 566–8, 1990

34 Cameron J L in *The Menstrual Cycle and its Disorders*, eds K M Pirke, W Wuttke and U Schweiger, Springer, Heidelberg, pp. 66–78, 1989

35  Barr S I, Prior J C and Vigna Y M, 'Restrained eating and ovulatory disturbances: possible implications for bone health' in *Am J Clinical Nutrition*, 59: 92–7, 1994

36  Wynn A H A and Wynn M, 'Slimming and Fertility' in *Modern Midwife*, 4 (6): 17–20, 1994

37  Kyo U C, Ishizuka J, Breame J, Townsend C M, Greeley G H, Byung P Y and Thompson J C, 'Changes in endocrine pancreatic function in short-term diet restriction' in *Nutrition*, 17: 425–9, 1991

38  Wynn A H A, Wynn M, *The Case For Preconceptual Care in Men and Women*, AB Academic Publishers, Bicester, p. 78, 1991

39  Coop I E, 'Effect of flushing on reproductive performance of ewes' in *J Agri Sci (Camb)*, 67: 305–23, 1966

40  Doyle W, Crawford M A, Wynn S W and Wynn A H A, 'Maternal nutrient intake and birthweight' in *J Human Nutri Diet*, 2: 415–22, 1989b

41  Brosens I A, Konnickx P R and Corveleyn P A, 'A study of plasma progesterone, oestradiol 17β, prolactin and LH levels and the luteal phase appearance of the ovaries in patients with endometriosis and infertility' in *British J of Obs. & Gynae*, 85: 246–50, 1978

42  Esch M W, Easter R A and Bahr J M, 'Effect of riboflavine deficiency on estrous cyclicity in pigs' in *Biol Reproduction*, 25: 659–65, 1981

43  Barnes B and Bradley S G, *Planning for a Healthy Baby*, Vermilion, London, 1990

44  Doyle W, Crawford M A, Wynn S W and Wynn A H A, 'Maternal nutrient intake and birth weight' in *J Human Nutri Diet*, 2: 415–22, 1989b

45  Wynn A H A and Wynn M, 'The need for nutritional assessment in the treatment of the infertile patient' in *J Nutri Med*, 1: 315–24, 1990

46  Le Fanu, J, 'Mother's Battle of the Bulge' in *The Times*, 30 March 1995

47  Smith N C, 'Detection of the foetus at risk' in *Europ J Clinical Nutrition*, 46 (supp 1): SI–S5, 1992

48  Hackman E, 'Maternal birth weight and subsequent pregnancy outcome' in *J Am Med Assoc*, Vol 250: 2016–19, 1983

49  Aherne W, Dunhill M S, 'Morphology of the human placenta' in *British Medicine Bulletin*, Vol 22 (1): 5–12, 1966

50  Hackman E, 'Maternal birth weight and subsequent pregnancy outcome' in *J Am Med Assoc*, Vol 250: 2016–19, 1983

51  Doyle W, Crawford M, Wynn A H A and Wynn M, 'The association of maternal diet and birth weight dimensions' in *J Nutri Med*, 1: 9–16, 1990

52  Committee to Study the Prevention of Low Birth Weight, *Preventing Low Birth Weight*, National Academy Press, Washington, 1985

53  Burke B S, Harding V V and Stuart H C, 'Nutrition studies during pregnancy' in *J Paediatrics*, 23: 506–15, 1943

54  Wynn A H A and Wynn M, 'The need for nutritional assessment in the treatment of the infertile patient' in *J Nutritional Medicine*, 1: 315–378, 1990

55 Bates G W, Bates S G and Whitworth N S, 'Reproductive failure in women who practise weight control' in *Fertility & Sterility*, 37: 373–8, 1982

56 Speroff L and Walllach E E, 'The changing face of infertility' in *Fertility*, pp. 8–23, 1987

57 Keen C L and Zidenberg-Cherr S, 'Should vitamin-mineral supplements be recommended for all women with childbearing potential?' in *Am J Clin Nutri*, 59 (suppl): 532S–539S, 1994

58 Ryan S, 'Scientists link falling sperm counts to chemicals in food' in *The Sunday Times*, 21 May 1995

59 Bentham P, 'VDV Terminal Sickness' in *Green Print*, pp. 27–35, 165, 1980

60 Whorton M D and Milby T H, 'Recovery of testicular function among DSCP workers' in *J Occup Med*, 22: 177–9, 1980 in Wynn and Wynn p. 35

61 Skakkebaek N and Keilding N, 'Changes in semen and the testes' in *British Medical Journal*, 309: 1316–17, 1994

62 Sharpe R M and Skakkebaek N, 'Are oestrogens involved in falling sperm counts and disorders of the male reproductive tract?' in *The Lancet*, 341: 1392–96,1993

63 Connor S, 'Mystery of the vanishing sperm' in *The Independent on Sunday*, 8 March 1992

64 Prasad A S, 'Is infertility linked to zinc deficiency?' in *Better Nutrition Magazine*, 8: 13–62, 1982

65 Tuormaa T E, 'Adverse effects of manganese deficiency on reproduction and health' in *J Orthomolecular Med*, 11: 3, 1996

66 Murray M T, *Male Sexual Vitality*, Prima Publishing, Rocklin, pp. 50–6, 1994

67 Colburn T, Myers J P and Dumanoski D, *Our Stolen Future*, Little, Brown, London, 1996

68 Link A, *Chlorine, Pollution and the Parents of Tomorrow*, Women's Environmental Network, London, 1991

69 Mormann R, *Endometriosis Association 10th Anniversary Handbook*, Milwaukee 1991

70 Urlocker K, 'Surviving infertility' in *Infertility Awareness*, 9 (2): 4–5, 1993

## CHAPTER 5

1 Kistner R W, 'The treatment of endometriosis by inducing pseudo-pregnancy with ovarian hormones: a report of 58 cases' in *Fertility and Sterility*, 10: 539, 1959

2 Grant E, *Sexual Chemistry*, Cedar Press, London, pp. 330–31, 1994

3 Hurst B S and Schalaff W D, 'Treatment options for endometriosis: Medical therapies' in *Infertility and Reproductive Medicine Clinics of North America Vol 2*, eds D Olive and W B Saunders, Philadelphia & London, 3: 645, 1992

4 Gunning J E and Moyer D, 'The effect of medroxyprogesterone acetate on endometriosis in the human female' in *Fertility and Sterility*, 18: 759, 1967

5  O'Connor D, *Endometriosis*, Churchill Livingstone, Edinburgh, p. 13, 1989

6  Barbieri R L, Evans S and Kistner R W, 'Danazol in the treatment of endometriosis analysis of 100 cases with a 4-year follow-up' in *Fertility and Sterility*, 37: 737, 1982

7  Holt J P and Keller D, 'Danazol treatment increases serum enzymes' in *Fertility and Sterility*, 41: 70, 1984

8  Hodgen G D, 'General applications of GnRH agonists in gynecology past, present and future' in *Ob Gyn Surv*, 44: 293, 1989

9  Luciano A A and Manzi D, 'Treatment options for endometriosis: Surgical therapies' in *Infertility and Reproductive Medicine Clinics of North America Vol 2*, eds D Olive and W B Saunders, Philadephia & London, 3: 657, 1992

10  'Hysterectomy prevalence and death rates for cervical cancer – United States' (editorial) in *Morb Mortal Wkly Rep*, 41(2): 17–20, 17 January 1992

11  Santow G and Bracher M, 'Correlates of hysterectomy in Australia, in *Soc Sci Med*, 34(8): 929–42, April 1992

12  Vessey M P, Villard-Mackintosh L, McPherson K, Coulter A and Yeats D, 'The epidemiology of hysterectomy: findings in a large cohort study' in *British Journal Obs & Gynae*, 99(5): 402–7, May 1992

13  Hurlbutt K, in Ballwegg M L, *Overcoming Endometriosis*, Congdon & Weed, New York, 1987

14  Tallo C P, Vohr B, Oh W, Rubin L P, Seifer D B and Haning R V Jr, 'Maternal and neonatal morbidity associated with in vitro fertilization' in *J Pediatric*, November 1995, 127 (50): 794–800

15  Venn A, Watson L, Lumley J, Giles G, King C and Healy D, 'Breast and ovarian cancer incidence after infertility and in vitro fertilization' in *The Lancet*, 16 December 1995, 243 (8990): 1627–8

16  Pouly J L, Canis M, Janny L, Vye-Pouly P, Zambrano R, Laurichesse H, Botroshvilli R and Boyer-Medeville C, 'The place of IVF in the treatment of endometriosis-related infertility' in *Endometriosis Today. Proceedings of the Vth World Congress on Endometriosis*, eds H Minaguch and O Sugimoto, Parthenon Publishing Group, New York & London, p. 443, 1997

17  Dmowski W P, Rana N, Michalowska J, Friberg J, Papierniak C and El-Roeiy A, 'The effect of endometriosis, its stage and activity, and of auto-antibodies on IVF and embryo transfer success rates' in *Fertility and Sterility*, 63: 555, 1995

18  Stolwijk A M, Zielhuis G A, Sauer M V, Hamilton C J and Paulson R J, 'The impact of the women's age on the success of standard and donor IVF' in *Fertility and Sterility*, 67: 702, 1997

19  Dmowski W P, Rana N, Michalowska J, Friberg J, Papierniak C and El-Roeiy A, 'The effect of endometriosis, its stage and activity, and of auto-antibodies on IVF and embryo transfer success rates' in *Fertility and Sterility*, 63: 555, 1995

20  Cornwell J, 'Why is this so difficult? Infertility' in the *Sunday Times Magazine*, 34–42, 11 November 1996

21  Syal R, 'Revealed: 30,000 embryos used in fertility experiments' in *The Sunday Times*, 3 May 1998

22  Davies S, 'Nutritional Medicine. Has it a role in handicap prevention and the medical treatment of infertility, including assisted ovulation, IVF and GIFT?' in *J Nutritional Medicine*, 1: 251–8, 1990

23  Whitworth N, 'IVF and Sperm Abnormalities' in *The Times*, 1996

24  Speroff L and Walsh E E, 'The changing face of infertility' in *Fertility*, 8–23, 1987

25  Masao Igarashi, 'Augmentative effects of ascorbic acid upon induction of human ovulation in clomiphene-ineffective anovulatory women' in *International J of Fertility*, 22(3): 168–75, 1977

26  Reuben C and Priestley J, *Essential Supplements for Women*, Thorsons, London, p. 190, 1991

27  *British National Formulary*, British Medical Association & Royal Pharmaceutical Society of Great Britain 32, 22: x, 1996

28  *British National Formulary*, British Medical Association & Royal Pharmaceutical Society of Great Britain 32, 22: 264, 1996

29  Mills D S, 'The Role of Nutrition in Preconceptual Care Within a Health Promotion Setting', Master of Arts Degree Investigative Study, University of Brighton, April 1996

30  *British National Formulary*, British Medical Association & Royal Pharmaceutical Society of Great Britain 32: 22, 1996

31  Hawkes N, 'Why grapefruit juice and drugs don't mix' in *The Times*, 24 November 1997

32  Oakley A, *From Here to Maternity – Becoming a Mother*, Penguin, Harmondsworth, p. 283, 1981

33  Freidson E, 'Dilemmas in the doctor/patient relationship' in *A Sociology of Medical Practice*, eds C Cox and A Mead, Collier Macmillan, London, 1975

34  Gilligan C, *In a Different Voice: Psychological Theory and Women's Development*, Harvard University Press, Cambridge, 1982

35  Wastell D and Macdonald V, 'Drug salesmen face jail over gifts to GPs' in *Sunday Telegraph*, 27 July 1997

36  Bequaert Holmes H and Purdy L M, eds, *Feminist Perspectives in Medical Ethics*, Indiana University Press, Bloomington & Indianapolis, p. 72, 1992

37  Ibid

38  Pellegrino E D and Thomasina D C, *For the Patient's Good*, Oxford University Press, New York, pp. 20–1, 1985

39  Phillips M, 'Losing our humanity at the embryo bank' in *The Sunday Times* p. 17, 6 December 1998

40  Lauersen N H and de Swann C, *Endometriosis Answer Book*, Fawset Columbine, New York, p. 197, 1988

41  'Too many hysterectomies in the UK' in *The Lancet*, 349: 1226, 1997

42  Lilford R J, 'Hysterectomy: Will it pay the bills in 2007?' in *British Medical Journal*, 314: 160–61, 1997

3 Lazarus K, Weinsier R L and Boker J R, 'Nutrition knowledge and practices of physicians in a family-practice residency programme: the effect of an education programme provided by physician nutrition specialists' in *Am J Clinical Nutrition*, 58: 319–25,1993

4 Green L W, Erikson M P and Schor E L, 'Preventive practices by physicians: behavioural determinants and potential interventions' in *Am J Preventative Med*, 4: 101–7, 1988

5 Null G, *No More Allergies*, Villard Books, New York,1992

6 Meldrum J M, 'A response to the health of the nation: a summary of the Government's proposals' in *J Nutrition Med*, 2: 415–21, 1991

## HAPTER 6

1 Berdanier C D, 'Nutrient-gene Interactions' in *Present Knowledge in Nutrition*, eds E E Ziegler and L J Filer Jr, ILSI Press, Washington, 1996 (7th ed)

2 Williams R J, *Biochemical individuality: The basis for the genetotrophic concept*, Wiley & Sons, New York, 1956

3 Null G, *The Complete Guide to Health and Nutrition*, Arlington Books, London, p. 499, 1984

4 Ibid

5 Quotes extracted from 'Human Reproduction' 10: 50–55, 1995, reproduced in *The Real Vitamin and Mineral Book*, S Lieberman and N Bruning, Avery Press, New York, p. 325, 1997

6 Ibid

7 Null G, *The Complete Guide to Health and Nutrition*, Arlington Books, London, 1984, p. 427

8 Griswold R E, 'The Health Tape', from *The Love Tapes*, Ediner, Minnesota, 1988

## HAPTER 7

1 Null G and Feldman M D, *Reverse the Ageing Process Naturally*, Villard Books, New York, 1993

2 Collins J K, O'Sullivan G and Shanahan F, 'Probiotics bacteria – interaction with the human immune system' in *Gut Flora and Health – Past, Present and Future*, The Royal Society of Medicine Press, pp 13–14, 1996

3 Rosenburg L E, 'Inborn errors of nutrient metabolism: Garrod's lessons and legacies' in *Genetic Factors in Nutrition*, eds A Valezquez and H Bourges, pp. 61–77, 1984

4 Vernon M V, personal communication, 1997

5 Thomas E J and Rock J A, *Modern Approaches to Endometriosis*, Kluwer Academic Publishers, Lancaster, p. 5, 1991

6 Dmwoski W P, Braun D and Gebel H, 'The immune system in endometriosis' in *Modern Approaches to Endometriosis*, E J Thomas and J A Rock, Kluwer Academic Publishers, Lancaster, p. 97, 1991

7 Meek J, *Immune Power*, Optima Macdonald, London, pp. 33–4, 1990

8 Ibid, p. 143

9 'Sugar and immunity' in *New York Time*, July 14 1987, quoted in G Null and M Feldman, *Reversing the Aging Process Naturally*, Villard Books, New York, p. 24, 1993

10 Meek J, *Immune Power*, Optima Macdonald, London, p. 34, 1990

11 Ibid, p. 33

12 Barlow D H, Kennedy S H, Fernandez-Shaw S and Starkey P M, 'Changes in humoral immunity in endometriosis' in *The Current Status of Endometriosis: Research & Management*, eds I Brosens and J Donnez, Parthenon, Lancaster, pp. 235–49, 1992

13 Kirkwood E and Lewis C, *Understanding Medical Immunology 2nd Ed*, John Wiley, Chichester, p. 26, 1994

14 Barnes B and Bradley S G, *Planning for a Healthy Baby*, Vermillion, London, p. 68, 1990

15 Null G and Feldman M D, *Reversing the Aging Process Naturally*, Villard Books, New York, pp. 90–3, 1993

16 Ibid

17 Thomas E J and Rock J A, *Modern Approaches to Endometriosis*, Kluwer Academic Publishers, Lancaster, p. 97, 1991

18 Meek J, *Immune Power*, Optima Macdonald, London, p. 139, 1990

19 Weir D M, *Immunology*, 6th ed, Churchill Livingstone, Edinburgh, p. 53, 1988

20 Halme J and Hammond M G, 'The role of growth factors in endometriosis' in *The Current Status of Endometriosis: Research & Management*, eds I Brosens and J Donnez, Parthenon Publishing, Lancaster, p. 211, 1992

21 Ibid

22 Ibid

23 Halme J K, 'Role of peritoneal information in endometriosis associated with infertility', (Congress papers) *Vth World Congress on Endometriosis*, p. 72 Yokohama, Japan, 1996

24 Evers J L H, 'The immune system in endometriosis: introduction' in *The Current Status of Endometriosis: Research and Management*, eds I Brosens and Donnez, Proceedings of the 3rd World Congress on Endometriosis Brussels, Parthenon Publishing, Lancaster, pp. 223–33, 1992

25 Odukoya O A, Wilson A P and Cooke I, 'The prevalence of endometria IgG antibodies in patients with endometriosis' in *Human Reproduction*, Ma 1: 10 (5) 1214–19, 1992

26 Vallatton M B and Forbes A P, 'Antibodies to cytoplasm of ova' in *The Lancet*, 2: 264–5, 1996

27 Braley J, *The Immuno Review* (newsletter), Immuno Laboratories, Fo

Lauderdale FLA, Vol 1: No. 1 & 2 Summer & Fall Issues, 1993 (Verbal communication ION Conference, 1995, London)

8   Singh A, Nery Danta Z, Stone S C, and Asch R H, 'Presence of thyroid antibodies in early reproductive failure: biochemical versus clinical pregnancies' in *Fertility and Sterility*, 63(2): 277–81, 1995

9   Howard S, 'Module 16: Current thinking in coeliac disease' in *Pharmacy Magazine*, CEI–CEVIII, February 1997

0   Toates F, *Stress – Conceptual and Biological Aspects*, John Wiley, Chichester, pp. 8, 65, 75, 76, 77, 83, 276, 1996

1   Null G, and Feldman M D, *Reverse the Ageing Process Naturally*, Villard Books, New York, p. 59, 1993

## CHAPTER 8

1   McCance X and Widdowson, 'A Comparison of Foods 1939 and 1991', 1991

2   McKeown T, *The Role of Medicine: Dream, Mirage or Nemesis?* Basil Blackwell, Oxford, 1979, quoted in *The Modern Rise of Population*, Arnold, London, 1976.

3   Lange T, 'The Food Programme', *BBC Radio 4 Food Choices*, 13 March 1997

4   'Ready-cooked meals account for 35 per cent of food bills' in the *Guardian*, 15 November 1994

5   Lipski E, *Digestive Wellness*, Keats Publishers, New Canaan, p. 29, 1996

6   Collins J K, O'Sullivan G and Shanahan F, 'Probiotic bacteria – interaction with the human immune system' in *Gut Flora and Health – Past, Present and Future*, pp. 13–19, 1996, Royal Society Med Press, London

7   Chaitow L and Trenev N, *Probiotics*, Thorsons, London, 1990

8   Collins J K, O'Sullivan G and Shanahan F, 'Probiotic bacteria – interaction with the human immune system' in *International Congress and Symposium Series*, 219, Royal Society of Medicine Press, London, pp. 13–18, 1996

9   Collins J K, O'Sullivan G and Shanahan F, 'Probiotic bacteria – interaction with the human immune system' in *Gut Flora and Health – Past, Present and Future*, eds A R Leeds, I R Rowland, Royal Society of Medicine Press, London, pp. 13–19, 1996

0   Lipski E, *Digestive Wellness*, Keats Publishers, New Canaan, p. 227, 1996

1   Office of Population and Census Statistics, *The Dietary and Nutritional Survey of British Adults*, HMSO, London, Monitor, 1991

2   Marks J, 'Current status and future prospects' in *Gut Flora and Health – Past, Present and Future*, eds A R Leeds, I R Rowland, Royal Society of Medicine Press, London, pp. 57–69, 1996

3   Gibson G R and Beaumont A, 'An overview of human colonic bacteriology in health and disease' in *Gut Flora and Health – Past, Present and Future*, eds A R Leeds, I R Rowland, Royal Society of Medicine Press, London, p. 57, 1996

14 Schiffrin F J, Rochat F, Link-Amster H, Aeschlimann J H and Donnet-Hughes A, 'Immune modulations of human blood cells following the ingestion of lactic acid bacteria' in *J Dairy Sci*, 78: 491–7, 1995

15 Crayhon R, *Health Benefits of FOS (Fructo-oligosaccharides)*, Keats Publishing, New Canaan, p. 28, 1995

16 Brostoff J and Gamlin L, *The Complete Guide to Food Allergy and Intolerance*, Bloomsbury Press, London, pp. 129, 230, 1989

17 National Institute of Health, Bethesda, *Food Allergy and Intolerance*, 1996

18 Hollander D and Tarnawski H, 'Ageing-associated increase in intestinal absorption of macromolecules' in *Gerontology*, 31: 133–7, 1985

19 Petres T J and Bjarnason I, 'Uses and abuses of intestinal permeability measurements' in *Can J Gastroenter*, 12(3), 1988

20 Ballweg M L, *Endometriosis Sourcebook*, Contemporary Books, Chicago, pp. 200–202, 1995

21 Feldman D, 'Steroid hormone systems found in yeast' in *Science Magazine*, August 1984

22 Edwards D A, 'Depression and Candida' in *J Am Med Ass*, 253: 340, 1995

23 Rivas V and Rogers T J, 'Studies on the cellular nature of *Candida albicans*-induced suppression' in *J Immunology*, 130: 376, January 1983

24 Null G, *The Complete Guide to Health and Nutrition*, Arlington Books, London, p. 129, 1984

25 Lamb K and Nichols T R, 'Endometriosis: A comparision of associated disease histories' in *Am J Preventive Medicine*, 2 (6): 324–9, 1986

26 Null G, *No More Allergies*, Villard Books, New York, p. 3, 1992

27 Golos N and Golos-Golbritz F, *If It's Tuesday It Must Be Chicken*, Keats Publishers, New Canaan, 1979

28 Null G, *Good Food, Good Mood*, St Martin's Press, New York, p. 13, 1998

29 Cohen R, 'The Health Dangers of Dairy Products' in *Nexus*, pp. 23–8, August 1998

30 Chaitow L and Trenew N, *Probiotics*, Thorsons, London, pp. 70–71, 1990

31 Councell C E, Taha A and Ruddell W S J, 'Coeliac disease and auto-immune thyroid disease' in *Gut*, 35: 844–6, 1994

32 Lindsay R S, Tift A D, 'Hypothyroidism' in *The Lancet*, 349, 8 February 1997

33 Wheetman A P, 'Hypothyroidism: screening and subclinical disease' in *British Medical Journal*, 314, 19 April 1997

34 Singh A, Dantas Z N, Stone S C and Asch R H, 'Presence of thyroid antibodies in early reproductive failure: biochemical versus clinical pregnancies' in *Fert & Steril*, 63(2): 277–81, 1995

35 Howard S, 'Current Thinking in Coeliac Disease' in *Pharmacy Magazine*, CEI–VII, February 1997

36 Sher K S and Mayberry J F, 'Female fertility, obstetric and gynaecological history in coeliac disease. A case control study' submitted for publication in Sher K S, Jayanthi V, Probert C S J, Stewart C R and Mayberry J F

'Infertility, obstetric and gynaecological problems in coeliac sprue' in *Digestive Diseases*, 12: 186–90, 1994

37 Councell C E, Taha A and Ruddell W S J, 'Coeliac disease and auto-immune thyroid disease' in *Gut*, 35: 844–6, 1994

38 Hemming W A, 'The entry into the brain of large molecules derived from dietary protein' in *Proc Royal Society London*, 200: 175–92, 1978

39 Maki M, Collin P, 'Coeliac disease seminar' in *The Lancet*, 349: 1755–9, 1997

40 Johnston S D, Watson R G P, McMillan S A, Sloan J and Love A H G, 'Prevalence of coeliac disease in Northern Ireland' in *The Lancet*, 349: 1370, 1997

41 Cronin C C and Shahan F, Insulin-dependent diabetes mellitus and coeliac disease, *The Lancet*, 349: 1096–7, 1997

42 Lark S, *Fibroid Tumors and Endometriosis: a Self-Help Book*, Celestial Arts, Berkeley, 1993

43 Fredericks C, *Guide to Women's Nutrition. Dietary Advice for Women of All Ages*, Perigree Books, New York, p. 32, 1989

44 Stock S, 'Nutrition and hormones' in *Nutrition Therapy Today*, 3: 4, Society for the Promotion of Nutritional Therapy, 1995

45 Ibid

46 Cowan D W et al, 'Breast cancer incidence in women with a history of progesterone deficiency' in *Am J Epidemiology*, 114: 209–17, 1981

47 Spallholz et al, 'Immunological responses of mice fed diets supplemented with selenite selenium' in *Proceedings Society Experimental Biology and Medical*, 143: 685–9, 1973

48 Stock S, 'Nutrition and hormones' in *Nutrition Therapy Today*, 3: 4, Society for the Promotion of Nutritional Therapy, 1995

49 Challem J J and Lewin R, 'Managing endometriosis through nutrition' in *Endo Association USA Newsletter*, 10(4), 1989

50 Devlin T M, *Textbook of Biochemistry with Clinical Correlations* (2nd ed), J Wiley, pp. 570–90, 1986

51 Lemon H M et al, 'Re: ethnic differences in estrogen metabolism in healthy women' in *J Nat Cancer Inst*, 89 (21): 1626–8, 1997

52 Lemon H M et al, 'A method for estimating catechol estrogen metabolism from excretion of noncatechol estrogens' in *Cancer*, 68 (2): 444–50, 1991

53 Goldin B R and Gorbach S I, 'The effect of milk and lactobaccillus feeding on human intestinal bacterial enzyme activity' in *Am J Clin Nutri*, 39: 756–61, 1984

54 Ockerman P A, Bachrack L, Glans S and Rassner S, 'Evening primrose oil as a treatment of premenstrual syndrome' in *Recent Advances in Clinical Nutrition*, 2: 404–5, 1986

55 Link A, 'Fertility and the environment' in *Nutrition Therapy Today*, Society for the Promotion of Nutrition Therapy, London, 3(3): 6–81, 1991

56 Vidal J and Cone M, 'Out for the count: do toxic chemicals reduce male

fertility' in the *Guardian*, 15 February 1995

57  McLachlin J A and Arnold S F, 'Environmental estrogens' in *American Scientist*, 84: 452–61, 1997

58  Ibid

59  Rier S E, Spangelo D C, Martin D C, Bowman R E and Becker J L, 'Production of interleukin-6 and tumor necrosis factor-alpha by peripheral blood mononuclear cells from rhesus monkeys with endometriosis' in *J Immunology*, 150: 49a, 1992

60  The Women's Environmental Leaflet: 'Living with dioxins', p. 15, 1993 in Hume Hall R 'New threat to public health: organochlorines and food' in *Nutrition and Health*, vol 8: 333, 1992

61  'Prostaglandins & Leukotrines March 1985 2nd International Congress on Essential Fatty Acids' quoted in Lieberman S and Bruning N, *The Real Vitamin & Mineral Book (2nd ed)*, Avery Books, New York, p. 315, 1997

62  Chaitow L and Trenev N, *Probiotics*, Thorsons, London, p. 47, 1990

63  Fredericks C, *Guide to Women's Nutrition: Dietary Advice for Women of All Ages*, Perigree Books, New York, p. 36, 1989

64  Messina M, Messina V and Setchell K, *The Simple Soyabean and Your Health*, Avery Publishing, New York, p. 73, 1994

65  Ibid

66  JEH Assessment on Phyto-oestrogens in the Human Diet, Final Report to the Ministry of Agriculture, Fisheries and Food, November 1997

67  Dees C et al, 'Dietary estrogens stimulate human breast cells to enter the cell cycle' in *Environmental Health and Perspectives*, 105(3), April 1997

68  'The Ice Cream Story' in *The Sunday Observer*, 29 May 1983

## CHAPTER 9

1  Walker C and Cannon G, *The Food Scandal*, Century Publishing, London, p. 68, 1984

2  Quoted in Doll R and Peto R, *Causes of Cancer*, Oxford University Press, Oxford, 1981

3  Silverberg E, 'Cancer Statistics, 1985' in *Cancer J for Clinicians*, 35(1): 19, 1985

4  Buss D H, 'Food patterns in the British Isles' in *Ann Nutri Metab*, 35 (Suppl 12–21, 1991

5  Badura B, Kickbish I, *Health Promotion Research: Towards a New Socia Epidemiology*, WHO Regional Publications, Copenhagen, European Serie: No. 37: 233, 1991

6  Lappalainen R, Saba A, Holm L, Mykkanen H and Gibney M J 'Perceived benefits of healthy eating among a nationally representativ

sample of adults in the European Union' in *European J Clin Nutri*, vol 51 (2): 247–57, 1997

7   Margetts B M, 'Basic issues in designing and interpreting epidemiological research' in *Design Concepts in Nutritional Epidemiology*, eds B M Margetts and M Nelson, pp. 22–4 Oxford University Press, New York, 1997

8   Nelson M M and Evans H M, 'Relation of thiamin to reproduction in the rat' in *Journal of Nutrition*, 55: 151–63, 1955

9   Brosens I A, Koninckx P R and Corveleyn P A, 'A study of plasma progesterone, oestradiol–17B, prolactin and LH levels and the luteal phase appearance of the ovaries in patients with endometriosis and infertility' in *British Journal of Obs. and Gynae*, 85: 246–50, 1978

10   HMSO Report 41: 'Dietary reference values for food, energy and nutrients for the United Kingdom' pp. 90, 94, 102, 146, 167, 1991

11   Lauersen N H and De Swann C, *Endometriosis Answer Book*, Fawcett Columbine, 1988

12   Esch M W, Easter R A and Bahr J M, 'Effect of riboflavine deficiency on estrous cyclicity in pigs' in *Biol Reproduction*, 25: 659–65, 1981

13   Ballweg M L, *Overcoming Endometriosis*, Congdon and Weed, 1987

14   Grant E, *Sexual Chemistry*, Cedar Press, London, 1992

15   Colgan M, *Hormonal Health*, Apple Publishing, Vancouver, 1996

16   Christianson R E, Oeshli F W and van den Berg B J, 'Caffeinated beverages and decreased fertility' in *The Lancet*, 1(8634): 378, 1989

17   Goldstein F, Goldman M B and Cramer D W, 'Infertility in women and moderate alcohol use' in *Am J Public Health*, 84 (9): 1429–32, 1994

18   Cited by Hope J, 'Just a little tipple can damage your fertility' in *Daily Mail*, 21 August 1998

19   Van Voorhis B J, Dawson J D, Stovall D W, Sparks A E and Syrop C H, 'The effects of smoking on ovarian function and fertility during assisted reproduction cycles' in *Obstet-Gynecol*, 88 (5): 785–91, 1996

20   Marks K, 'Women smokers leave daughters a deadly legacy' in the *Daily Telegraph*, 3 February 1994

21   Derbyshire D, 'Babies "poisoned" by mothers who smoke' in *Daily Mail*, 24 August 1998

22   Passwater R A and Cranton E M, *Trace Elements, Hair Analysis and Nutrition*, Keats Publishing, New Canaan, 1983

23   Zeigler E E and Filer L J Jr, *Present Knowledge in Nutrition (7th edition)*, ILSI Press, Washington, p. 316, 1996

24   Joo S J and Betts N M, 'Copper intakes and the consumption patterns of chocolate foods as sources of copper for individuals in the 1987–1988 nationwide food consumption survey' in *Nutrition Research*, 16(1): 41–52, 1996

25   Null G, *No More Allergies*, Villard Books, New York, p. 3, 1992

21   Lieberman S and Bruning N, *The Real Vitamin and Mineral Book 2nd Ed*, Avery Books, New York, p. 315, 1997

27 Yudkin J, 'Objectives and methods in nutrition education: let's start again' in *J Human Nutrition*, 1981

## CHAPTER 11

1 Gudice L C, 'Insulin-like growth factor and other endometrial modulators in endometrial development and endometriosis' in *Endometrium and Endometriosis*, eds M Diamond and K Osteen, Blackwell Science, Cambridge, pp. 24–31, 1996

2 Osteen K G, Bruner K L and Sharpe-Timms K L, 'Steroids and growth factor regulation of matrix metalloproteinase expression and endometriosis' in *Seminars in Reproductive Endocrinology*, 14: 247–55, 1994

3 Osteen K G, Bruner K L and Eisenberg X, 'Progesterone and transforming growth factor beta co-mediate matrix metalloproteinase expression in a model of endometriosis' in *Endometriosis Today. Proceedings of the Vth World Congress on Endometriosis*, eds H Minaguchi and O Sugimoto, Parthenon Publishing Group, New York, 13: 210–15, 1994

4 Lessey B A, Sastelbaum A J, Sawin S J, Buck C S, Schinnar R and Wilkins B, 'Aberrant integrins expression in the endometrium of women with endometriosis' in *J Clin Endo Metab*, 79: 643–9, 1994

5 Ibid

6 Haney A F, Muscanto J J and Weinberg J B, 'Peritoneal fluid cell populations in infertility patients' in *Fert Steril* 25: 696–700, 1981

7 Halme J, Becker S, Hammond M G, Raj M H G, Raj S, 'Increase activation of peritoneal macrophages in patients with endometriosis', in *Am J Obstet Gynecol*, 148: 85–90, 1983

8 Olive D L, Montoya I and Schenken R M, 'Macrophage-conditioned media enhanced endometrial stromal cell proliferation in vitro' in *Am J Obstet Gynecol*, 164: 953–8, 1991

9 Nothnick W B and Vernon M W, 'Immunomodulation of endometriotic implants' in *Endometriosis Today. Proceedings of the Vth Congress on Endometriosis*, eds H Minaguchi and O Sugimoto, 13: 107–17, Parthenon Publishing Group, New York, 1997

10 Sharpe, K L and Vernon M W, 'Polypeptides synthesized and released by endometriotic tissue differ from those of the uterine endometrium in culture' in *Biol Reprod*, 48: 1334–40, 1993

11 Knight J, 'Far from the madding cows' in *New Scientist*, 24 January 1998

12 Mills D, 'Endometriosis: possible nutritional strategies' in *Lamberts Nutrition Bulletin*, 2: 1–12, 1992

13 O'Connor D, *Endometriosis*, Churchill Livingstone, Edinburgh, p. 145, 1989

14 Coutinho E M, 'Progress in the management of endometriosis' in *The Proceedings of the 4th World Congress on Endometriosis 28 May 1994*, Parthenon Press, London, p. 1, 1994

# Glossary

| | |
|---|---|
| Abdomen | Belly. The area of the body below the lungs and above the hips. Internally known as the peritoneal cavity. (*see* Peritoneal cavity) |
| Acute | Describes a disease of rapid onset, severe symptoms and brief duration. Acute abdomen as with ectopic pregnancy or ruptured ovarian cysts. (*see* Pain) |
| Adhesions | Used in medicine to describe the abnormal attachment of organs to each other by fibrous scar tissue. Caused usually by trauma to tissue from an injury or surgery. Endometriosis causes adhesion formation in the peritoneal cavity from the congealed sticky blood strands. (*see* Endometriosis *and* Peritoneal cavity) |
| Adipose tissue | The fat storage tissue of the body. |
| Aflotoxins | A poisonous substance in the spore of fungus which affects peanuts. |
| Allergy | A hypersensitive immune response acquired by some individuals to environmental substances. These environmental substances are called allergens, the most common of which are pollen, dust and animal dander. With foodstuffs the most common allergens are wheat, dairy and citrus fruits. (*see* Immune system) |
| Amenorrhoea | The absence of the menstrual period (monthly bleeding). (*see* Menstrual cycle *and* Menstrual period) |
| Amino acid | The fundamental chemical constituents of all proteins. The digestive tract breaks down proteins into amino acids in order for that portion to be absorbed into the bloodstream. Used as building blocks by the body to produce hormones, enzymes, prostaglandins, etc. (*see* Proteins) |
| Anabolic hormones | Hormones which stimulate the formation of the larger chemicals of the body from the smaller precursor chemicals. For instance, an anabolic hormone stimulates the building up of body proteins, like muscle proteins, from amino acids. Testosterone is an anabolic hormone which is formed from oils hormones) and stimulates the build-up of muscle proteins, which is why it has been used by some athletes to increase their muscle size. |

| | |
|---|---|
| Analgesic | A drug that relieves pain. |
| Anaemia | A condition in which the blood has a deficiency of red blood cells (RBCs) or haemoglobin, the iron-based molecule in RBCs that carries oxygen in the blood. Anaemia may be caused by deficiencies of iron, copper, B12 or B6. (*see* Red blood cells). |
| Anorexia nervosa | An illness common in female adolescents, in which the patients starve themselves or use other techniques, such as vomiting or taking laxatives, to induce weight loss. Motivated by a false perception of their bodies as fat. Linked to deficiencies in iron and zinc. Zinc is used by 20 enzymes in the brain and by the hypothalamus, the seat of appetite control. |
| Anovulation | No ovulation occurs during the menstrual cycle. (*see* Luteinizing unruptured follicle syndrome) |
| Antagonist | A substance such as a vitamin, mineral or hormone whose action opposes that of another substance. Thus taking zinc at the same time as iron can cut down the absorption of both. They should be taken at different times. |
| Antibiotics | Drugs that inhibit the growth of micro-organisms. Prolonged use may disrupt gut flora and oestrogen excretion. Using probiotics after taking a course of antibiotics will replace the bifido bacteria. (*see* Probiotics) |
| Antibody | A Y-shaped protein produced by the immune system B lymphocytes that attacks matter that is 'alien' to the body. (*see* Immune system) |
| Antigens | Substances that are 'alien' to the body and which elicit an immune response when they enter the body, e.g. virus and bacteria. (*see* Immune system) |
| Antihistamine | A drug which inhibits the release of histamine in the body. This effect can dampen pain and allergic reaction. Some antihistamines make the user drowsy and unable to operate machinery or drive. |
| Antioxidants | These are comprised of vitamins, minerals and compounds found in food which can neutralize the damaging effects of free oxidizing radicals. Antioxidants prevent cells from ageing too rapidly. |
| ART | Assisted reproductive technology. The use of processes like IVF, GIFT and ICSI to help infertile couple conceive. (*see* In vitro fertilization, Gamete intrafallopian transfer, Intracytoplasmic sperm injection). For endometriosis the success rate is below 10 per cent. |

| | |
|---|---|
| Ascorbic acid | *see* Vitamin C |
| Auto-immune disease | When the immune system wrongly attacks its own tissue and treats it as if it were 'alien' matter. A false recognition pattern seems to evolve. |
| Bacteria | A loosely used term that refers to micro-organisms that are usually rod-shaped and are not viruses or fungi. Some bacteria, such as the bifido bacteria in our gut, are beneficial. Other types of bacteria are dangerous to health, e.g. salmonella. |
| Bifido bacteria | These bacteria prevent the colonization of the intestine by harmful pathogenic bacteria and yeasts. They protect the integrity of the mucosal barrier which prevents harmful substances from entering the bloodstream. They also assimilate B vitamins and promote bowel movements. |
| Biochemistry | The chemistry of living organisms. |
| Bioflavinoids | Give colour to leaves and plants. Used to be called vitamin P. Strengthen capillary walls and help prevent bruising. Found in fruits and vegetables. |
| Blastocyst | An early stage of embryonic development that occurs at 7–8 days after fertilization. A blastocyst consists of a hollow ball of cells with a localized thickening that will develop into the embryo. (*see* Embryo *and* Zygote) |
| Bonds | In chemistry, the physical, magnetic, electrical and chemical forces that keep atoms of a molecule attached to each other. |
| Bone marrow | Cells found in the centre of the long bones (e.g. femur) that manufacture most of the blood cells. |
| Boron | Boron is an element which works very much like oestrogen to prevent loss of minerals from the bone and osteoporosis. Synergy with vitamin D and calcium. Modulates immune and inflammatory processes.. |
| Brain | The highly developed mass of nervous tissue that forms the upper end of the central nervous system. Encased in the skull. It sends nervous ganglia throughout the body to receive and send messages. Two-thirds of the brain is made of oils. It relies on nutrients to pass messages across gaps, and the neurotransmitters are based on proteins. |
| Bulimia | Insatiable overeating, due to neurological causes. The hypothalamus may be at fault. |

| | |
|---|---|
| Butyric Acid | Liberated in a healthy large intestine. Helps the acidophilus and bifido bacteria to stick to the gut membrane, thereby protecting it. Required as a primary source of energy for all cells on the intestinal wall, which renew themselves every three days. Aids the natural healing of the gut membrane after antifungals have been used to eradicate *Candida albicans*. Plays a supporting role in the release of immunoglobulins from the gut mucosa. |
| Caffeine | An alkaloid drug, obtained from coffee, chocolate, coke and tea, that has a stimulant action, particularly on the central nervous and reproductive systems. |
| Calcium | Metallic element essential for the normal development and functioning of the body, muscle function and constituent of bones and teeth. Its uptake is facilitated by vitamin D. Works in the immune and nervous systems. |
| Calorie | A unit of measure used to determine the amount of energy in foodstuffs. It is equal to the amount of energy that would be able to raise the temperature of one gram of water one degree Centigrade. |
| Cancer | Malignant growth of abnormal cells which may invade and spread to other parts of the body and can cause death. |
| *Candida albicans* | A genus of yeast (fungus) that is commonly found in the human gut flora. In some individuals *Candida albicans* will overwhelm the digestive and immune system. If a yeast infection develops, it can lead to food intolerances and disrupt normal hormonal regulation. |
| Carbohydrate | A group of compounds, including the sugars, starch and fibres (non-starch polysaccharides), that contain carbon, hydrogen and oxygen. Used by the body for energy production, but excess intake is converted to fat and stored in adipose tissue. Fibre is essential to health and should be eaten daily. |
| Carcinogenic | A substance or action that causes cancer, e.g. benzene, chemicals, pesticides. |
| Catabolic hormones | Hormones which stimulate the breakdown of the larger chemicals of the body to form smaller precursor chemicals. For instance, some catabolic hormones stimulate the breakdown of body proteins, like muscle proteins, into amino acids (muscle wasting). The opposite to anabolic hormones. |
| Cataracts | Clouding of the lens of the eye resulting in blurred vision. |

| | |
|---|---|
| Cell | The basic unit of all living organisms, which can reproduce itself exactly using the DNA blueprint at its core. A group of cells is referred to as a tissue. The body is made up of many different types of cells – nerve, immune, sperm, connective tissue, fat cells, etc. |
| Cell-mediated immunity | This involves free-floating white cells in the bloodstream which neutralize 'alien' invaders. |
| Cell membrane | The phospholipid layer which protects the cell organelles from damage, allowing substances to move in and out. Made up from oils. (*see* Cytoplasm) |
| Cellulose | A fibrous carbohydrate consisting of linked glucose units that can not be digested by the human. It passes through the body unchanged, but is able to absorb water, cholesterol and oestrogens. It speeds up excretion time and helps the body rid itself of harmful toxins. The cell walls of all fruits, vegetables, cereals, nuts and seeds are made of cellulose. |
| Cervix | The small opening of the uterus into the vagina. (*see* Uterus *and* Vagina) |
| Chelate | A chemical substance which attaches in a claw-like manner to metals and can prevent the metals, especially heavy metals such as lead, mercury and cadmium, from hurting the body. |
| Chemotactic | Movement of a cell or organism in response to a stimulus – a chemical change. |
| Chemotoxins | Chemicals which have a toxic effect in the body. |
| Chlamydia | A virus-like bacteria which can causes damage to the reproductive system leading to infertility. Studies show 81.7% of women under 25 years of age to be infected. |
| Cholecalciferol | *see* Vitamin D |
| Choriocarcinoma | Highly invasive malignant tumour that can develop from the chorion, a membrane that surrounds the fetus. Hydatioiform mole occurs when the blastocyst turns cancerous. (*see* Chorion) |
| Chorion | The embryonic membrane that totally surrounds the embryo and serves as a protective barrier while in uterus. (*see* Embryo) |
| Chromium | Needed for glucose tolerance factor along with vitamin B3. Used for fatty acid synthesis. Deficiency leads to heart disease. Normalizes blood sugar levels. |
| Chromosomes | Thread-like structures in the cell nucleus that carry genetic |

|  | information. The human has 46 chromosomes – 23 from the father, 23 from the mother. (*see* Gene *and* DNA) |
|---|---|
| Chronic | Describes a disease of long duration, involving slow changes. (*see* Endometriosis *and* Pain) |
| Cis fatty acid | The natural form in which oils exist. Builds a strong cell membrane. Found only in cold-pressed oils. |
| Clomiphene | A synthetic non-steroidal compound used in IVF that stimulates the pituitary to produce hormones (FSH and LH) that induce follicular growth and egg development by the ovary. (*see* Follicle-stimulating hormone, Lutenizing hormone *and* Ovarian follicle) |
| Codeine | An analgesic derived from morphine but less potent as a painkiller and sedative, and is less toxic. |
| Coenzymes | Non-protein organic compounds such as vitamins and minerals that, as part of an enzyme, play an essential role in a chemical reaction. (Without sufficient supplies of the coenzyme the reaction could not take place.) |
| Collagen | The main supportive protein of the skin, tendons and bone. It relies on uptake of vitamins A and C, essential fatty acids and zinc for its formation. |
| Complementary medicine | Systems of healing which complement orthodox medicine, including homeopathy, herbal remedies, acupuncture, osteopathy, chiropractic, naturopathy, hydrotherapy and faith healing. |
| Conception | The process of fertilization of the egg when the egg and sperm collide and new life begins. (*see* Fertilization *and* Pronuclei) |
| Congenital | From birth. |
| Constipation | Difficult, incomplete, or infrequent evacuation of the bowel. Insufficient fibre is being eaten which reduces water uptake. This leads to a build-up of harmful toxins and reduced excretion of cholesterol and oestrogens. Related to some food intolerances. Wheat, bananas, cheese and eggs can trigger constipation. Vitamin C and magnesium are known to soften stools. |
| CoQ10 | Aids the heart muscle in its uptake of oxygen. Has strong antioxidant properties which are protective to all body cells. Also works within cells in process of energy production. |
| Corpus luteum (CL) | The structure that forms from the follicles of the ovary after ovulation. The corpus luteum produces the hormone |

| | |
|---|---|
| | progesterone which supports the pregnant state. (*see* Ovary, Ovulation *and* Progesterone) |
| Cytoplasm | The fluid matrix inside the living cell which surround all the organelles. (*see* Cell) |
| Department of Health | A department of central government in the UK that supports the Secretary of State for Health in meeting his obligations which include the National Health Service, and the prevention and control of infectious diseases. |
| Dermatitis | Infection or irritation of the skin. |
| D-gamma linolenic acid (DGLA) | An omega 6 essential fatty acid found in evening primrose oil. |
| Diabetes mellitus | An endocrine disease caused by insufficient insulin production by the pancreas. Blood sugars, like glucose, are not used properly by the body cells of people with diabetes mellitus. There is a new research link between high insulin levels and polycystic ovaries. (*see* Pancreas) |
| Diet | The mixture of foods that a person eats. A balanced diet contains adequate quantities of all the macro- and micro-nutrients. As we are all unique individuals, our needs will vary. |
| Diethylstilboestrol (DES) | A synthetic oestrogen used as a drug replacement for natural oestrogen. DES given to pregnant women in the 1960s to prevent abortion was found to cause abnormal development of their growing baby's reproductive tract. |
| Dietitian | A trained dietitian looks at a person's calorie intake and assesses which foods should be eaten if they are ill, underweight or overweight. |
| Dioxins | A powerful toxin used in industrial processes and as an aerial herbicide. Used in 'agent orange' during the Vietnam war. Known to damage the reproductive system due to its oestrogenic effect on body cells, and thought to be a carcinogen. Stored in body fat so care must be taken when dieting to go slowly. Powerful immunosuppressants. |
| DL phenylalanine (DLPA) | Phenylalanine is an amino acid that occurs as two mirror images, the L and D form. The L form occurs naturally in nature, and the D form is man-made. DL phenylalanine is a mixture of the L and D forms and is used for pain relief, as an appetite suppressant and works an anti-depressant. |
| DNA | Deoxyribonucleic acid. The scientific name for the chemical that our genes are made of. It is found in all living cells and acts as a blueprint for cell reproduction and |

renewal. If part of the DNA is corrupted, then cell mutations can occur. (*see* Gene *and* Chromosomes)

Dopamine               A hormone which is found in the adrenal glands and brain.

Dyspareunia            Painful or difficult sexual intercourse experienced by a woman. Can be caused in endometriosis if adhesions stick organs together, or if there are large ovarian cysts or internal inflammation.

Ectopic pregnancy      The development of a pregnancy in an area of the body other than the uterus. An ectopic pregnancy in the Fallopian tubes may lead to the death of the mother after eight weeks if it is not found and removed. A major obstetric problem.

Eczema                 A non-contagious inflammation of the skin that is characterized with redness, itching and sometimes sores. May be related in some to dairy intolerances and low fatty acid intake.

Embryo                 The first cells of the newborn from fertilization to about 8 weeks of development.

Embryology             The study of the growth and development of the embryo.

Endocrine system       The body's control system that involves interactions between hormones. The word endocrine means internal secretions which act as messengers. Includes the hypothalamus, hypocampus, thyroid, parathyroid, thymus, adrenal glands, ovaries, testes pituitary, pancreas, liver, and placenta.

Endocrinology          The study of the endocrine glands and the substances they secrete (hormones). (*see* Hormones)

Endogenous             Contained or produced in the body.

Endometriosis          The disease condition where endometrium develops and grows in areas and organs of the body other than where it belongs. The endometrium is normally found lining the uterus. Endometriosis may cause pain and infertility. (*see* Uterus *and* Endometrium)

Endometriotic          The pieces of endometrium that develop outside the wombs
implants               of women who have endometriosis, i.e. on the bowel, bladder, ovaries and appendix. (*see* Endometrium)

Endometrium            The inner lining of the uterus that is the surface where the blastocyst/embryo implants during pregnancy. The endometrium is the tissue that is lost during the menstrual period and it is also the source of tissue for endometriosis formation. It relies on oestrogen for its growth. (*see* Uterus *and* Endometriosis)

| | |
|---|---|
| Endorphins | Small molecules secreted by the pituitary gland in the brain that act as a natural analgesic to control pain. They are thought to be concerned with controlling the activity of the endocrine glands. Thiamine is known to be used by endorphins. |
| Enzyme | An organic chemical, usually a protein, that speeds up biochemical reactions or causes the breakdown of large molecules into smaller molecules. They act as catalysts as the reaction does not change them. The co-factors used to create enzymes are vitamins and minerals. Each enzyme is very specific. They are vital for body function. |
| EPA (Eicosapentaenoic acid) | An omega 3 EFA found in fish liver oils. The body metabolizes EPA to form anti-inflammatory prostaglandins, and to keep blood thin. Important in prevention of heart disease, PMS and cancers. |
| Epididymis | The collecting tube on the side of each testis that stores sperm before ejaculation. (*see* Testes, Sertoli cell *and* Sperm) |
| Epithelial cells | The surface cells that usually cover the outer or innermost layers of an organ. |
| EPO (Evening primrose oil) | Gamma-linolenic acid (GLA). The precursor to anti-inflammatory prostaglandins. A useful addition to the diet with conditions such as endometriosis, arthritis, asthma, PMS, eczema and heart disease. Stops blood becoming sticky. Should not be used by those with epilepsy or manic depression. (*see* Precursor) |
| Essential amino acid (EAA) | Amino acid that is essential for normal growth and development but cannot be synthesized by the body. Amino acids are the smallest part of a protein. Used for tissue renewal, enzymes, hormones, etc. |
| Essential fatty acid (EFA) | A fatty acid that is essential for normal growth and development but cannot be synthesized by the body. Used in brain cells and cell membranes. |
| Embryo transfer (ET) | The placement of embryos into the uterus at the end of an IVF cycle. (*see* In vitro fertilization *and* Uterus) |
| Enzyme saturation | When all cells are replete with all the nutrients which they require in order to work at their optimum level. |
| Estrogen/oestrogen | The female sex hormone secreted in large concentrations by the ovary and placenta. Responsible for the female secondary sex characteristics. (*see* Ovary *and* Placenta) It comprises a large family of steroid hormones that includes oestriol, oestrone, oestradiol. Small amounts are produced by the adrenal cortex, fat cells and testes. |

| | |
|---|---|
| Fallopian tubes | Two tubes attached at each corner of the uterus which stretch out towards the ovaries. They are the passageways used by eggs to meet the sperm and the place of fertilization. The newly formed embryo can then enter the uterus. Also known as the oviducts. (*see* Uterus) |
| Family planning | The use of contraception to limit or space out the numbers of children born to a couple. To maintain the woman's health one child every two years is felt to be optimum. |
| Fertility rate | The number of live births occurring in a year per 1,000 women of child-bearing age (usually 15–44 years of age). |
| Fertilization | The fusion of a sperm and an ovum. (*see* Sperm *and* Ova) |
| Fetus | Baby before birth. (*see* Pregnancy) |
| Flatulence | Gas that forms in the gastrointestinal (GI) tract. An excess of gas can be formed when the bacteriodes bacteria become overgrown as the bifido bacteria are destroyed by antibiotics, the pill, HRT and stress. |
| Folic acid | B vitamin essential for preventing fetal abnormalities. Reduced by the pill and stress. The metabolic role of folic acid is interdependent with that of zinc and vitamin B12 (both are required by rapidly dividing cells) and a deficiency in one may lead to a deficiency in the other. |
| Follicle | *See* Ovarian follicle. |
| Follicle-stimulating hormone (FSH) | The hormone released by the anterior pituitary gland that stimulates the ovary to produce follicles and mature eggs. Released in the first 14 days of the cycle. In anovulation, FSH is deficient. (*see* Pituitary, Ova *and* Ovary) |
| Free radicals | Small singlet oxygen molecules that have a high capacity to react chemically with other molecules. They are highly unstable as they only have one electron and try to steal another from a normal cell membrane or its DNA. This chemical reaction can be destructive, especially to protein molecules. Also known as free oxidizing radicals (FoRs). |
| Fructo-oligosaccharides (FOS) | *See* Prebiotics. |
| Gamete | A mature sex cell; the egg of the female or the sperm of the male. Gametes are haploid, containing half the normal number of chromosomes, 23 chromosomes in an ova and 23 in a sperm, so that when they join, the embryo has a full 46. (*see* Sperm, Ova, Chromosomes *and* Gamete) |
| Gastrointestinal (GI) | Pertaining to the stomach and intestine; the digestive tract/system. |

| | |
|---|---|
| Gene | The basic unit of genetic material, which is found at a unique place on a chromosome, e.g. a damaged P53 gene is known to be responsible for cancer formation. (*see* Chromosome *and* DNA) |
| General practitioner (GP) | A doctor who is the main agent of primary care, through whom patients make first contact with medical services. The majority have had no training in nutrition. |
| Germ cells | The precursor cells that have the potential to develop into sperm or eggs. (*see* Precursor, Sperm *and* Ova) |
| Gestation | The duration of a pregnancy. (*see* Pregnancy) |
| GIFT (Gamete intrafallopian transfer) | A form of assisted reproduction in which ova are mixed with the partner's sperm and then introduced into a Fallopian tube where fertilization takes place. (*see* Ova, Sperm *and* Fertilization) |
| GLA (Gamma-linolenic acid) | An EFA abundant in evening primrose oil. (*see* Essential fatty acid *and* EPO) |
| Glycoprotein | Large protein molecules that also contain sugar (carbohydrate) molecules. (*see* Proteins) |
| Glucose | A simple sugar used by cells in energy production. Two teaspoons are the norm in the body's eight pints of blood. (*see* Carbohydrate) |
| Gonadotrophins | The hormones (LH and FSH) released from the pituitary gland which stimulate the ovaries to produce follicles and undergo the process of ovulation. (*see* Pituitary, Lutenizing hormone *and* Follicle-stimulating hormone) |
| Gonadotrophin-releasing hormone (GnRH) | Hormone produced in the hypothalamus that stimulates the pituitary to produce and secrete gonadotrophins. Its production is dependent on absorption of zinc and vitamin B6. (*see* Pituitary gland, Lutenizing hormone *and* Follicle-stimulating hormone) |
| Graafian follicle | A mature follicle on the ovary prior to ovulation, containing a large fluid-filled cavity that distends the surface of the ovary. The oocyte develops inside the follicle attached to one side. (*see* Ovarian follicle, Ovary *and* Ovulation) |
| Gram | A unit of weight equal to 0.035oz. |
| Granulosa cells | The cells that line the inside of the Graafian follicle. They produce large amounts of oestrogen and the fluid of the follicle. They also supply nutrients to the egg and, as a result of this role, are also called 'nurse cells'. (*see* Ovary, Ovarian follicle *and* Oestrogen) |

| | |
|---|---|
| Growth factor | A polypeptide (small protein) that is produced by tissue that stimulates cells to proliferate. |
| Gynaecologist | Doctor specializing in women's reproductive illnesses. |
| HCG (Human chorionic gonadotrophin | Hormone produced by the placenta during pregancy, used as the basis for pregnancy test. HCG maintains the secretion of progesterone by the corpus luteum of the ovary as the secretion of pituitary LH is blocked during pregnancy. Poor placental formation will lead to poor HCG secretion and the pregnancy will not be maintained. (*see* Pregnancy *and* Placenta) |
| Health centre | A building owned or leased by a district health authority, that houses personnel or services from one or several sections of the National Health Service. |
| Health education | Persuasive methods used to encourage people to adopt life-styles that the educators believe will improve health, and to reject habits regarded as harmful to health. Disease prevention. |
| Health promotion | A programme of surveillance planned on a community basis to maintain the best possible health and quality of life of the members of that community, both collectively and individually. |
| Histamine | A chemical that can cause blood vessels to dilate. It is secreted at the site of a wound and is one of the major factors that cause the wound to become red. It is also secreted by the immune system during an immune response to antigens. Involved in anaphelactic shock. Vitamin C is antihistamine. (*see* Immune system *and* Antigens) |
| Holistic | Viewing the body as a whole unit which works together when considering matters of health and healing. Prevention being better than cure. |
| Homeostasis | The tendency of the body to always strive to maintain a stable or uniform state. |
| Hormones | The body's chemical messengers that are secreted by the endocrine glands. |
| Hormone receptors | Special proteins on or in cells to which hormones attach. Attachment (binding) of the hormone to the receptor will cause the endocrine effect of the hormone. Can be disrupted by exogenous hormones. (*see* Endocrinology *and* Hormones) |

| | |
|---|---|
| Hormone replacement therapy (HRT) | The administration of oestrogen and progesterone to replace these hormones in women who have no ovarian function due to menopause or surgery. Natural menopause should not be a problem if a woman is well nourished. (*see* Menopause, Oestrogen, Progesterone *and* Ovary) |
| Hyperventilation | Rapid deep breathing. Lowers the carbon dioxide in the blood and can lead to unconsciousness, dizziness and 'spaced out' feelings. Low oxygen supply to cells causes malfunction. |
| Hypoglycaemia | Low amounts of glucose sugar in the blood. This can lead to irritability, weakness, fatigue, excessive sweating. The body relies on insulin and glucose tolerance factor (B3 and chromium-based) to control blood sugar levels. (*see* Diabetes mellitus) |
| Hypothalamus | Part of the base of the brain that is connected to the pituitary gland. Secretes hormones that control the production and secretion of the pituitary hormones. The seat of appetite control. Also controls body temperature. Integrates hormone control and nervous system activity. (*see* Pituitary gland) |
| Hypothyroid | A condition where the thyroid secretes insufficient amounts of thyroid hormones T3, T4, which affect TSH from the pituitary. Causes constipation, skin coarseness, sluggishness, lethargy, dull brain, loss of outer third of eyebrows. (*see* Thyroid) |
| Hysterectomy | Surgical removal of the uterus. Should only be essential if diseased. Removal of the uterus has been seen to shorten life by five years, and lead to strokes and heart disease. (*see* Uterus) |
| Humoral immunity | The fluid and hormonal (i.e. humors) system of the body. The immune system depends upon antibodies produced by B lymphocytes circulating via the bloodstream. |
| Iatrogenic condition | A condition that results from medical treatment, as either an unforeseen or inevitable side effect, e.g. hair loss with chemotherapy, gut flora disruption with antibiotics. |
| Intracytoplasmic sperm injection (ICSI) | The injection of a single sperm directly into an ova, done by an endocrinologist. The resulting zygote is then transferred back into the woman's uterus. (*see* Ova *and* Sperm) |
| Immune | Having a natural resistance to harmful substances. |
| Immune system | The defence system of the body that helps fight off infections from bacteria, viruses and other 'alien' substances. |

| | |
|---|---|
| Immunoglobins | Immune cells are produced by B lymphocytes, which form antibodies against 'alien' bacterial protein material. |
| Infant mortality rate (IMR) | The number of deaths of infants under one year of age per 1,000 live births in a given year. |
| Infertility | Inability of a couple to induce conception after 12–18 months of unprotected sexual intercourse. |
| Inflammation | The body's response to injury, which may be acute or chronic. It is associated with a local increase in temperature and the activation of the immune system. Histamines are released. (*see* Immune system) |
| Integrins | The 'adhesive' material which enables one cell to 'stick' to another in order to form the structure of the body. Forms the connective tissue collagen. |
| Interferon | Produced by macrophages and T lymphocytes. Protects cells from damage by shutting down the mitochondria, the energy production site, in order to stop the virus from reproducing itself. Needs choline, manganese and vitamin C. Our ability to produce interferon is damaged by pesticides. |
| Interleukins | Regulating chemicals secreted by the white blood cells (leukocytes) e. g. interleukin 2 stimulates T lymphocytes and is used in the treatment of cancer. (*see* White blood cells) |
| In vitro fertilization (IVF) | The fertilization of the egg outside the body, usually in a dish in a specially designed incubator. |
| Iron | A metallic element essential to the process of respiration and therefore life. It stimulates immunity, boosts physical performance and allows blood to carry oxygen to cells for energy production. |
| Lactation | The production and release of milk from the breast. (see Prolactin *and* Pituitary gland) |
| Laparoscope | A fibre-optic surgical instrument that can be inserted through a small incision in the belly button to view the contents of the peritoneal cavity. |
| Laparoscopy | A surgical procedure for the examination of the peritoneal cavity using a laparoscope. Also called 'belly-button' surgery. |
| Laparotomy | A surgical procedure for the examination of the peritoneal cavity using a longer incision in the abdominal wall (belly). |
| Leaky gut | Where the gut membrane has been eroded or breached, and toxins can enter the bloodstream and set up intolerances and toxic feelings. Autointoxification. |
| Leukotrines | Form a sub-group of series two (PG2). They increase |

inflammation and blood clotting. Responsible for bronchial constriction (as in asthma), and inflammatory processes.

| | |
|---|---|
| Lindane | A powerful insecticide which has oestrogenic properties. Found in chocolate and milk, and linked to breast cancer. |
| Linoleic acid | An omega 6 polyunsaturated cis fatty acid. We cannot make this and depend upon good oils in foods. Found in vegetable oils such as sunflower and safflower oils. |
| Linolenic acid (LA) | An omega 3 cis fatty acid. We cannot make this and depend upon food intake. The alpha form is found in fish oils and linseeds. (*see* EFA) |
| Lipids | Water insoluble substances which have a greasy feel. They include neutral fats, fatty acids, steroids and waxes. |
| Luteinizing hormone (LH) | Hormone produced by the pituitary which stimulates ovulation and the corpus luteum to produce progesterone. Released from day 14 to day 28 in the normal cycle. (*see* Pituitary gland *and* Progesterone). |
| Luteinizing unruptured follicle syndrome (LUFS) | The condition where a woman appears to have a normal menstrual cycle but the egg does not ovulate (pop) out of the ovarian follicle. (*see* Anovulation) |
| Lymph | A transparent to yellow-coloured liquid found in lymphatic vessels. It carries lymphocytes and bathes tissues. (*see* Lymphatic system) |
| Lymph glands | Structures found in the lymphatic system that filter the lymph and are part of the immune system. Found in the neck, groin, armpit. They prevent 'aliens' from entering the bloodstream. (*see* Immune system) |
| Lymphatic system | A system of tubes (lymph vessels) that drain lymph from various organs and return the lymph to the blood. Part of the immune system. (*see* Immune system *and* Tonsils) |
| Lymphocyte | A type of white blood cell that originates from the lymph glands. |
| Lysosome | A particle inside cells which helps break down 'alien' invaders. |
| Lysozyme | Contained by T-cells. This is a deadly enzyme which kills germs and our own cells once released by these immune cells. Vitamin C provides some protection, 'mopping up' any excess. |
| Macrophage | A wandering cell that is found in tissue and blood that can phagocytize (eat) bacteria and other 'alien' matter that makes its way into the body. (*see* Phagocytize, White blood cells *and* Immune system) |
| Magnesium | A white metallic element that is an essential nutrient. |

|  |  |
|---|---|
|  | Magnesium deficiency can lead to impaired nerve and muscle function. Marginal magnesium deficiency is becoming common. It causes loss of appetite, nausea, diarrhoea, confusion, muscle tremors and spasms, lack of co-ordination. Useful with PMS and abdominal cramps. |
| Malabsorption | When the intestines are malfunctioning and nutrients from foods are not absorbed effectively into the bloodstream. It can be due to coeliac problems when gluten damages the villi, or if the gut mucosa is damaged by drugs or constant stress. It may be corrected by slippery elm, butyric acid and NAG. |
| Medical | Of or relating to medicine; the diagnosis, treatment and prevention of disease. |
| Medicine | The science or practice of the diagnosis, treatment and prevention of disease. |
| Melatonin | A hormone secreted by the pineal gland in the brain. Excess melatonin hampers fertility and raises the levels of prolactin. Modern life causes imbalances in light and dark cycles which affect melatonin production. Zinc is vital in this process as is natural daylight. Exposure to electromagnetic fields reduces melatonin levels. Blocks oestrogen from binding to oestrogen receptors of cells, e.g. breast cancer cells (*see* Pineal gland) |
| Menarche | Start of menstrual cycles. Usually from the age of 12 to 17. (*see* Menstrual cycle *and* Menstrual period) |
| Menopause | The end of the monthly menstrual cycle that results from the use of all the eggs of the ovary. Usually starts between 44 and 55 years of age and takes 7 years to occur naturally. (*see* HRT, Ova *and* Menstrual cycle) |
| Menstrual cycle | The reproductive cycle of women that lasts for approximately one month. The menstrual cycle is controlled by the hormones of the pituitary, ovary and uterus. During the menstrual cycle, the endometrium of the uterus thickens in preparation for pregnancy. If pregnancy does not occur, the endometrium is sloughed off as the menstrual period (flow) and the cycle is repeated. (*see* Uterus, Pituitary gland, Ovary *and* Endometrium) |
| Menstrual period | That part of the menstrual cycle that is associated with the flow of blood out of the vagina. Also referred to as 'menstruation' or 'menstrual bleeding'. Should be pain-free and symptomless in healthy individuals. The nutrients B6, zinc, chromium, magnesium and vitamin C are known to play a role. (*see* Menstrual cycle) |
| Metabolism | The biochemical reactions of the body that are involved in |

the maintenance of life. The thyroid gland and hypothalamus are related to the metabolic rate at which foods are burnt to provide energy. Iodine and selenium are important for this process.

| | |
|---|---|
| Microgram | One-millionth part of a gram. |
| Milligram | One-thousandth part of a gram. |
| Miscarriage | The tragic premature loss of a fetus due to natural causes. |
| Mitochondria | A small organelle found inside all cells that makes the energy of the cell. Exercise promotes the formation of more mitochondria. |
| Morula | An early embryo with approximately 16–200 cells. (*see* Embryo) |
| Mutagen | A substance which can cause changes in the DNA of cells of the body. (*see* DNA *and* Gene) |
| Mutation | A change in form, structure or characteristics of an organism due to alterations in the DNA of the nucleus. (*see* DNA *and* Gene) |
| Myometrium | The thick muscle layer of the uterus. It contracts during the birthing process to expel the baby. Menstrual cramps are the pain signals transmitted to the brain during myometrial contractions. In PMS these cramps can be alleviated by use of magnesium supplements. (*see* Uterus) |
| NAG | N acetyl glucosamine is an integral part of the 'glue' which holds cells together, especially the mucous membranes lining the intestines (*see* Integrins). It helps normal intestinal mucosa growth and helps to protect it from acids, enzymes and organisms. It is an amino sugar which occurs naturally in a healthy body. |
| Naturopathy | A system of medicine that relies upon the use of only natural substances for the treatment of disease. |
| Neural tube defects (NTD) | Defects of the nervous system, such as spina bifida. Attributed to deficiencies in folic acid and zinc. |
| Neurotransmitters | The chemicals produced at the end of a nerve that transmit to the next nerve or muscle, or produce an excitatory signal within the brain. They inhibit or excite a response. Serotonin, acetylecholine and the catcholamines depend upon tryptophan, choline and tyrosine, respectively. |
| Neutrophil | A type of white blood cell found in the blood that is part of the immune system. (*see* Immune system) |

| | |
|---|---|
| Nicotinic acid<br>Niacin<br>Nicotinamide | Vitamin B3 which aids lowering of blood cholesterol and protective against heart disease. Reduces high blood pressure. |
| Nutrients<br>(niacin) | Food substances that are nourishing and which are the supply of materials for body metabolism. Vitamins, minerals and fatty acids are micro-nutrients, and fats, carbohydrates and proteins are macro-nutrients. |
| Nutritionist | A trained nutritionist or nutrition consultant assesses a person's illness and works with that person to correct individual body biochemistry imbalances and improve nutrient intake from the diet. Tests can be done to assess vitamin and mineral levels, gut fermentation, etc. |
| Obstetrician | A doctor who specializes in pregnancy and childbirth. |
| Oedema | Swelling, retention of fluid in spaces between cells. Oedema is spelled edema in America. |
| Oestrogen | The female sex hormone secreted in large concentrations by the ovary and placenta. Responsible for the female secondary sex characteristics. (Oestrogen is spelled estrogen in America.) Also produced in the adrenal glands, fat cells and testes. |
| Oral contraceptive | Orally administered drugs derived from ovarian steroids which interfere with the reproductive process and induce infertility. They disrupt blood chemistry causing vitamin A and copper levels to be raised, while lowering levels of B vitamins and zinc. |
| Organelles | The structures within each cell which allow the cell to function. |
| Organochlorines | Organic compounds containing chlorine, including chloroform, DDT, dioxins and other pesticides. |
| Oocyte | Same as ova. (*see* Ovary *and* Ova) |
| Oophorectomy | Surgical removal of the ovary. (*see* Ovary) |
| Ova and ovum | The unfertilized egg produced in the ovary. Ovum is singular (one egg) and ova more than one. (*see* Ovary) |
| Ovarian cysts | A fluid-filled sac, one or more of which can develop in the ovary. Most are non-malignant but can reach a very large size and cause gross swelling and pain. In endometriosis chocolate cysts filled with stale dark-brown blood are common. With polycystic ovaries, many follicular cysts develop. High copper levels are related to cyst formation. The pill increases blood copper levels. |
| Ovarian follicle | The cyst-like structure that forms on the ovary during the |

menstrual cycle and which contains the developing egg and granulosa cells. (*see* Ovary, Ova *and* Granulosa cells)

| | |
|---|---|
| Ovary | Paired almond-shaped organs lying in the pelvis that produce hormones (oestrogen and progesterone) and eggs. (*see* Oestrogen, Progesterone *and* Ova) |
| Ovulation | The process of expulsion of the egg from the ovarian follicle to the Fallopian tube. Occurs around the 14th to 15th day of a normal cycle. (*See* Ova, Ovary *and* Fallopian tube) |
| Oxytocin | A protein-derived hormone secreted by the posterior pituitary that stimulates uterine contractions during the birthing process and the release of milk from the breast. |
| Pain | Suffering, distress of body or mind. Usually caused by disease or injury, but can be emotional pain from trauma. |
| Pancreas | The gland that is located under the liver that functions as both an endocrine and exocrine gland. As an endocrine gland the pancreas secretes insulin and glucogon to control the concentration of blood sugar and as an exocrine gland the pancreas secretes digestive enzymes into the intestine (*see* Diabetes mellitus *and* Endocrine system). |
| Pelvic inflammatory disease (PID) | A general infection in the peritoneal cavity that can be caused by a variety of bacteria that gain entrance into the peritoneal cavity through the female reproductive tract from poor hygiene or infected male sperm. The disease is associated with flu-like symptoms and adhesions, leading to infertility. (*see* Peritoneal cavity, Chlamydia *and* Adhesions) |
| Peristalsis | Rhythmic muscular contraction in the intestines which pushes food through the digestive system. The process is involuntary. Bifido bacteria and fibre encourage peristalsis. |
| Peritoneal cavity | The lower abdomen (belly) which contains the reproductive tract, bladder, kidneys and adrenals, small and large intestine, liver, pancreas and stomach. |
| Peritoneal fluid | The fluid found in the peritoneal cavity. (*see* Peritoneal cavity) |
| Petechia | A small red to purplish-red area on the surface of the skin or an organ that is caused by small broken blood vessels. |
| Petechial implants | Endometriotic implants that are red and have the appearance of a petechia. These are the most active implants and cause the most inflammation and pain. May be producing their own oestrogens. |
| Peyer's patches | Clusters of cells found on the small intestine that are involved in the immune system. They act as testing stations for 'alien' food particles, bacteria, parasites, chemicals, etc. |

| | |
|---|---|
| Phagocytize | The ability to ingest (eat) micro-organisms or other foreign matter. The process whereby white blood cells ingest micro-organisms. (*see* Macrophage, Immune system *and* White blood cells) |
| Phytochemicals | Substances found in plants and not in animals, which have an effect upon body biochemistry. |
| Phyto-oestrogens | Oestrogens present in plants. Isoflavones, lignans, coumestans which are structurally similar to oestradiol. They have an oestrogen-modulating effect. Lower binding activity than endogenous oestrogens. Found in soya, wheat, citrus, seeds, pulses and grains. |
| Phthalates | Phthalic acid diesters are organic chemicals used in industry as plasticizers. They are found in low levels in foods which are wrapped in plastics. Some researchers feel that these levels are high enough to have profound effects on reducing human fertility. Oestrogenic in action. |
| Pineal gland | Gland found in the middle of the brain that secretes the hormone melatonin. Controls the seasonal changes in the reproductive system and hair growth in seasonal animals (e.g. sheep and horses). (*see* Melatonin) |
| Pituitary gland | Endocrine gland at the base of the brain that secretes a variety of hormones, many of which affect other endocrine glands. The major hormones of the pituitary that affect the reproductive system are follicle-stimulating hormone (FSH), luteinizing hormone (LH) and prolactin. The pituitary is divided into the anterior (front) and posterior (back) pituitary. Known to use vitamin B6 and zinc. |
| Placebo | An inactive substance or other pretend 'medicine' administered to a patient usually to compare its effects with those of a real drug or treatment, but which may help to relieve a condition because of the patient's belief that it will cure him/her. 'Works' by psychosomatic suggestion. |
| Placenta | The tissue that connects the developing fetus to the uterus of the mother. This organ has to develop over the space of one month, so nutrient intake is crucial to its healthy formation. (*see* Fetus) |
| Platelets | Blood cells that are important in blood clot formation. If they become too sticky they cause heart disease problems. Vitamins C, E and garlic and root ginger thin blood. Vitamin K is necessary for blood to clot. Sugar causes blood to become sticky. |
| PMS/PMT | Premenstrual syndrome/premenstrual tension. The build- |

up of symptoms before a period is due. May be related to faulty nutrition or malabsorption of nutrients. Responds to the use of B complex, B6, magnesium, zinc, chromium, vitamins C and E, and esential fatty acids.

| | |
|---|---|
| polychlorinated phenyls (PCBs) | Toxic chemicals commonly used in electrical components and industrial processes. Thought to be damaging to the reproductive system. Stored in body fat, so care must be taken when dieting to go slowly. |
| pouch of Douglas | The blind pouch that makes the bottom of the peritoneal cavity. It lies between the vagina and the colon and below the ovaries. Also called the 'cul-de-sac' area of the peritoneal cavity. It is a prime site for endometriotic implants. (*see* Peritoneal cavity) |
| precursor | One that precedes another. |
| pregnancy | The condition of having a developing embryo or fetus in the body for nine months' gestation. (*see* Embryo *and* Fetus) |
| premarin | Conjugated oestrogens obtained from the urine of pregnant mares used for HRT. (*see* Oestrogen) |
| premenstrual | A few days before a menstrual period. PMS symptoms such as bloating, irritability, headaches, anxiety etc., often build up from day 14–28 of the cycle. (*see* Menstrual period) |
| prebiotics | Fructo-oligosaccharides that encourage growth of bifidobacteria in the gut flora. 15mg per day is optimum. |
| probiotics | Replenish the bifido factor bacteria which inhabit a healthy gut. The growth of these friendly bacteria encourages oestrogen clearance. If they are not present in healthy quantities, the oestrogen is reactivated and sent back into circulation to cause havoc. Also support immunoglobins. |
| progesterone | Female steroid sex hormone which prepares the endometrium of the uterus for pregnancy and is required for the maintenance of pregnancy. Secreted by the corpus luteum in the ovary once conception has taken place to prepare the womb lining and placenta. Maintains the pregnancy and prevents release of further eggs from the ovary. (*see* Ovary *and* Corpus luteum) |
| prolactin | Pituitary hormone which stimulates milk synthesis. It also stimulates the production of progesterone by the corpus luteum of the ovary. Excess melatonin causes an increase in prolactin, which lowers zinc and prostaglandins. (*see* Pituitary gland *and* Lactation) |

| | |
|---|---|
| Pronuclei | The two nuclei that form in the egg after fertilization. One nucleus contains the genes of the egg (mother) and the other nucleus contains the genes of the sperm (father). |
| Prostaglandin (PG) | A lipid hormone found in many cells of the body. Some are pro-inflammatory while others are anti-inflammatory. |
| Proteins | A group of complex organic nitrogen-containing compounds found throughout the body. They are composed of sequential strands of amino acids and are used for body building and repair, for hormones and enzyme production. |
| Pseudo | Superficial resemblance, false. |
| Pyridoxine | Vitamin B6. Required for more than 60 enzymes and essential for DNA and protein synthesis. It influences the nervous and reproductive systems and plays a vital role in immunity and avoidance of PMS symptoms. Aids infertility along with zinc. |
| Quercetin | A flavinoid which acts as as antioxidant. Helps prevent water retention and leaking capillaries. Acts as a phyto-oestrogen and helps the body to convert oestradiol to oestriol – the safe form of oestrogen. |
| Red blood cells | The major cell type found in the blood. Its main function is to transport oxygen throughout the body. Also called erythrocytes. |
| Retrograde | To move backwards. Endometriosis may be a result of retrograde menstruation, that is, menstrual flow into the peritoneal cavity via the Fallopian tubes instead of into the vagina. |
| Riboflavin | Vitamin B2, part of the body's antioxidant mechanism. Needed for correct thyroid function. Used alongside B5 in the reproductive system. |
| Scurvy | A disease condition that develops as a result of vitamin C deficiency. People with scurvy have anaemia, weakness, spongy gums and a tendency to bleed. (*see* Anaemia) |
| Selenium | A non-metallic element resembling sulphur. Small amounts of selenium are required for normal metabolism. Major antioxidant. Needed for thyroid function alongside iodine. Significant in sperm motility. |
| Seminal fluid | The fluid in the ejaculate that contains sperm. High levels of zinc in each ejaculation, 1.5mg. (*see* Sperm *and* Testes) |
| Sertoli cell | The cells of the testes that surround the developing sperm. They supply nutrients to the developing sperm and secrete |

fluids that help push the sperm out of the testes and into the epididymus. (*see* Sperm, Testes *and* Epididymis)

| | |
|---|---|
| rotonin | A neuro hormone produced in large amounts in the pineal gland of the brain. It is also found in other tissues of the body, including blood platelets and intestinal walls. It is believed to play a role in inflammation. Features in the process of sleep, prevention of depression, anxiety and mood disorders. |
| x steroids | Lipid-soluble steroid hormones involved in the reproductive process. They include: oestrogen, progesterone and testosterone. Good quality cis fatty acids are essential for their formation. (*see* Steroids, Oestrogen, Progesterone *and* Testosterone) |
| DS | Sudden infant death syndrome. |
| ppery elm | A herb which soothes irritated tissues especially mucous membranes such as those in the digestive tract. |
| erm | The male reproductive cell produced in the testes and which contains the genes of the father. The head and tail of the sperm depend upon zinc. (*see* Testes *and* Seminal fluid) |
| ermatogenesis | Formation of sperm in the testes. (*see* Sperm *and* Testes) |
| ermatozoa | Same as sperm. |
| eroids | A group of lipid-soluble biochemical substances which chemically resemble cholesterol. Cholesterol is the precursor of all steroid hormones. Vitamin D is also closely involved. The atoms of steroids are arranged in four rings. The major steroid-producing organs of the body include: the ovary, testis, adrenal gland and placenta. |
| lboestrol | Synthetic non-steroid oestrogen, known as DES (diethyl-stilboestrol) in America. Causes cancer. (*see* DES) |
| llbirth | When a child is dead at birth. |
| peroxide smutase (SOD) | A highly reactive enzyme that neutralizes free oxidised radicals (FoRs). (*see* Free radicals) |
| nergism | Working together for the good of each other. |
| mbiotic ationship | When two organisms work together for the benefit of both organisms. |
| cells | A type of cell that helps the immune system. Also known as T-helper cells, which switch the immune system on and T-suppressor cells which switch the immune system off. (*see* Immune system) |

| | |
|---|---|
| Teratogen | A substance, agent or process that induces the formation of developmental abnormalities in a fetus, e.g. excess vitamin A, alcohol, thalidomide and measles. (*see* Fetus) |
| Teratogenesis | The process leading to developmental abnormalities in the fetus. |
| Testes | The paired organs located in the scrotum under the penis. The site of production of sperm and testosterone. (*see* Sperm *and* Testosterone) |
| Testosterone | Major masculinizing hormone produced in large amounts by the male testes. Dependent upon vitamin E and zinc for its manufacture. |
| Thymus | A ductless gland that is found under the breastbone. Doubles in size by puberty and shrinks thereafter. Functional tissue is replaced by fatty tissue. Involved with the early development of the immune system and the main production site for T lymphocytes which migrate from bone marrow to mature in the thymus (white blood cells associated with antibody production). Zinc-dependent organ. (*see* Immune system) |
| Thyroid | The endocrine gland that controls the overall level of metabolism in the body. It is located in the neck and secretes the hormone thyroxine. For temperaure regulation (*see* Metabolism, TSH *and* Thyroxine) |
| Thyroid-stimulating hormone (TSH) | The hormone secreted by the pituitary that stimulates the thyroid gland to produce thyroxine. (*see* Thyroid *and* Thyroxine) |
| Thyroxine | The major hormone secreted by the thyroid. Thyroxine regulates general metabolism. Iodine dependent. Requires riboflavine, vitamin B2, selenium, tyrosine and vitamin E for its formation. Antagonistic with oestrogen. If oestrogen is too high, thyroxine will be low and vice versa. (*see* Thyroid) |
| Tocopherol | *see* Vitamin E. |
| Tonsil | A small almond-shaped mass on the back of the mouth that is composed mostly of lymphoid tissue. It is believed to be a source of the white blood cells that phagocytize (eat) the bacteria that enter the mouth and nose. (*see* Lymphatic system, Phagocytize *and* White blood cells) |
| Transit time | In reference to the digestive system, transit time is the time that foodstuffs spend in the gastrointestinal tract from the time of ingestion to defecation. Should be 12–24 hours.(*see* Gastrointestinal) |

| | |
|---|---|
| Uterus | The organ of the reproductive system where pregnancy occurs. Also called the womb. It is a muscular organ that is about the size of a small fist that has an inner lining of mucus-like tissue called the endometrium. Magnesium aids relaxation of uterine muscles. (*see* Endometrium) |
| Vagina | The lower part of the female reproductive tract that connects the cervix of the uterus to the exterior. (*see* Uterus *and* Cervix) |
| Villi | Finger-like projections in membranes of the gut which can be damaged by gluten grains in susceptible people. The villi increase the surface area for nutrients to be absorbed, so damage leads to malabsorption. |
| Vitamins | A general term for a group of unrelated biochemical substances that occur in food in small amounts and are required for normal metabolic functioning of the body. They may be either water-soluble or fat-soluble substances. |
| Vitamin A | A vitamin found primarily in fish liver oils and some yellow and dark green vegetables, functioning in normal cell growth and development. Deficiency causes roughening and hardening of the skin, night blindness and deterioration of mucous membranes in the lung etc. Exists in two forms: vitamin retinol (animal) and beta carotene (plant-based). Excess amounts of vitamin A retinol are toxic. |
| Vitamin B1 | Thiamine. Deficiency can cause learning defects. |
| Vitamin B2 | Riboflavin. Deficiency can cause limb defects. |
| Vitamin B3 | Nicotinamide or niacin. Deficiencies can cause harelip or cleft palate. |
| Vitamin B5 | Pantothenic acid. The anti-allergy vitamin. Needed for reproduction. Aids memory. |
| Vitamin B6 | Pyridoxine. Most commonly deficient especially in pill, HRT or other sex hormone takers because of their abnormal amine metabolism. Lowered by the pill. Deficiency can cause depression, urinary tract cancer or dermatitis. Precursor of progesterone. |
| Vitamin B12 | Cyanocobalamine. Often deficient in smokers or vegetarians. Only found in animal produce. |
| Vitamin B complex (other) | Water-soluble vitamins found primarily in yeast, liver, eggs, and certain vegetables. Taking too much of one B vitamin can cause shortages of the others. Lowered by the pill. Also produced in the small intestine by bifido bacteria.<br>**Folic acid.** Lowered by the pill, HRT and fertility |

stimulants. Taking the pill causes localized folate deficienc
of the cervix, which may trigger cervical cancer. Extra
required during pregnancy. Deficiency can cause anaemia
and spina bifida. Aspirin, anaesthetic gas, sulfasallzine
interfere with folate absorption. Has oestrogenic propertie
(*see* Anaemia *and* HRT)

**Choline**. Important in the synthesis of phosphatidylcholine
(lecithin) and other phospholipids, DNA and RNA.
Insecticides inactivate choline-enzymes which prevent the
uptake of manganese in plants, which is then linked to a fall
in manganese absorption. Choline and inositol are importan
in liver enzyme function, for aiding the degrading of
oestrogens so that they can be excreted safely by the body.

**Inositol**. Aids choline in oestrogen degradation in the
liver. Involved in the synthesis of phospholipids so is
essential for the digestion and absorption of fats and their
uptake by cells.

**Biotin**. Not a true vitamin as it is made by the bifido
bacteria in the gut. Prevents overgrowth of yeast in the
intestines. Biotin deficiency resembles Alzheimer's disease
Drugs like antibiotics cause a deficiency.

| | |
|---|---|
| Vitamin C | Ascorbic acid. Water-soluble vitamin present in citrus fruits, rosehip powder and chilli peppers. Lowered by pill hormones, smoking and tetracyclines. Antiviral, antibacterial, antihistamine. Smokers are deficient as each cigarette burns up 25mg vitamin C. |
| Vitamin D | Fat-soluble vitamin that is produced in response to skin exposure to the sun. Also found in fish oils. Deficiencies in vitamin D cause rickets. A precursor to cholesterol and thought to be a hormone in its own right. Deficiency may cause problems in hormone formation. |
| Vitamin E | Fat-soluble vitamin that belongs to the tocopherol family and found in wheat germ oil, cereals, egg yolk. Rats fed a vitamin E-deficient diet have fertility problems. Importan in preventing sticky platelets and blood clots. |
| Vitamin K | A fat-soluble vitamin. Has two forms: phytomenadione (plant origin) and menaquinone (animal origin) and is required for normal blood clot formation. Found in alfalf spinach, cabbage, fish meal, egg yolk. |
| White blood cells | Free-floating cells found in the blood that help the immun system. Also called leukocytes. (*see* T-cells *and* Macrophag |
| Womb | *see* Uterus. |

eno-oestrogens    Oestrogens from outside the body. They are oestrogens
which are metabolized in the body from synthetic man-
made chemicals. They disrupt normal hormone profiles.
Body fat stores these chemicals and releases them as weight
is lost. High exposure to these pesticidal chemicals can
disrupt oestrogen levels and may be related to
endometriosis.

inc    Metal co-factor necessary for the correct functioning of
reproduction and the immune system. Lowered by the pill.
Available in oysters and red meat. (*see* Sperm *and* Vitamin B6)

ygote    The newly fertilized ovum before cleavage begins. (*see*
Fertilization)

# Recommended reading

**Endometriosis**
Ballweg, Mary Lou, *The Endometriosis Sourcebook*, The Endometriosis
    Association/Contemporary Books, 1995
Hawkridge, Caroline, *Living with Endometriosis*, Vermilion, London, 1996
Henderson, Lorraine, Robyn Riley and Ros Wood, *Explaining Endometriosis*,
    Allen and Unwin, Sydney, 1991
Wittgenstein, Kate, *Living with Endometriosis*, Addison Wesley Longman,
    Harlow, 1987


**Fertility**
Barnes, Belinda and Suzanne G. Bradley, *Planning for a Healthy Baby*, Vermilion
    London, 1994
Bradley, Susan Gail with Nicholas Bennett, *Preparation for Pregnancy*, Argyll, 199
Leese, Henry, *Human Reproduction and in vitro Fertilization*, Macmillan Education
    Ltd, London, 1989
Wynn, Margaret and Arthur, *The Case for Preconceptual Care in Men and Women*,
    A B Academic Publishers, Bicester, 1991


**Digestion and absorption**
Brostoff, Dr Jonathan and Linda Gamlin, *The Complete Guide to Food Allergy and
    Intolerance*, Bloomsbury, London, 1989 (reissued in 1998)
Chaitow, Leon and Natasha Trenev, *Probiotics*, Thorsons, London, 1990
Connolly Pat and Price-Pottenger, *The Candida Albicans Yeast-Free Cookbook*,
    Nutrition Foundation/Keats Publishing, New Canaan, 1985
Lipski, Elizabeth, *Digestive Wellness*, Keats Publishing, New Canaan, 1996
MacDonald Baker, Sidney, *Detoxification and Healing*, Keats Publishing, New
    Canaan, 1997
Murray, Michael and Joseph Pizzorno, *Encyclopaedia of Natural Medicine*, Optim
    MacDonald, London, 1990
Trattler, Ross, *Better Health Through Natural Healing*, Health, 1987

## Foods, vitamins, minerals and essential oils

Carper, Jean, *The Food Pharmacy*, Simon & Schuster Ltd, London, 1990
——*Food, Your Miracle Medicine*, Simon & Schuster Ltd, London, 1995
Chaitow, Leon, *The Stone Age Diet*, Optima MacDonald, London, 1988
Cherry Hills, Hilda, *Good Food, Milk Free, Grain Free*, Keats Publishing, New
    Canaan, 1980
Coffey, Lynette, *Wheatless Cooking*, Ten Speed Press, California, 1984
Cousins, Barbara, *Cooking Without*, Moorside Natural Healing Clinic, 1989
Cox, Peter and Peggy Brusseau, *Secret Ingredients*, Bantam Books, London, 1997
Erasmus, Udo, *Fats that Heal, Fats that Kill*, Alive Books, Burnaby BC, 1996
Graham, Judy, *Evening Primrose Oil*, Thorsons, London, 1993
Hendler, Dr Sheldon Saul, *The Doctor's Vitamin and Mineral Encyclopaedia*, Arrow
    Books, London, 1991
Lieberman, Shari and Nancy Bruning, *The Real Vitamin and Mineral Book*, 2nd
    edition, Avery Press, New York, 1997
Null, Gary, *The Complete Guide to Sensible Eating*, 4 Walls 8 Window, New York,
    1990
——*The '90s Healthy Body Book*, Health Communications Inc, Florida, 1994
Null, Gary with Dr Martin Feldman, *Good Food, Good Mood*, St Martin's Press, New
    York, 1988


## Environmental issues

Buist, Robert, *Food Chemical Sensitivity*, Prish, Dorset, 1986
Colburn, Theo, John Peterson and Dianne Dumanoski, *Our Stolen Future*, Little
    Brown, London, 1996
Millstone, Erik, *Food Additives*, Penguin, Harmondsworth, 1986
Mumby, Dr Keith, *Complete Guide to Food Allergies*, Thorsons, London, 1993
Philpott, William H and Dwight K Kalita, *Brain Allergies*, Keats Publishing, New
    Canaan, 1987
Van Straten, Michael and Barbara Griggs, *Superfoods*, Dorling Kindersley,
    London, 1990
Virtue, Doreen, *Constant Craving*, Hay House, Carlstad, CA, 1996
Wunderlich Jr, Ray C, *Sugar and Your Health*, Good Health Publications,
    Florida, 1982


## Medical ethics

Bequaert Holmes, Helen and Laura M Purdy, *Feminist Perspectives in Medical
    Ethics*, Indiana University Press, Bloomington and Indianapolis, 1992
Lipton, Dr Sampson, *Conquering Pain*, Methuen, London, 1994

Miles, Agnes, *Women, Health and Medicine*, Open University Press, Buckingham, 1991

**Pain management**
Sadler, Jan, *Natural Pain Relief*, Element Books, Shaftesbury, 1997

**Miscellaneous**
Anderson, Greg, *50 Essential Things to Do When the Doctor Says It's Cancer*, Plume, New York, 1993
Carter, Jean and Michael, *Sweet Grapes: How to stop being infertile and start living again*, Perspective Press,
Colgan, Dr Michael, *Hormonal Health*, Apple Publishing, Vancouver, 1996
Fredricks, Carton, *Guide to Women's Nutrition*, Pedigree Books, New York, 1989
Grant, Dr Ellen, *Sexual Chemistry*, Cedar Press, London, 1994
Jones, J, *The Unofficial Guide to Smart Nutrition*, IDG Books, New York, 2000
Kenton, Leslie, *Ageless Ageing*, Arrow Books, London, 1987
Kübler-Ross, Elizabeth, *On Death and Dying*, Tavistock/Routledge, London, 197'
Langer, Stephen E and James F Scheer, *Solved the Riddle of Illness*, Keats, New Canaan, 1984
Meek, Jennifer, *Immune Power: Health and the Immune System*, Optima Macdonald 1990
Null, Gary and Martin Feldman, *Reverse the Ageing Process Naturally*, Villard Books, New York, 1996
Pizzorno, Joseph, *Total Wellness*, Prima Publishing, Rocklin, CA, 1996
Reynolds, Siimon, *Become Happy in Eight Minutes*, Plume, Middex, 1996
Worwood, V A, *Endometriosis and Aromatherapy* (booklet), The Earth Garden Clinic, 2 Fairview Parade, Romford, Essex RM7 7HH

# Useful addresses

## ACUPUNCTURE

The American Association of
Acupuncture and Oriental Medicine
433 Front Street
Catasauqua
PA 18032
USA

Council for Acupuncture
38 Mount Pleasant
London WC1X 0AP UK

## AROMATHERAPY

The American Alliance of
Aromatherapy
PO Box 750428
Petalumo
CA 94975
USA

International Federation of
Aromatherapists
4 Eastmearn Road
West Dulwich
London SE21 8HA
UK

National Association of Holistic
Aromatherapy
219 Carl Street
San Francisco
CA 94117
USA
Phone: 415 564-6785

## CANCER

Women's National Cancer Control
1 South Audley St
London W1Y 5DQ UK
Phone: 0171 729 2229

## CHIROPRACTIC

The American Chiropractic
Association
1701 Clarendon Boulevard,
Arlington
VA 22209
USA

Anglo-European College of
Chiropractic
13–15 Parkwood Road
Bournemouth BH5 2DF
UK
Phone: 01202 436200

The British Chiropractic Association
Premier House
10 Greycoat Place
London SW1P 1SB
UK

Chiropractors' Association of
Australia
PO Box 241
Springwood
New South Wales 2777
Australia
Phone: 61 47 515 644

Chiropractic Association (Singapore)
Box 23 Tanglin Post Office
Singapore
Phone: 65 293 9843/734

The International Chiropractors'
Association
110 N. Glebe Road
Suites 1000
Arlington
VA 22201
USA

New Zealand Chiropractors'
Association
PO Box 7144
Wellesley Street
Auckland
New Zealand
Phone: 64 9 373 4343

## COUNSELLING

British Association for Counselling
37a Sheep Street
Rugby
Warwickshire CV21 3BX
UK
Phone: 01788 578328

## ENDOMETRIOSIS GROUPS

Association Brasileira Endometriosis
Rua Francisco de Mello Palheta
203 CEP 06410-120
Barueri, S. P.
Brazil

Endometriosis Association
(Victoria) Inc
37 Andrew Crescent
South Croydon
Victoria 3136
Australia

Endometriose Foreningen
c/o Gynaekologisk-Obstetrisk Afd G
Herlev Amtssygehus
2730 Herlev
Denmark
Phone: 2172 4300

Endometriosforeningen
Box 6004
151 06 Södertalje
Sweden
Phone: 08 550 10245

Endometrioseforeningen
Postboks 1012 LURA
4391 Sandnes
Norway
http:\\www.endonorge.tsx.org/

Endometrioosiyhdistysry
PL 142
00531 Helsinki
Finland
Phone: 050 380 6715

Endometriose-Vereinigung
Deutschland e.V.
Bernhard-Goring-Str 152
04277 Leipzig
Germany
Phone: 0341 306 5304

Endometriosis Association
International Headquarters
8585 N. 76th Place
Milwaukee
WI 53223-2600
USA
Helpline: 800 992 3636
Phone: 414 355 2200
Fax: 414 355 6065
www.endometriosisassn.org
(For information on drugs, surgery
and complementary medicine.)

The Irish Endometriosis Association
Carmichael House
4 North Brunswick Street
Dublin 7
Ireland
Phone: 353 1 873 5702

JEMA
Japanese Endometriosis Association
5-60-2-302
Nakan
Nakano-ku
Tokyo 164-001
Japan
Phone/Fax: 81 3 3228 9960

National Endometriosis  Society
50 Westminster Palace Gardens
Artillery Row
London SW1P 1RL
UK
Helpline: 0171 222 2776 (7-10pm)
(For information on drugs and
surgery.)

SHE Trust
(Simply Holistic Endometriosis)
Red Hall Lodge, Red Hall Drive
Bracebridge Heath
Lincs LN4 2JT
UK
Phone/Fax: 01522 519992
www.endometriosis.co.uk
www.endometriosis.uk.org
(For information on drugs, surgery
and complementary medicine.)

New Zealand Endometriosis
Foundation
PO Box 1683
Palmerston North
New Zealand

**ENVIRONMENTAL MEDICINE**

Citizens for a Better Environment
Suite 505, 942 Market Street
San Francisco
CA 94102
USA

Environmental Action
1525 New Hampshire Avenue NW
Washington DC 20036
USA

Environmental Air Systems
Martin Wells
Sandyhill Cottage
Sandy Lane, Rushmore
Tilford, Farnham
Surrey GU10 2ET
UK

Friends of the Earth
530 7th Street SE
Washington DC 20003
USA
Phone: 202 543-4312

Greenpeace USA
1611 Connecticut Ave NW
Washington DC 20009
USA

Healthy House
Cold Harbour
Ruscombe, Stroud
Gloucestershire GL6 6DA
UK
Phone: 01453 752216

Hyperactive/Autism/Ausbergers
Child's Support Group
71 Whyke Lane
Chichester
Sussex PO19 2LD
UK

National Coalition Against the
Misuse of Pesticides
530 7th Street
Washington DC 20003
USA
Phone: 202 543 5450

PEX
The Pesticide Trust
Eurolink Centre
49 Effra Road
London SW2 1BZ
Phone: 0171 274 8895

Society for Environmental Therapy
Mrs H Davidson
521 Foxhall Road
Ipswich IP3 8LW
UK

## FERTILITY

Foresight
The Charity for Preconceptual Care
28 The Paddock, Godalming
Surrey GU7 1XD
UK
Phone: 01483 427839

Infertility Network Exchange
PO Box 204
East Meadow
NY 11554
USA
Phone: 516 794 9772

Issue (the National Fertility
Association)
509 Aldridge Road
Great Barr
Birmingham B44
UK
Phone: 0121 344 4414
Fax: 0121 344 4336

Maternity Alliance
45 Beech Street
London EC2P 2LX
UK
Phone: 0171 588 8582

National Childbirth Trust
Alexandra House
Oldham Terrace
Acton, London W3 7NH
UK

Natural Family Planning
Fertility Trust
Mrs Colleen Norman
218 Heathwood Road
Heath, Cardiff CF4 4BS
S Wales
Phone: 01222 754628

Resolve Inc.
1310 Broadway Avenue
Somerville
MA 02144
USA
Phone: 617 623 1156
Website:
http://www.makingbabies.com

## HEALING

Breath Fellowship
Chilston Mead
Pembury Road
Tunbridge Wells
Kent
UK

The Divine Healing Mission
Crowhurst
Bexhill-on-Sea
East Sussex
UK
Phone: 01424 830266

## HEALTHY EATING

American College of Health Science
6600-D Burleson Road
Austin, TX 78744
USA

American Vegan Society
501 Old Harding Highway
Malaga, NJ 08328
USA

Center for Science in the Public
Interest
Americans for Safe Food
1501 16th Street, NW
Washington
DC 20036
USA
Phone: 202 332 9110

The Centre for the Study of
Complementary Medicine
51 Bedford Place
Southampton
Phone: 01703 334752

FACT
Food Additives Campaign Team
23-25 Western Park
London N8 9SY
UK
Phone: 0181 348 9195

Food Commission
94 Whitelion Street
London N1 9PF
UK
Phone: 0171 837 2250

Friends of the Earth
26–28 Underwood Street
London N1 7JQ
UK
Phone: 0171 490 1555

Freshwater Filters
Carlton House
Aylmer Road
Leytonstone
London E11 3AD
UK
Phone: 0181 558 7495

Good Gardeners Association
Pinetum Lodge
Churcham
Gloucestershire GL2 8AD
UK

Greenpeace
5 Caledonian Road
London N1
UK
Phone: 0171 713 1269

Henry Doubleday Research
Association
Ryton-on-Dunsmore Organic
Gardens
Coventry
Warwickshire CV8 3LG
UK
Phone: 01203 303517

Institute for Optimum Nutrition
(ION)
12–13 Blades Court
London SW15 2NV
Phone: 020 8877 9993
for 1hour Consultations with Dian

The Hale Clinic, 7 Park Crescent
London W1B 1PF
Phone: 020 7637 3377
for 1hour Consultations with Dian
emails: Dian@endometriosis.co.uk

McCarrison Society
c/o Institute of Brain Chemistry and
Human Nutrition
Hackney Hospital, Hackney Road
London E2 8PS
UK
Phone: 0181 510 5555

The Natural Medicine Society
Regency House
97–107 Hagley Road
Edgbaston
Birmingham B16
UK

North American Vegetarian Society
PO Box 72
Dolgeville, NY 13329
USA

Organic Growers Association
Aeron Park
Lampeter
Dyfed, Wales
Phone: 01570 423280

Organic Information
PO Box 1503
Poole
Dorset BH14 8YE
UK
Phone: 01202 715130

Soil Association
86 Colston Street
Bristol BS1 5BB
UK
Phone: 0117 929 0661

Wholefood
24 Paddington Street
London W1M 4DR
UK
(For organic food and books.)

Wholelife
89 Fifth Avenue
Suite 600
New York
NY 10003
USA

## HERBALISM

The American Herb Association
PO Box 673
Nevada City
CA 95959
USA

Canadian Holistic Medical
Association
491 Eglington Avenue West,
Apt 407
Toronto
Ontario M5N 1A8
Canada
Phone: 1 416 485 3071

National Herbalists' Association
of Australia
Suite 305, BST House
3 Smail Street
Broadway
New South Wales 2007
Australia
Phone: 61 2 211 6437

National Institute of Medical
Herbalists
56 Longstock Street
Exeter EX4 6AH
UK

North American Herbalists' Guild
PO Box 1683
Sequel
CA 95073
USA

The College of Practitioners of
Phytotherapy
Bucksteep Manor
Bodle Street Green
Near Hailsham
Sussex BN27 4RJ
UK
Phone: 01323 834 800
Website:
www.blazeweb.com/phytotherapy/

## HOMEOPATHY

American Foundation for
Homeopathy
1508 S Garfield
Alhambra, CA 91801
USA

Australian Institute of Homeopathy
21 Bulah Heights
Berdwra Heights
New South Wales 2082
Australia

British Homeopathic Association
27a Devonshire Street
London W1N 1RJ
UK
Phone: 0171 935 2163

British Institute of Homeopathy and
College of Homeopathy
520 Washington Boulevard, Suite 423
Marian Del Rey
CA 90292
USA
Phone: 310 306 5408

Hahnemann Society
Hahnemann House
15 Clerkenwell Close
London EC1R 0AA
UK
Phone: 0171 566 7800

The International Foundation for
Homeopathy
2366 Eastlake Avenue
East/Suite 801
Seattle
WA 98102
USA

National Center for Homeopathy
801 N Fairfax Street, Suite 306
Alexander
VA 22314
USA
Phone: 703 548 7790

The Royal London Homeopathic
Hospital
Great Ormond Street
London WC1N 3HR
UK
Phone: 0171 837 8833

Society of Homeopaths
4a Artizan Road
Northampton NN1 4HU
UK
Phone: 01604 621400

## HYDROTHERAPY

The American Board of
Hydrotherapy
16842 Von Karman Avenue
Suite 475
Irvine
CA 92714
USA

Aquatic Exercise Association
PO Box 1609
Nokomis
FL 3427
USA
Phone: 1 813 486 8600

UK College of Hydrotherapy
515 Hagley Road
Birmingham B66 4AX
UK

## HYPNOTHERAPY

British Society of Experimental and
Clinical Hypnosis
Psychology Department
Middlewood Hospital
Sheffield S6 1TP
UK

British Society for Medical and
Dental Hypnosis
151 Otley Old Road
Leeds LS16 6HN
UK

New World Music
Freepost
Paradise Farm
Westhall
Halesworth
Suffolk IP19 8BR
UK
(For tapes on relaxation, pain, sleep,
health by Robert E Griswold. From
the series 'The Love Tapes' by
Electronic Music Research Inc.)

The Society for Clinical and
Experimental Hypnosis
University of Colorado Medical
Center
Colorado
USA

## INTERNET ADDRESSES

http://www.endometriosis.co.uk
http://www.nutrition-health.co.uk
http://www.obgyn.net
http://www.fert.net/na/pub/links.htm

http://makingbabies.com
(Many libraries have the facility for
you to use a computer to surf the
Internet as do some cybercafes in
many towns and cities.)

## IMMUNE AND ALLERGY EFFECTS

Action Against Allergy
PO Box 278
Strawberry Hill Road
Twickenham TW1 4QQ
UK
Phone: 0181 892 2711

American Liver Foundation
1425 Pompton Avenue
Cedar Grove
NJ 07009
USA
Phone: 800 223 2550
Phone: 201 256 2550

British Society for Allergy and
Environmental Medicine
PO Box 28
Totton
Southampton
UK
Phone: 01703 812124

Candida Research Information
Foundation
PO Box 2719
Castro Valley
CA 94546
USA
Phone: 415 582 2179

Chronic Fatigue Syndrome
Foundation
PO Box 220398
Charlotte
NC 28222 0398
USA
Phone: 704 362 2343

Gluten Intolerance Group
26604 Dover Court
Kent
WA 98031
USA

Intestinal Disease Foundation Inc
1323 Forbes Ave, Ste 200
Pittsburgh
PA 15219
USA
Phone: 412 261 5888

ME Action Campaign
4 Dean's Court
St Paul's Churchyard
London EC4V 5AA
Phone: 0171 329 2211

National Society for Research Into
Allergy
PO Box 45, Hinckley
Leicestershire LE10 1JY
UK
Phone: 01455 851546

## MAIL ORDER SUPPLEMENTS AND FOODS

Allergy Care Catalogue
Pollards Yard, Wood Street
Taunton
Somerset TA1 1UP
UK
Phone: 01823 325022
(For allergy-free foods.)

Anglo-German Homeopathic Centre
11 Atlay Street
Westfields
Hereford HR4 9PF
UK

Biocare Nutritional Supplements
54 Northfield Road
Kings Norton
Birmingham B30 1JH
UK
Phone: 0121 433 3727

Britannia Health Products Ltd
41–51 Brighton Road
Redhill
Surrey RH1 6YS
Phone: 01737 773741
Fax: 01737 762672
(Homeopathic tinctures for
endometriosis.)

Health Plus Ltd
Nutritional Supplements
Lushington Road
Eastbourne
East Sussex BN 21
UK
Phone: 01323 737374

Helios Pharmacy
Homeopathic Supplements
92 Camden Road
Tunbridge Wells
Kent TN1
UK
Phone: 01892 537254

Higher Nature Nutritional
Supplements
Burwash Common
East Sussex TN19 7LX
UK
Phone: 01435 882880

Homeopathic Education Services
2124 Kittredge Avenue
Berkley
CA 94704
USA
Phone: 800 359 9051

Nutrition Information
Lamberts Library Trust
1 Lamberts Road
Tunbridge Wells
Kent TN2 3EQ
UK
Phone: 01892 552116
Fax: 01892 540597/540699
http://www.nutrition-library.co.uk
(Public enquiry £5.00)

Larkhall Natural Health
White Horse Business Park
Trowbridge
Wiltshire BA14 XQ
UK

Lifestyle Gluten-free Foods
Centenary Business Park
Henley-on-Thames
Oxfordshire RG9 1DS
Phone: 01491 411767
Fax: 01491 571 704
Website: www.glutenfree.co.uk
(Fresh food, home delivery service.)

Metagenics
917 Calle Negocio
San Clemente
CA 92673
USA
Phone: 714 366 0818
Fax: 800 692 9400

Nature's Best Nutritional Supplements
1 Lamberts Road
Tunbridge Wells
Kent TN2 3EQ
UK
Phone: 01892 552120

The Nutri Centre
7 Park Crescent
London W1N 3HE
UK
Phone: 0171 436 5122
(Mail order bookshop on site.)

Nutricology Inc
Allergy Research Group
PO Box 489
San Leandro
CA 9477
USA
Phone: 510 639 4572
Fax: 800 545 9960

Professional Botanicals
PO Box 9822
Ogden
UT 94409
USA
Phone: 801 621 3450
Fax: 800 824 8181

Quest Vitamins
140 Arrowood Lane
San Mateo
CA 94403
Phone: 415 345 1233

Solgar Vitamin and Herb Co
World Headquarters
500 Willow Tree Road
Leonia
New Jersey 07605
USA

pecialist Herbal Supplies
 Burton Villas
love
ussex BN3 6BR
JK
hone: 01273 202401

he Village Bakery
ledmerby Ltd
enrith
'umbria CA10 1HE
hone: 01768 381515

**1ASSAGE**

he American Tantric Massage
herapy Association
636 Lake Lawford Court
uite 100, Lake Sherwood
A 70816–4421
JSA

he London College of Massage
 Newman Passage
ondon W1P 5PF
JK
hone: 0171 323 3574

he Northern Institute of Massage
00 Waterloo Road
lackpool
ancs FY4 1AW
'K
hone: 01253 403548

**ATUROPATHY**

merican Association of
laturopathic Physicians
O Box 20386
eattle
'A 98102
'SA
hone: 1 206 323 7610

Australian Natural Therapists
PO Box 308
Melrose Park
South Australia
Phone: 61 8 371 3222

British College of Naturopathy and
Osteopathy Register of Naturopaths
Frazer House
6 Netherhall Gardens
London NW3 5RR
UK
Phone: 0171 435 6464

Canadian Naturopathic Association
205, 1234 17th Avenue
South West
PO Box 3143
Station C, Calgary
Alberta
Canada
Phone: 1 413 244 4487

**NUTRITIONAL TESTING**

Biolab Medical Unit
The Stone House
9 Weymouth Street
London
W1N 3FF
UK
Phone: 0171 636 5959

Diagnostech
4501 Sunbelt Drive
Addison
TX 75248
USA
Phone: 972 250 6410

The Doctors Laboratory Plc
58 Wimpole Street
London W1M 7DE
UK
Phone: 0171 480 4800

Great Smokies Diagnostic Laboratory
63 Zillcoa Street
Ashville 28801–1074
North Carolina
USA
European link:
Health Interlink Ltd.
1a Crown Street
Redbourn
Herts AL3 7JX
UK
Phone: 01582 794097 (Med referral)

Trace Elements Inc
Dallas Texas
USA
Phone: 972 248 4896
(Hair mineral analysis.)

## OSTEOPATHS

General Council and Register of
Osteopaths
56 London Street
Reading
Berkshire RG1 4SQ
UK

Naturopathic and Osteopathic
Association
Frazer House
6 Netherhall Gardens
London NW3 5RR
UK

## OSTEOPOROSIS

National Osteoporosis Society
Barton Meade House
PO Box 10
Radstock
Bath
Avon BA3 3YB
UK
Phone: 01761 471771

## PAIN

American Chronic Pain Association
PO Box 850
Rocklin
CA 95677
USA
Phone: 916 632 0922

California Center for Pelvic Pain and
Fertility
780 Welch Road
Suite 206
Stanford Professional Center
Palo Alto
CA 94304
USA
Phone: 650 833 7900

Input Clinic
St Thomas's Hospital
Westminster
London SE1 7EH
UK
Phone: 0171 928 9292 ext.8107
(For the relief of chronic pain.)

The National Association for Back
Pain
31 Park Road
Teddington
Middlesex TW11 0AB
UK

## PMS

National Association for Premenstrual
Tension
PO Box 72
Sevenoaks
Kent TN13 1XQ
UK
Phone: 01227 763133
Helpline: 01227 763133

## REFLEXOLOGY

The British Reflexology Association
Monks Orchard
Whitbourne
Worcester WR6 5RB
UK
Phone: 01886 821207

The International School of
Reflexology
PO Box 12642
St Petersburgh
FL 33733
USA

## SYSTEMIC KINESIOLOGY

Academy of Systemic Kinesiology
39 Browns Road
Surbiton
Surrey KT5 8ST
UK
Phone: 0181 399 3215

## SURGERY

Community Health Council
(Redress for poor treatment – your
local branch.)

Consumers for Ethics in Research
PO Box 1365
London N16 0BW
UK

Family Health Services
(Medical Records Access
Your local branch)

Hysterectomy Support Group
40 Longleat Gardens
New Milton
Hants BH25 5XF
UK
Phone: 01425 620438

Hysterectomy Support Network
3 Lymne Close
Green Street Green
Orpington
Kent BR6 6BS
UK
Phone: 0181 856 3881

Medical Records
Medical Information Bureau
Consumer Info Office
PO Box 105
Essex Station
Boston
MA 02112
USA
Phone: 617 426 3660

Medical Self Care
Box 717
Inverness
CA 94937
USA
Phone: 415 663 8462

The Patients' Association
18 Victoria Park Square
Bethnal Green
London E2 3PF
Phone: 0181 981 5676

## WOMEN'S HEALTH

Communities for a Better
Environment
500 Howard Street
Suite 506
San Francisco
CA 94105
Phone: 413 243 8373

Menopausal Helpline
Send an sae:
228 Muswell Hill Broadway
London N10 3SH
(Offers natural alternatives to HRT
drugs)

Pelvic Inflammatory Disease
Support Group
C/O Women's Health
52 Feather Stone Street
London EC1 8RT
UK
Phone: 0171 251 6580

Association for Post Natal Depression
25 Jerdan Place
Fulham
London SW6 1OE
UK
Phone: 0171 386 0868

Stillbirth & Neonatal Death Society
(SANDS)
28 Portland Place
London W1N 4DE
UK
Phone: 0171 436 5881/7940

Support for Termination after
Abnormalities
(SAFTA)
29 Soho Square
London W1V 6JB
UK

Women's Environmental Network
87 Worship Street
London EC2A 2BE
UK
Phone: 0171 247 3327

Women's Health Network
224 7th Street, NE
Washington
DC 20003
USA
Phone: 202 543 9222

## YOGA

The American Yoga Association
513 South Orange Avenue
Sarasota
FL 34236
USA
E-mail: Am Yoga Assn@aol.com.

Yoga Biomedical Trust
PO Box 140
Cambridge CB4 3SY
UK

# Index

Hormones, 18, 19, 26, 32, 34, 35, 49, 60, 67–9, 99, 150, 151, 185, 189, 195, 200, 201, 217, 244, 245, 249
Hormonal messengers, 9, 18
Hormone replacement therapy (HRT), 105–6, 161, 175, 178, 221, 329
Hot flushes, 296
Hydrotherapy, 130, 353
Hygiene, 86, 157
Hyperthyroidism, 185, 200
Hyperventilation, 45–6
Hypnotherapy, 41
Hypoglycaemia, 83
Hypothalamus, 10, 18–20, 60, 77, 80, 124, 155, 191, 221, 329
Hypothyroidism, 13, 62, 161, 184, 185, 200–1, 206
Hysterectomy, 105–6, 114, 329

Immune system, 4, 35, 40, 45, 47, 55, 58, 72–3, 97, 135–54, 159–61, 170, 175, 222, 236, 242, 245, 247, 251–2, 282–3, 380
 cell-mediated, 140, 245
 humoral immunity, 144
Indoles, 198
Infertility
 abnormal ovulation, 70, 80, 94, 243, 335
 adhesion induced, 67, 94
 digestion/diet, 155, 161, 184, 186
 endometriosis and, 29, 37, 68, 69, 85, 93
 fertilization, 70–1, 78, 94
 immune system, 29, 72–3, 85, 184, 186
 implant proteins, 55, 69
 incidence , 22, 30, 66, 86, 94
 miscarriage, 68, 71, 73, 75, 78,

 94, 184, 196, 333
 prostaglandins, 55, 68–9
 support groups, 93, 350
 thyroid disease, 62, 184, 200
 treatments, 2, 7, 76, 82
Inflammation, 7, 27, 34, 35, 39–40, 48, 49, 54–9, 61 96, 143, 145, 207, 219, 250, 285, 330
Informed consent, 112, 291
Inositol, 191, 197, 224
Institute for Optimum Nutrition (ION), 236, 237
Insomnia, 296
Insulin, 216, 221
Integrins, 281–2, 330
Intercourse, sexual 19, 66, 92, 102, 105, 207
Interleukins, 40, 148, 330
Interferon, 40, 142, 144–5, 151, 330
International Endometriosis Association, 4, 7, 174, 193, 239, 278
Intestine, 24, 136, 155, 160–2, 164–6, 169, 171, 173, 180, 190–1, 205
Intrautrine insemination (IU), 107
In vitro fertilization (IVF), 70, 107–10, 124, 230, 330
Iodine, 78, 80, 88, 93, 191, 200, 222, 254–5
Iron, 21, 33, 36, 55, 80, 136–7, 140, 144, 147, 149, 185, 195, 224, 226, 237, 242, 252, 260, 295, 297, 330
Irritability, 63
Irritable bowel syndrome, 27, 28, 29, 204, 231
Irvine Allsa, 41
Isoflavins, 197–8

Kidney, 23, 29, 136, 191
Kresch, Dr. Arnold, 42–3, 64